Health Education Films in the Twentieth Century

Rochester Studies in Medical History

Senior Editor: Theodore M. Brown
Professor of History and Preventive Medicine
University of Rochester

Additional Titles of Interest

Intrusive Interventions: Public Health, Domestic Space, and Infectious Disease Surveillance in England, 1840–1914
Graham Mooney

The Antivaccine Heresy: "Jacobson v. Massachusetts" and the Troubled History of Compulsory Vaccination in the United States
Karen L. Walloch

Healthy Boundaries: Property, Law, and Public Health in England and Wales, 1815–1872
James G. Hanley

Psychiatry and Racial Liberalism in Harlem, 1936–1968
Dennis A. Doyle

Childbirth, Maternity, and Medical Pluralism in French Colonial Vietnam, 1880–1945
Thuy Linh Nguyen

Setting Nutritional Standards: Theory, Policies, Practices
Edited by Elizabeth Neswald, David F. Smith, and Ulrike Thoms

Technological Change in Modern Surgery: Historical Perspectives on Innovation
Edited by Thomas Schlich and Christopher Crenner

The History of the Brain and Mind Sciences: Technique, Technology, Therapy
Edited by Stephen T. Casper and Delia Gavrus

Reasoning against Madness: Psychiatry and the State in Rio de Janeiro, 1830–1944
Manuella Meyer

Fit to Practice: Empire, Race, Gender, and the Making of British Medicine, 1850–1980
Douglas M. Haynes

A complete list of titles in the Rochester Studies in Medical History series may be found on our website, www.urpress.com.

Health Education Films in the Twentieth Century

Edited by Christian Bonah,
David Cantor, and Anja Laukötter

University of Rochester Press

FONDATION BROCHER

The University of Rochester Press gratefully acknowledges generous support from the Brocher Foundation.

First published 2018

University of Rochester Press
668 Mt. Hope Avenue, Rochester, NY 14620, USA
www.urpress.com
and Boydell & Brewer Limited
PO Box 9, Woodbridge, Suffolk IP12 3DF, UK
www.boydellandbrewer.com

ISBN-13: 978-1-58046-916-6
ISSN: 1526-2715

Library of Congress Cataloging-in-Publication Data

Names: Bonah, Christian, editor.
Title: Health education films in the twentieth century / edited by Christian Bonah, David Cantor, and Anja Laukötter.
Description: Rochester, NY : University of Rochester Press, 2018. | Series: Rochester studies in medical history, ISSN 1526-2715 ; v. 43 | Includes bibliographical references and index.
Identifiers: LCCN 2017044657 | ISBN 9781580469166 (hardcover : alk. paper)
Subjects: LCSH: Health education—Audio-visual aids—Europe—20th century. | Health education—Audio-visual aids—North America—20th century. | Mass media in health education.
Classification: LCC RA440.55 .H434 2018 | DDC 613.071—dc23 LC record available at https://lccn.loc.gov/2017044657

To the memory of Elizabeth Lebas (1947–2014)

Contents

Part Three: International Reorganization

Part Four: Constructing Audiences

A selection of the films discussed in this book can be viewed at http://medfilm.unistra.fr/wiki/health_education_films.

Acknowledgments

This book began life as a symposium funded by the Brocher Foundation, and held at its spectacular conference center in Hermance, Switzerland, on the shores of Lake Geneva, May 26–27, 2011. The editors would like to thank the Foundation, and in particular Marie Grosclaude, for their superb organization. The University of Strasbourg and the Research Unit SAGE (UMR 7363), the Agence Nationale de la Recherche (Grant ANR-10-BLAN-2004 MedFilm), and the Max Planck Institute for Human Development Berlin (Center for the History of Emotions) helped with the funding of this conference. The book has received support from the Excellence Initiative of the University of Strasbourg funded by the French government's Future Investments program.

Several other people have helped. Jean-Yves Bart undertook significant work of translation and copyediting. Leonard Keutner, Monja Schünemann, and Nancy Schumacher provided copyediting of the final versions of the chapters. Therese Vicente has given administrative support to the organization. David Cantor would like to acknowledge the support of the staff at the Office of History, National Institutes of Health, especially the late Robert L. Martensen.

Finally, the editors would like to acknowledge the Brocher Foundation for an additional grant supporting the publication of this volume. The Brocher Foundation's mission is to encourage research on the ethical, legal, and social implications of new medical technologies. Its main activities are to host visiting researchers and to organize symposia, workshops, and summer academies. More information on the Brocher Foundation program is available at www.brocher.ch.

Introduction

CHRISTIAN BONAH, DAVID CANTOR, AND ANJA LAUKÖTTER

The twentieth century was to have been the age of the motion picture. For many of its proponents, film was a revolutionary technology that would entertain, document, instruct, and transform a mass audience in much the same way that moveable type had transformed medieval Europe. In the fields of medicine and public health, doctors, educators, and health advocates seemed especially enthusiastic about the potential uses of the motion picture in public health education.[1] From the silent era onward, they wrote, directed, acted in, and produced films on a broad range of medical and health-related topics. To enthusiasts, movies promised an unrivaled means of transforming public health behaviors and of managing public anxieties and hopes about health, illness, and medical interventions. The public health education message of the future, they claimed, would be printed on celluloid, not paper.

But not everyone shared such optimism. For some critics, film was not a help but a hindrance, even a dangerous threat to public health goals. These commentators argued that commercial movie theaters were often dens of vice, and that entertainment films often encouraged risky behaviors, from sex to smoking. Even the humble public health education film could work against the very messages it was supposed to promote. Some feared that by modeling themselves on commercial films, public health education films tended to entertain more than educate. Others worried that these films were likely to undermine public health education efforts by promoting irrational hopes and fears, by lulling audiences into torpor, or simply by confusing them with mixed messages.[2]

One of the aims of this book is to capture some of the many, and at times conflicting, uses and meanings of the health education film in North America and Europe from the 1910s to the 1960s.[3] We use the terms *health film*, *public health film*, and *public health education film* interchangeably with the term *health education film*. We define these films as "utility"[4] or "message" films. They were produced with the intention of reforming or reinforcing public health beliefs and practices, and they have to be understood in terms of specific instrumental purposes—including the varied and sometimes conflicting purposes of the organizations and individuals that sponsored, created, collected, distributed, or exhibited them. Chapters in this book will explore the many different purposes and messages of public health education films, what they meant to the various stakeholders involved with the film (sponsors, collectors, distributors, filmmakers, and exhibitors), how the public responded to the messages put out by these films, and how public responses shaped and reshaped these films. As the opening paragraphs of this chapter suggest, film could be seen in very different ways by different groups and individuals.

In using the term *utility film*, this book expands on Thomas Elsaesser's influential approach to the subject. Reacting against what he calls essentialist approaches within film history, Elsaesser suggests that utility films must be seen within the context of their production and use—the key questions, he suggests, are "who commissioned the film?," "what was the occasion for which it was made?," and to "what use was it put or to whom was it addressed?"[5] The problem, from our perspective, is that in practice such questions have tended to focus on the perspectives of those who commission the film (in our case a wide range of groups and individuals—physicians, public health officials, pharmaceutical companies, film companies, government organizations, insurance companies, medical organizations, and health advocacy groups, among others). But sponsors are only one stakeholder in public health films. Chapters in this book broaden the approach to look at a variety of other stakeholders (filmmakers, collectors, distributors, exhibitors, educators, and audiences) and how all of these interact at various occasions in the life of a film (its commissioning, production, distribution, exhibition, and collection in film libraries). We suggest that the historian's task is to differentiate and explain the various occasions in which a film may be used, the various perspectives of the different stakeholders at different points in the life of a film, and how each stakeholder at these various points uses the film and imagines its message and who it is addressed to.

In using the term *utility film*, we also distinguish our point of view from those that focus on "ephemeral" or "orphan" films:[6] films that had a short life, and which in the case of orphan films often lack "either clear copyright holders or commercial potential"[7] to pay for their preservation, or which were in other ways neglected. Such labels have been adopted by those who seek to promote the preservation of films that otherwise might be neglected. However, these two categories do not serve our analytic purpose. Many of the films explored in this collection were ephemeral (they did not last much longer than the purposes for which they were commissioned, and too many no longer exist) and some (though by no means all) may be classed as orphans, without a parent organization to ensure their preservation. Yet our interest in them is not primarily in helping to ensure their preservation, though we hope this book helps toward that end. Rather, our attention focuses on explaining how and why they were made, how they were distributed and screened, how they were received, and (in some cases) why they disappeared. The valuable work undertaken by various organizations seeking to preserve and make available orphan or ephemeral films rarely extends to providing significant historical context to their films beyond rudimentary information about them: production dates, directors, or circumstantial information about their origin and use.[8]

Two other distinctions might be made. First, our interest is not in the "Hollywood" portrayal of health and illness—the focus of most histories of medical film to date[9]—except to show the blurry boundary between theatrical and nontheatrical (as health education films were sometimes classed) films in the twentieth century, and how theatrical film production shaped conventions in and aspirations of public health education films. Nor is our interest in documentary film—a genre that includes health films—except, as with entertainment film, to show the overlapping boundaries between health education and documentary films and how they have shaped each other. Indeed, a growing body of literature on documentary film has begun to distance itself from the older historiography that focused on the visions of documentary filmmakers and to explore the complex meanings and uses of documentary film, a literature that informs this volume.[10]

While several recent books have explored the history of medicine in film, none have focused significant attention on noncommercial health education films. Thousands of these films were made during the twentieth and early twenty-first centuries in Europe and North America. They were shown in an enormous variety of places: schools; universities; mobile projection cars; movie theaters; museums; and many other places, outdoors and indoors. Yet because of their ephemeral nature they are very difficult to find, and they have been so far marginal to the interests of both film and medical history. One of the aims of this volume is to shape the newly emergent field of health related "utility" films by bringing together for the first time European and North American scholars who are working on these types of films from the perspectives not only of the history of medicine and science, but also of film and media studies.

The book aims to contribute to a broader understanding of efforts to instruct, educate, and promote medical and scientific knowledge of health, disease, and risk to the general public and, crucially, to transform public behaviors. It does not seek to be comprehensive but to suggest how—by looking at production, dissemination, and exhibition—organizations and individuals sought, and still seek, to shape public beliefs and practices and the social, cultural, and political structures and assumptions that shape these efforts. By looking at the public's responses to public education we intend to examine the ways in which audiences have themselves shaped medical and scientific knowledge and how organizations have sought to promote it. In short, we see movies as a valuable tool for exploring how the conditions of production, dissemination, exhibition, and reception come together to shape efforts to communicate ideas and practices about health, disease, and risk. As such the book should be of value not only to (medical) historians and film scholars, but also to experts in public health and health education.

The Corpus

In terms of output, health education films are a prolific format or genre, perhaps more prolific than entertainment films that touch on health-related issues. Yet they can be extraordinarily difficult to study. These films are scattered in many locations: national and university libraries, hospitals, governmental and corporate archives, and philanthropic and international organizations such as the American Cancer Society and the World Health Organization. The titles, production information, and whereabouts of many of these films are not easily available or accessible to researchers. Many, perhaps most, films have been lost: the only record of these is in published reviews, catalogues, brochures, or the internal documents of the organizations that produced, collected, distributed, evaluated, or exhibited them. And sometimes these records do not correspond with what could be seen on screen—films might be screened in limited geographical areas; they might be available for only a limited length of time; or they might be shown under particular circumstances such as a circumscribed institutional setting like a workplace. For researchers, this makes it difficult to understand the scope, politics, cultural meaning, and context of public health educational filmmaking, distribution, and exhibition. There is a growing body of historical work on health education films, but it is often difficult to know to what extent these accounts are representative of the format or genre, since we know little about the thousands of films that have not survived.

This book suggests that one of the ways in which we can begin to address this issue of representativeness is to focus not on individual films but on corpuses of films. There are some rich accounts of individual films that explore what they were commissioned for, how they were made, and the response of viewers to them. But focusing on a corpus allows us to ask questions that are not always possible for an individual film—for example, how stylistic and rhetorical patterns may recur from film to film, or how new technologies such as sound or color, styles of editing, camera techniques, and so on were taken up (or not) by health education films.[11] Such questions can only be asked, though, through comparative analysis of many films. Only then is it possible to determine, for example, the extent to which the before and after narrative often used to portray the benefits of a new medical or public health intervention can be said to be a defining feature of the public health film; the relationship between the mutable human forms found in many health education films, and related figures in other industrials and educationals; or the use of scenes from one film later cut and taped into others. Serial analysis of many films also provides insight into strategies and styles of public health communication and what changes and what does not over time. It is a form of comparative history that is not possible to undertake with only one film.[12]

We are not the first to focus on such corpuses. Indeed, in recent years there have been several efforts to develop corpuses of films to facilitate historical enquiry and to help film librarians develop collections policies. Perhaps the most ambitious of these were efforts in the mid-to-late 2000s to develop censuses of all health education films in North America and Europe since the early twentieth century. Essentially such censuses would have created databases of health education films—both lost and surviving—founded on surveys of online and printed filmographic databases, searches through journals and newspapers known to have reviewed medical films, and research in archival collections. But they turned out to be immense, complicated, and often unwieldy projects. The American effort would have taken years and involved a substantial staff, and there were difficult questions about what types of film to include in the census. It was quite unclear how to draw the line between the health education film and the vast range of related formats and genres—research and clinical films, medical training films, accident prevention films, social service films, ecological films, documentary films, entertainment films, and so on. The American effort did not get beyond a prototype,[13] while the European one has mutated into an academically edited media wiki—the Medfilm database.[14]

In the absence of such all-encompassing censuses and the corpuses that they would have created, this book focuses on smaller, more manageable corpuses and methodological reflections on how to constitute them. In the first place, it explores corpuses of films produced by a variety of organizations and individuals concerned with health issues—film production/distribution companies (Cantor), film directors (Lowy and Cantor, Sumpf), national governments, local authorities (Lebas), pharmaceutical companies (Bonah), international organizations (Ostherr), and antidisease voluntary associations and their campaigns, among others. A focus on such organizations can have an advantage of allowing the historian to use records of or about that organization to identify the films it produced, collected, distributed, or exhibited—both ones that have survived and the often many more that have not—and so to say something about the situatedness and representativeness of particular films or groups of films within that corpus. More broadly, it also allows the historian to situate these films within the aims and objectives of these organizations and to set out the meanings of these films to various stakeholders at various occasions in their life, and the relation of these meanings to the aims and objectives of the organization that produced, collected, distributed, or exhibited the films.

In the second place, this book also explores corpuses organized around particular subjects. To some extent this may overlap with an organizational focus. Many organizations produced corpuses of films around particular subjects such as tuberculosis, alcoholism, or venereal disease (Posner, Laukötter, Sumpf), and a focus on organizations can show how corpuses emerge in response to particular social or health issues. But some subjects can also be followed through a variety of films, produced by a variety of organizations, some of which may not properly be regarded as health education films. Put another way, public health issues may be raised in films that are produced for other reasons than public health, and a corpus can be created by following this subject through the variety of formats or genres of film in which it appears. For example, cancer, diabetes, tuberculosis, and venereal diseases among other health conditions have been the subject of many different film treatments (in public education films, scientific films, medical training films, and entertainment films) and comparison of their treatment in these different genres or forms of film will entail the historian building a corpus of such film treatments. Such a corpus may help to understand the relationship of the health education film to other genres and formats and what happens to a subject when it travels from one form of film to another.

In the third place, this book also aims to explore corpuses organized not only around organizations or health subjects, but also around aspects internal to the film itself—aesthetics, techniques of production, narrative tropes, or visual imagery, sound, or music, for example (von Keitz, Ostherr, Sumpf). All these can be followed through a variety of different formats and genres, much like following a trail of breadcrumbs through a variety of difficult landscapes. One of the advantages of such an approach is that it allows us to destabilize the category of the health education film by exploring how elements of the health education film cross boundaries of genre and format.

The Story of Wendy Hill (1949)[15] (an American antidiabetes film) illustrates the ways in which individual films can fit into a variety of corpuses. The film tells the tale of Wendy Hill, who is hit by a truck one day on her way home from work. Her family physician witnesses this from his office and rushes her to the hospital. Although her injuries are not serious, a routine laboratory check in the hospital indicates diabetes, and the rest of the film shows the wonders of insulin treatment, the stigma associated with the condition, and public ignorance about it.

The film itself was produced jointly by the United States Public Health Service (USPHS) and the American Diabetes Association. It could be situated in a corpus of diabetes films produced by either or both organizations, or perhaps it could be part of a corpus of health films produced by the film production company Warner News, Inc. In the case of the USPHS or the ADA, one might wish to compare the educational strategies used in *Wendy Hill* with those of other USPHS or ADA films. Was *Wendy Hill* a typical USPHS or ADA film, did it draw on the lessons of earlier films, or did it inform later ones? In the case of Warner, one might wish to show how techniques developed in other Warner films were deployed in *Wendy Hill* or vice versa.

If it fits into a corpus organized around the institutions that produced it, it might also fit into corpuses organized around elements of the movie. The narrative of the film includes a conversion story in which Wendy Hill and her husband are converted to medical understandings of and approaches to diabetes, so it could be used in a comparative account of conversion stories in health education films, a common device in such films.[16] The film also borrows from the genre of the melodrama, often used in American public health films to target female audiences, and could be part of an account of the use of melodrama as a tool of health education films. It could also fit into other corpuses: stories in which the doctor is narrator, stories in which the doctor is also the patient, stories in which folk knowledge is denigrated, and stories in which traffic accidents provide the opportunity for other messages. Minor traffic accidents in health education films often seem to be the prelude to the discovery of something medically more serious.[17]

The Emergence of the Health Education Film

The health education film first emerged in the United States in the 1910s, notably as part of a series of reform films such as films concerning drunkenness and tuberculosis. This is not to say that movies did not deal with health subjects before then. In fact, almost from the beginning of cinema in the late nineteenth century, a wide variety of subjects that might be classed as health were screened—including films about sneezing, giving a child a morning bath, fire engines responding to a morning alarm, bodybuilding, and the various activities of the Red Cross in war.[18] There are several points to note about these films. They are very short, sometimes only a few seconds. Some don't tell a story, or provide only a glimpse of a narrative, or subordinate the story to efforts to engage an audience through spectacle, using narratives as containers for a bag of tricks and illusions. They aimed to elicit a reaction from the audience such as laugher, admiration, emulation, and shock, sometimes to the discomfort of doctors.[19] They are not health education films of the sort that will emerge in the 1910s, though health films would later try to engage with audiences in such ways, hoping to encourage admiration, emulation, and sometimes shock and laughter.

These early films may be part of a corpus of films that the historian Tom Gunning has called the cinema of attraction(s). According to Gunning, the cinema of attractions was a form of film unto itself, distinguished from later emphases on storytelling because it actively sought to attract a viewer's interest by means of overt display: "This is a cinema that displays its visibility, willing to rupture a self-enclosed fictional world for a chance to solicit the attention of the spectator."[20] Other historians, such as Charles Musser, have questioned Gunning's account of the early film, suggesting, for example, that where early cinema did produce a narrative, it was not the sole product of film producers.[21] Exhibitors might string together a series of actualities to make a story, or use other devices such a lecturers, lantern slides, and skits to contextualize the films and create a narrative.[22] It is not impossible that some of these early films may have been given a health twist by the speaker or organizer of a health event.

What differentiated the health education film as it emerged in the 1910s from these earlier films was that its makers and sponsors imagined it as a storytelling medium, one with a moral or message within it. In addition, this story would be embedded in the film itself, so that the producers of film had begun to challenge the storytelling role of the exhibitor. This is not to say that producers entirely replaced the exhibitors as storytellers, for even when filmmakers themselves created a narrative, it was always possible that the exhibitors might rearrange or recut the footage to tell their own stories. In addition, filmmakers continued to have trouble making their stories clear to audiences, and some theaters persisted in hiring lecturers to explain the events on the screen.

One key transformation, according to Gunning, was the development of what he calls a narrator system, a series of filmic devices through which the director could integrate the narrator into the film. In Gunning's view, a crucial figure here was the director D. W. Griffith. Gunning argues that Griffith helped create a narrator system by focusing on three categories of "filmic discourse": profilmic elements (those elements placed before the camera—actors, lighting, set design, and so on); the enframed image (the way the camera presents the image); and editing. For example, Gunning uses *The Drunkard's Reformation* (1909) to show how Griffith employed editing to convey the psychological development of the main character and, in the final shot, directional lighting to intensify the effect of the family reconciliation following the drunkard's epiphany.[23]

The *Drunkard's Reformation* was one of a number of temperance movies created in the late 1900s and early 1910s as part of an effort by the film industry to move away from "obscene films" to "high-class drama" following the censorship crackdown on New York City movie theaters on Christmas Eve of 1908. "High-class dramas" like *A Drunkard's Reformation* can be considered the industry's response to fears of censorship and an expression of its efforts to expand the moviegoing audience, especially to include the middle class, women and children, and the higher returns and economic stability they promised. A consequence was that the industry began regulating itself, and one of the results of this was a slew of films that told a moral lesson, often one of reform. Thus, films such as *The Drunkard's Reformation* were reform films in two senses of the term. They told stories of personal reform, and they were also about reforming the film industry.[24]

According to Gunning, reform films such as *The Drunkard's Reformation* were a key moment in a shift from "a 'cinema of attractions,' which was more interested in the display of curiosities, to a cinema of narrative integration which subordinates film form to the development of stories and characters," including from 1908 onward the melodrama, a leading form of film.[25] This helped to create a narrative template that would be adapted by many health films—the conversion narrative.[26] Borrowing from older temperance literature and drama and from religious discourses of conversion, the film tells the story of a drunkard who undergoes a conversion as a consequence of seeing his own actions enacted on the stage and, crucially, of how he reforms his behavior and so saves his family.

Similar stories were mobilized later in many health education films, where a character realizes the errors of his or her ways and is persuaded to follow the advice of the agency that sponsored the film.[27] And in this volume, Vincent Lowy and David Cantor highlight the continuing connections between the conversion narratives and social and film reform in the 1930s. But the use of conversion narratives in such films also helps to highlight the limitations of integrating the narrator into the film. The problem for those that sponsored films was that such integrated narratives did not always promote the desired effect; they constantly worried that audiences did not adopt the lessons set out in the films. The consequence was that, in their efforts to ensure that films did the work they were intended to do, such sponsors reintroduced the external narrator or lecturer. Public health films were often introduced by a lecturer providing extra information, explaining certain aspects or even repeating the health message of the film.[28] The lecturers would also answer questions when the film was over.

Ironically, if D. W. Griffith helped to usher in a period where film narration dispensed with the need for exhibitors or lecturers to make movie stories understandable to the public, public health campaigners in the United States and Europe would reintroduce the lecturer as a means of ensuring that audiences adopted the lessons of the film.

In Europe the story is slightly different. Although there, too, there is a shift from a cinema of attractions to one of narrative integration, and while there are also periodic efforts at reform of the film industry that are reflected in the format of films, the periodization is often different to that in the United States and often varies from one European country to another. In France, for example, the first theatrical health education films had appeared by 1902, notably the anti-alcoholism film *Victimes de l'alcoolisme/Victims of Alcoholism* (1902) produced by Pathé. In Germany, by contrast, such films appeared much later, during the World War I. Richard's Oswald's 1916/17 release *Let There be Light* (*Es werde Licht*) is a key example here, the success of which led to the release of three more episodes.[29] Russia provides another example of the complex periodization of health education films in Europe and the interconnections between different European countries. Thus, the presence in Russia of Pathé and Gaumont meant that French models of film were influential before the war, for example, in the popular and critical success of Aleksandr Khanzhonkov's *Drunkenness and its Consequences* (1913). Then, during World War I, homegrown productions grew as film imports from France and Scandinavia, massive before the war, dried up.[30] As Alexandre Sumpf notes in this volume, German *Kulturfilm* would gain particular attention in Russian health education films after the war, a paradoxical shift in influence given that Germany and Russia had been at war and France—the prewar influence on Russian health films—had been an ally of the Russians.

A similarly complex picture emerges for other aspects of the European tale. As in the United States, conversion stories emerged as a key narrative form in European health films, and although the periodization is slightly different from country to country, it was a common means of getting a health education message across by the early 1920s. In addition, Europeans seem to have had similar doubts about the ability of film narratives—including conversion narratives—to get the health message across. Just as Americans turned to lecturers to ensure that the message of the film got across to their audiences, so too did the Europeans from the 1910s. In some countries, Europeans seem to have been very cautious about film. In Britain, for example, health education films were greeted with some suspicion by a number of doctors and public health officials, part of a more general suspicion of public health education. Regarding cancer, for example, while the first American health education films were released in the 1920s, the first British ones did not appear until much later, in part because the British feared that public health education would create undue pressure on physicians. For many in Britain the key was to funnel health education through the patient's doctor rather than directly to the patient him or herself.[31] A similar reluctance about public health education is also evident in the Netherlands.[32]

Such differences reflected, in part, very different attitudes toward managing the public.[33] For example, critics in Britain and the Netherlands worried that American-style efforts to promote self-examination might encourage the public to self-diagnose disease, and so undermine programs of disease control, challenge the authority of the doctor, and blind the public to any educational message by inducing either a paralyzing fear of an illness or an undue optimism about the possibility of a cure that would eventually be disappointed as the expected cure failed to materialize. Such concerns led British and Dutch cancer agencies to adopt a much more cautious, paternalistic attitude toward public education, as did related fears that such programs might overwhelm general practitioners with trivial complaints from their patients or undermine efforts to persuade the public to support cancer research or treatment. Educational efforts in these countries tended to focus less on the public than on the profession, and where they did focus on the public, they tended to stress local (and often low-key) rather than national efforts.

A further difference between European and American approaches to film and health education might also be noted. Pre–World War I European health education films had roots in scientific and popular science films that are not so evident in health education films in the United States of the same period. In particular, visual devices employed in scientific and medical films—the use of x-rays, recordings of dysfunctions of body movements, surgical procedures, and micro-cinematography, sometimes combined with time-lapse techniques—began to appear in European films aimed at the wider public shortly after the turn of the twentieth century. As we shall discuss later in this introduction, this provided a means of offering viewers a vicarious insight into the otherwise hidden worlds of the body, the clinic, and the operating room. Film was thus a virtual witnessing technology that helped to give a veneer of scientific authenticity to European films that is not so evident in American health films until the World War I.

Finally, although we have emphasized the contrasts between early American and European health education films, it is also important to stress their interconnections. Films produced on one continent could be shown on another, though versions of a film, their distribution, and audience reactions could vary from continent to continent and from country to country. Such transnational connections seem to have grown especially after World War I, leading to struggles over what styles of film might dominate. Thus, while American health education films became more common in Europe after 1918, they did not dominate.[34] In some counties, they found themselves competing with and often losing to films and film styles from other European countries such as Russia, where health filmmakers were influenced by German filmmaking. The Weimar Republic was the only European nation that allowed film commerce with the Communist Soviet Union, and Russian filmmakers became one of the routes by which German Kulturfilm reached other countries. Thus, following the popular and critical reception of German Kulturfilm in Russia, Russian film directors were hired for films like *Frauennot-Frauenglück* (Women's misery—women's happiness; Eisenstein/Tissé, 1929) that were screened in several European countries and the film *Feind im Blut* (1929) (*Enemy in the Blood*), that was screened in Europe and the United States.

The Health Campaign

The emergence of the health education film was shaped not only by developments in film, but also by developments in public health, notably the health campaign. Many of the earliest films were part of such campaigns: antifly campaigns, efforts to promote dental hygiene or eugenics, or crusades to prevent accidents (at work and in the street), tuberculosis, venereal disease, hookworm, cancer, alcoholism, and a range of other public health and safety issues. Some were organized by state agencies, which had been a driving force behind the development of the field of public health in the nineteenth century, but others were the creations of voluntary agencies and commercial organizations such as pharmaceutical and medical instrument companies. Most had multiple stakeholders: partnerships between state and voluntary organization, advertisers and marketing corporations, educational and health bodies, and the many other organizations and individuals concerned with health and illness. Such campaigns had roots in the nineteenth century but came into their own in the twentieth, orchestrating a range of media to reach a mass audience: posters, pamphlets, exhibitions, lectures, theatrical performances, newspaper and magazine articles, lantern slides, and later film and radio.

Film was thus only one of a range of media technologies deployed in such campaigns. It never replaced any of them but was one of many methods employed to ensure that the campaign message reached a mass audience, and in ways that campaign organizers hoped were appropriate to different segments of that audience. Indeed, such organizers often saw posters, newspaper and magazine articles, and talks by local physicians and public health officials as crucial to the success of a film, since these were the ways by which films were advertised and audiences directed to the screening. Others might be shown to captive audiences, in the workplace, in school classrooms and assemblies, in the military, or perhaps as part of the educational schedule of a clinic, or a woman's or workman's club, or in international and national fairs and exhibitions.

At times, the other media choreographed by these public campaigns served to make up for perceived weaknesses in film. Lecturers were often used along with film to ensure that audiences understood the message of the movie (as noted above, not always a given, even after producers integrated the narrative into a film), to address their questions, and counter any unexpected or unwanted reactions. Pamphlets might reinforce a film's message, while local physicians and health officials were often given crib notes so that they could answer questions that patients and the public might bring to them after viewing a movie. A particular concern was that film might generate unwanted emotions that could undermine the goals of a campaign—excessive fear of a disease, pessimism about the possibility of a cure or prevention, undue hope in particular treatments or preventive measures. And there were concerns that a movie designed to prevent venereal disease might promote promiscuity or, just as bad, sexual abstinence in married couples. By coordinating a mix of media, campaign organizers hoped to counter such untoward effects and to create an intense media effort that reached into every dark corner of the public sphere.

Some of the perceived shortcomings of film were a consequence of a sponsor's ambivalence about movies. Early and mid-twentieth-century health agencies saw that the power of film came largely from its ability to entertain, to pleasure the audience. But the commissioning agencies, while completely aware of this, even motivated by it, were often reluctant, given the serious subjects with which they concerned themselves, to fully commit to making films that were entirely pleasurable. And even if they were committed, they often found themselves incompetent to produce pleasurable films (or employed filmmakers who were not competent). The psychologist L. L. Thurstone noted (mocking those who wanted no entertainment in an educational film) that "a film may be of the very highest educational value as a teaching tool, even if it is extremely boring and uninteresting to the casual onlooker."[35] Choreographing a range of media productions thus had its limits in making up for perceived weaknesses in film. Some weaknesses were self-inflicted.

If sponsors and makers worried about the limitations of film, they also argued that movies had a particular power to influence audiences. Like the lantern slide, the images produced by film were projectable (assuming the availability of projectors, a problem at times and in some parts of the world), which made it possible to show audiences things that would be impossible otherwise: new approaches and technologies brought to bear against disease; campaigns to eradicate illness in remote parts of the country and globe; the world of the hospital and public health department; the microbes that caused ills; and the wonders of the internal workings of the body and the damage that disease did to it. But film did more than the lantern slide. Its ability to record the randomness of the natural world gave it a documentary function, while techniques such as cinemicrophotography, time-lapse photography, and x-ray cinematography allowed filmmakers to show audiences aspects of the world around and in them that were otherwise invisible. Such techniques, combined with film's documentary function, allowed some physicians and public health officials to argue that part of the power of film was its ability to substitute for the real thing—be it disease or the interventions against it. The viewer was to be a virtual witness to such events.

Virtual witnessing did not begin with the movies: scientists had long relied on literary and visual technologies to enable other scientists to witness their experiments without having to travel to their laboratories or field stations to see the results themselves. In effect, direct witnessing came to be unnecessary to convince scientists of the validity of observations and experiments. And not only scientists. In the nineteenth century, roving public lecturers and demonstrations allowed those outside of the scientific community to directly witness natural and experimental phenomena, but increasingly most people witnessed science through newspapers and magazines, which in effect became virtual witnessing technologies. In the late nineteenth and (especially the) twentieth centuries, the movies provided a further means of allowing audiences to witness, virtually, natural phenomena, or the results of experimental manipulation.[36]

Virtual witnessing through the movies became a way of educating the public, but it also often blurred into showmanship. For example, Charles Urban produced some of the most successful early films by attaching a camera to a microscope. His "Unseen World" series, which included pioneering microphotographer F. Martin Duncan's classic 1903 film *Cheese Mites*, revealed a hidden natural world that audiences were unaware of and had never before had the chance to see. Urban's and Duncan's scientific revelations were too revealing for some; the British cheese industry had the film censored because the industry was afraid it would negatively impact the public's perceptions of their product.[37]

Movies thus did much more than document. Sponsors and filmmakers argued that their ability to tell dramatic, often melodramatic, stories of the sorts used in public health films from the 1910s gave added power to the medium. They allowed the dry facts of science to be wrapped in an engaging tale that would help persuade the viewer of the value of scientific, medical, and public health approaches to health and illness. They also allowed physicians and public health officials to counter public anxieties about disease and its treatment or prevention by offering a story of hope or by using the narrative to downplay disturbing aspects of their subject that might undermine the willingness of the public to seek help—surgery in cancer, the pneumothorax operation in tuberculosis, and so on. At the same time, the use of animation could also be used to downplay the horribleness of an intervention or to counter the tendency of photographic film to provide too much information: techniques of animation could highlight those parts of the natural world the sponsor wanted to target.

At the heart of this debate were assumptions about how film affected an audience. In *The Photoplay: A Psychological Study* (1916), the Harvard psychologist Hugo Münsterberg set out to challenge the moral condemnation of moviegoing, and especially the idea that cinematic escapism undermined the work ethic.[38] In his view, the medium had a unique capacity to bypass voluntary effort—such as thinking, remembering, and physical effort such as eye movement—which made it more effective at reaching audiences than the theater. Furthermore, he claimed that film communicated directly with involuntary mental functions and emotions and more closely resembled the functioning of the human brain than other media. Cinematic techniques (such as the close-up, flashback, and parallel cutting), he claimed, formed closer approximations to inner mental processes and emotions than the theater could achieve.[39] Münsterberg's concern with the power of film for social influence, both good and bad, would help inform debates about its role in education and set the stage for the burgeoning of psychological studies of audience responses to educational film from the 1920s (see Laukötter this volume).

The campaign approach underwent great development during World War I. Public health and military establishments came to share a common vocabulary (campaigns, mobilizations, officers, enemies, containments, crusades, surveillance, evacuation, battles, wars, victories, tactics, strategies, logistics) and a common organizational model: the disciplined, deployable, hierarchical service; command and control; and a common obsession with scientific and technological innovation, including new media such as film, the telephone, and radio. This is not to say that health films were only used in health and safety campaigns. Some were used to document the work of a health department, clinic, hospital, voluntary organization, or philanthropic agency or to record (and promote the interests of) commercial organizations such as pharmaceutical or medical instrument corporations and life insurance companies. All these turned to film in the belief in its transformative power and its ability to document and to reach audiences that other media could not. Nevertheless, the campaign movie was one of the major uses of film within a public health setting throughout the period covered by this book, from its deployment in the 1910s to the post–World War II period by authoritarian regimes and democratic regimes alike, and to its use by multiple international organizations.

Physicians and public health officials thus turned to film for a variety of reasons. It promised to reach audiences that other media could not reach; to show them things that other media could not, and to do so in an engaging way, often as part of a mass campaign that orchestrated a variety of media. Crucially, they turned to film because it allowed them to represent themselves as modern, and in two ways: by the use of film itself, a quintessentially modern technology, and by using film to represent modern approaches to public health. In addition, by portraying key events, achievements, and anxieties, the public health movie invited audiences to participate in the rapidly changing public health world that was working for them: to go to their physicians at the first sign of an illness, to avoid (nonmodern) quacks and folk remedies, and to understand the dangers of microbes and microscopic changes in the body and what to do to prevent them turning into something hazardous to health. Paradoxically, such films also became a means of highlighting the perils of modernity. From the silent era onward, public health films showed the dangers of the development of modern ways of moving people and goods (traffic accidents, the threat posed to public health by international trade and immigration). They also showed the dangers of modern manufacturing and its products (factory fires, explosives) and of modern ways of living and the city: the problems of infectious disease in crowded cities, the lack of proper sanitation, and infestation with insects and rats.

Edison's Tuberculosis Films

The origins of the campaign film are well illustrated by the six films about tuberculosis made between 1910 and 1915 by Thomas Edison's film company in collaboration with the National Association for the Study and Prevention of Tuberculosis (NASPT).[40] They were often called the Red Cross Seal films after the annual Christmas Seal campaign, an important source of income for the NASPT. During the Christmas Seal campaign, thousands of volunteers from schoolchildren to fraternal organizations sold the stamps, which each year featured a different illustration.

The films were part of a much broader effort by the NASPT to promote what historian Nancy Tomes calls the "gospel of germs" about tuberculosis.[41] Robert Koch's discovery of the tubercle bacillus in 1882 redefined tuberculosis as a bacterial disease. It also laid a foundation for vast educational programs to persuade the public that tuberculosis was a contagious disease and to abandon habits such as spitting that might spread the disease. These programs employed a wide range of activities including public lectures and demonstrations; the publication of posters, cartoons, drawings, and charts; the construction of exhibits and models; and efforts to promote the campaign through newspapers and magazines. As in many campaigns, film did not replace these older forms of public education. Rather, films joined them, often as part of carefully coordinated publicity events that mixed older marketing methods with newer ones. These films and campaigning methods were exported to Europe at the end of World War I, notably under the Rockefeller mission: a liaison office in Paris that coordinated touring mobile projection units in France and promoted TB prevention programs that in the mid-1920s became the basis for the French anti-TB committee, the National Defense against Tuberculosis Committee (CNDT).[42]

The NASPT's reasons for turning to film anticipated and echoed the reasons why many other disease campaigns began to see film as an educational tool at this time. In its view, film was a particularly powerful medium for instructing the public about tuberculosis and what could be done to detect, treat, and prevent it.[43] It not only provided a unique mix of storytelling and visuals, but it also attracted enthusiasm that traditional educational methods did not: the screening of a movie was an event in itself, reported in local newspapers and magazines, the focus of broader publicity and education programs. Thus Edison's films seemed to be screened almost everywhere, on the walls of churches, factories, schools, libraries, clinics, clubhouses, and tenement buildings, the usual places where public health educational films would be screened from the 1910s onward. The label "educational" film did not yet mean "nontheatrical," and in the 1910s it was quite normal for theaters to screen pictures about topics that would later be more often encountered elsewhere. Edison's tuberculosis films shared the schedule with actualities (nonfiction films), scientific films, and fictional dramas and comedies.

The NASPT's interest in sponsoring films also highlights the reformist impulses illustrated by contemporary films such as *The Drunkard's Reformation.* It coincided with concerns in the young movie industry about a growing censorship movement, and film producers and exhibitors in the 1910s were determined to raise the social prestige of motion pictures. To this end, they increasingly turned to progressive and benevolent organizations such as the NASPT for storylines and moral messages and began to make films about social problems such as poverty, usury, and crime as well as public health, hoping to broaden the audience for film to include the middle classes, women, and children. There was thus a commercial rationale for producing films for the Christmas Seal campaign. They targeted the sorts of audiences that the movie industry was hoping to reach, helped to stave off the possibility of censorship, and promised a financial return as well. Given that the films entered general release, producer-distributors like Edison earned income from rentals on the film. These films were thus not only a corpus in themselves, they were part of other overlapping corpuses—health education films, reform films, and entertainment films—a mix of corpuses that later film entrepreneurs such as Frank Tichenor (see Cantor in this volume) would also seek to blur.

A Shape Shifting, Hybrid Format

As the above suggests, the health education film is a shape-shifting, hybrid format or genre. Not only may the message of a film may mean something very different to different stakeholders, but the film itself may contain elements of other forms of film (actualities, entertainment films, medical training films, research films, clinical observation films, documentaries, industrials, accident prevention films, occupational safety films, newsreels, and advertisements, among others). While health education films may be distinguished by their subject matter, they borrow from and inform the aesthetics, techniques of production, narrative tropes, visual imagery, sound, or music of many other forms of film.

The hybrid nature of the health film can be illustrated by Edison's tuberculosis films. Like the contemporary anti-alcohol films, they appeared before the category of the health education film emerged, mixed older modes of cinematic storytelling with newer forms of narration, and crossed boundaries that would emerge later between theatrical and nontheatrical film.[44] For Edison these films were part of a broader effort to defend against threats of government regulation and censorship by linking films to efforts of moral and health reform. Edison himself forecast that films would wipe out "narrow-minded prejudices" based on ignorance and create a "feeling of sympathy and a desire to help the down trodden people of the earth."[45] In his view, showing films about tuberculosis and other health and social issues in movie theaters alongside comedies, features, and other entertainment films was a key to attaining such goals. These films entered general release, and audiences in the 1910s would likely have not seen anything exceptional in their inclusion in the theatrical program. Social problem films, scientific films, and actualities often shared the program with emergent feature and comedy entertainment films.

But such hopes and uses for the health film were short-lived in the United States. By the mid-1910s and especially in the 1920s, theater owners came to exclude educational films—including health education films—from their programs, fearful that audiences did not want to pay for them and that the subject matter of some made theatrical screening problematic.[46] While some film entrepreneurs and public health officials continued to argue that well-made films could find a place in commercial movie theater programs, and indeed that people paid more attention to films that they paid for, such films were increasingly shown outside of these venues in soldiers' camps, women's clubs, libraries, workplaces, exhibitions, traveling shows, and so on, frequently at more than one of these places. Movie theaters might be hired for a special showing of a health education film. But by and large such films tended to be excluded from a regular theatrical event, with the exception of short "spots"—perhaps thirty seconds or a minute—that might be shown along with advertisements.[47]

In Europe a similar tendency to separate out health education films from theatrical films also emerged.[48] In France and Germany, for example, state censorship—or the threat of state censorship—was a moving force behind this separation. But the separation was never as complete as in the United States, and kulturfilms with a public health theme continued to be shown in movie theaters as part of the regular theatrical show. Health education films may also have benefited from European efforts to protect their industries from American domination: European health films sometimes remained in the theatrical event as theater owners sought to fill the gaps in the regular cinema program. In Switzerland, Austria, France, and Germany educational films were often screened as prefilm before feature films because such screening allowed theater owners to obtain tax reductions or to reduce ticket prices for feature-length film. A further reason was that these films could be very difficult to distinguish from entertainment films, so that films could easily cross the boundary between education and entertainment.[49] In the USSR, there were political reasons for the inclusion of the health film in the regular program: Lenin argued that an ideal film show should comprise a documentary, a cartoon film, and a fiction film; in this way he hoped both to satisfy public expectations for entertainment and at the same time to instruct and educate audiences. But such hopes were never realized. In practice, health education films were mainly shown in special events to captive audiences (the military, schools, trade unions) or to invited test audiences for their feedback. Attempts to create specialized movie theaters for educational films failed in the USSR, as did efforts to attract audiences to health education film shows by keeping admission prices low.

Despite their increasing exclusion from or marginalization in theatrical venues, health educational films often included components of theatrical films. Their health messages were often wrapped in a dramatic narrative that paralleled and sometimes informed or derived from commercial cinema, and camera, editing, animation, and other film and sound techniques developed in commercial film filtered into health education film production, as for example during World War II, when the American government hired commercial film producers to develop public and military education and training films as part of war mobilization. It should come as no surprise then that health education films from the 1910s to the 1960s regularly plundered genres such as the melodrama, German expressionism, the woman's film, film noir, crime and gangster movies, and cartoon comedies. These films were often intended to entertain as well as to educate, despite the naysayers who, on the one hand, doubted that educational films could be entertaining or, on the other hand, wondered whether entertainment did more to attract an audience than to educate it.

Generally, health education films were not as well financed as entertainment films, and so the technical development of the health education film is often different from that of the entertainment film. For example, sound was generally adapted much later in education films than in entertainment films, and some "sound" educational films were in fact silent films with a sound track added later—perhaps a narrator, and some canned music—a cheaper way of making a sound movie. (Only well-financed educational films had music specially composed for them.) Nevertheless, it should not be supposed that health education film events were entirely silent, even in the silent era. Event organizers often hired a pianist to accompany the film and physicians and other experts commented on the film and its subject matter before, during, or after the show. And this is to say nothing of the fidgeting of audiences, their comments, questions, laughter, and perhaps the (humorous) interjection of a sound effect.

If health education films came to incorporate elements of the entertainment film, they also incorporated elements of other types of film.[50] One was the use of film in scientific or clinical experiment or observation. Physicians and scientists, for example, had turned to film almost the moment it came about. They used it to extend observational powers, as a means of training other physicians, and as a form of self-advertisement.[51] But these sorts of films were often regarded as inappropriate for the public. Their subject matter could be too gruesome or too technical for a popular audience, and it was also the case that the messages that might be appropriate for physicians were not deemed appropriate for the public.[52] Despite such reservations, however, some medical films came to gain a popular following. For example, the films of cells dividing in tissue culture produced by the pathologist R. G. Canti at the Strangeways laboratory in Cambridge, England, proved—to the surprise of sponsors—to be highly popular with nonspecialist audiences.[53] This was also the case with the Steinach film, a 1922–23 Universum Film AG (UFA) production directed by Curt Thomalla and Nicholas Kaufmann on the theoretical and practical work of the Austrian physiologist and endocrinologist Eugen Steinach (1861–1944) and his rejuvenation experiments. In this case, the film was screened in two versions: a "scientific" version and a version for the wider public, which became a widely acknowledged success.[54] In other cases, sequences shot originally as part of an experiment might later be cut out of the footage of the experiment and incorporated into a health education film. Thus, the Soviet *kulturfil'my* of the 1920s, in contrast to many popular science films, were hybrids that mixed—sometimes by means of montage—fiction, life action scenes, and sequences of scientific technique including microphotography.

Health education films also blurred other categories. Some borrowed techniques and scenes from the newsreel, a genre that had emerged during the World War I: newsreels sometimes touch on medical themes, while health films also incorporated newsreel footage or formats and techniques.[55] Similarly, as essays in this collection will demonstrate, the public health education film borrowed from documentary film genres, advertising film, Kulturfilm, and the industrial film. The public health film was for these reasons a hybrid format, distinguished by its subject matter, but incorporating a wide range of other genres and formats.

Finally, it needs to be said that public health film was not only a hybrid format but—as artifacts—these films were not a stable category. The films themselves might be printed and reprinted over time, with minor changes to the texture of the film, depending on the film stock that was used. They could also be cut and recut, so that fragments of films appeared in others.[56] Indeed, some films were designed to be cut so that an educator could choose the most appropriate scenes for instructional purposes.[57] Other films seem to have been modified during their lives, taking quite different forms in different places and times.

An example of the last of these is *Frauennot-Frauenglück* (1929) (Women's misery–women's happiness) (Eisenstein/Tissé, 1929), commissioned by Lazar Wechsler, the director of the Swiss Präsens-Film corporation.[58] The film was a highly successful and controversial pro-abortion silent film produced against the backdrop of political debates in Europe about the decriminalization of abortion after World War I.[59] Half fiction, half documentary the one-hour commercially distributed black and white picture stages in successive and parallel montage four case histories of women and why abortion might be a solution to their problems.[60] Initially distributed in Switzerland, the film was quickly adapted for distribution in Austria, Germany, France, Brazil, England, the United States, Mexico, and Finland.[61] Crucially, the message of each of these different versions depended on the status of the discourse on abortion within each country. For example, a French version released in 1930 under the title *L'Appel de la vie* (The call of life) turned the original pro-abortion film into one that was pro-life. Such a reversal of message might be extreme in the history of the health education film, but it serves to highlight the point that film was (and is) a highly adaptable medium and that the first release of a film is not necessarily its final form. It is something that can be (and has been) adapted to fit different purposes and the introduction of new technologies: *Frauennot-Frauenglück*, like many other silent films, was later rereleased with an added sound track.

Adolf Nichtenhauser

This book is indebted to the pioneer film historian, Adolf Nichtenhauser, whose unpublished book manuscript on the history of historical medical films has in many ways not been surpassed in the sixty plus years since he wrote it.[62] Based on an impressive range of sources, Nichtenhauser showed how motion pictures became a research tool within the field of medicine shortly after the invention of film technology in the United States and Europe, and how from the 1910s it was transformed into an educational tool targeted at the wider public. This manuscript, and the related Nichtenhauser manuscript collection at the US National Library of Medicine (NLM) at Bethesda, Maryland, have provided key sources for many historians of medicine and film.[63]

Nichtenhauser raised several points that our volume builds upon. First, he highlighted the importance of war—especially the two world wars—as key moments in the history of the health education film. Nichtenhauser showed that in both world wars the health education film gained mass military and civilian audiences, increased funding, and a key role in campaigns against a variety of public health threats. The ways in which this happened varied from country to country, sometimes spearheaded by government, sometimes by private philanthropic or commercial organizations, and sometimes by physicians and public health officials, among others. But Nichtenhauser did not believe that war was an unequivocal boon to the health film. Government funding was often temporary (as in the United States, France, and Germany in and shortly after World War I) and could dry up after hostilities ended. Nevertheless, there are also hints in his manuscript about how military interest in health films persists outside of war, and how wartime and peacetime uses of film are not easily separated. Such a focus is further developed in this volume, where we suggest that war and the health film must be studied as constitutive of the societies and cultures in which they were set. Film was often part of "campaigns" and "wars" against disease in "peacetime" (Ostherr, Lowy and Cantor), sometimes organized on military lines, and could portray the body as a site of war as in the French film *Syphilis Public Enemy N° 1* (1939) or the World War II production *L'ennemi secret/ The secret enemy* (1945).

Second, Nichtenhauser also highlighted the importance of national histories of the health education film. In his account, the development of the health film, including during the two world wars, happened in very different ways in different countries.[64] Overall, Nichtenhauser presents a complicated and changing picture of the history of the health education film with numerous institutions and individuals involved in promoting it, sometimes collaborating, sometimes competing, and the importance of each to the health film changing over time within each country and across different countries. Part of our rationale for looking at health films in North America and Europe is to capture something of this complexity.

Third, if Nichtenhauser emphasizes the importance of national histories, he also emphasizes the importance of an international perspective. At times in his narrative, he traces the importance of international scientific and medical meetings to the promotion of film, how films were seen by some as a tool for promoting international exchange,[65] how national organizations like the American Film Centers in the 1930s became international information and consultation centers about film,[66] and how before World War II a variety of international organizations emerged: such as the International Institute of Educational Cinematography; the International Federation of Students; the International Teaching Film Chamber; and perhaps most importantly, the League of Nations.[67] The NLM dates this book manuscript to 1950, and Nichtenhauser does not trace history of medical film into the postwar period. There is no mention of the United Nations, WHO, or other post World War II international organizations involved with health education films. Nor does he situate the health education film within the emergent Cold War. Some of the chapters in our collection begin this work, notably those by Ursula von Keitz and Kirsten Ostherr.

Fourth, Nichtenhauser highlights the importance not only of the conditions of producing films, but also of screening, collecting, and distribution. Nichtenhauser undertook an immense amount of research into the various government, philanthropic, and commercial organizations that produced and sponsored films; the development of film libraries, including those for health education films; and where and how films were shown. He is also interested in how audiences responded to film and how their responses were assessed. In addition, he provides considerable detail on technologies involved in especially film production and screening (the evolving technologies of the camera, the projector, and the film medium), and how these influenced what was filmed, how it was shown, and how audiences (might have) experienced the film. Nichtenhauser's manuscript can tell us much about the distribution of film technologies, and there is more in his manuscript collection, including figures on the geographical distribution of film projectors and how the combination of technology, distribution, skill of operator, and the conditions of the screening venue shaped the experience of viewing films.

Fifth, Nichtenhauser is interested in understanding what counts as a good film. Nichtenhauser tends to mean two different things by this. On the one hand, he refers to what contemporaries meant by a good film. Thus, for example, at various points in the manuscript he highlights complaints about how the poor quality of films undermined their value to audiences, a problem compounded by the poor conditions under which films were often screened. In addition, he is able to show how such concerns were linked at times to efforts to evaluate and improve the quality of films or to efforts to compare certain national styles of filmmaking, or the filmmaking of various organizations, governmental, commercial, and voluntary. On the other hand, Nichtenhauser also tends to offer his own assessments of the quality of films—indeed, at times his own comments seem to blur seamlessly into the comments of others. It is important in this respect to note that Nichtenhauser is himself a player in this story. He is part of a small group of people in the 1940s and 1950s who were interested in promoting the use of film in medicine, including health education, and concerned about the profusion of poor quality films. This volume was in part an effort to help contextualize then-contemporary efforts to improve film production and use. At the same time that this book was being written, Nichtenhauser and the Medical Film Institute of the Association of American Medical Colleges were providing reviews of the quality of educational and training films to help readers/viewers identify quality films. Some of these reviews were published, others survive in the Nichtenhauser papers at the NLM.[68] Nichtenhauser's manuscript is part of this story.

Finally, Nichtenhauser is also interested in what today might be called visual culture. He argues that the problem of motion picture filmmaking was not primarily "one of equipment, photographic technique and finances but one of thinking in a visual language which has its own particular grammar, syntax and logic."[69] Yet, Nichtenhauser devotes little space to the grammar, syntax and logic of the film, nor does he give much attention to analysis of aesthetics, narratives, and techniques of persuasion of these films. And where he does, it is as someone who is involved in the 1940s and 1950s in trying to shape that visual culture. The numerous reports on the films collected in his papers show Nichtenhauser and his colleagues struggling to explain what makes a film work, and part of the explanation is whether it follows film's grammar, syntax, and logic. Nichtenhauser, the historian and the promoter of films, recognizes that this grammar, syntax, and logic has to be created for the new medium and that it evolves over the course of the late nineteenth and early twentieth centuries. Nichtenhauser, the promoter of film, tends to measure the success or otherwise of a film against an almost timeless grammar, syntax and logic.

Our book builds upon these insights, but it also differs from his. Nichtenhauser tends to regard what counts as a good film as independent of audience response and national/regional context. It is almost intrinsic to the film itself. In addition, he tends to regard the corpus of health education films as somewhat unproblematic. This book argues, by contrast, that what counts as a "good" film depends on context—the views of different stakeholders in a film may differ (sponsor, producer, audience, etc.). And it may vary according to national/cultural/institutional context. In addition, as we have already noted, our book also problematizes the corpus. A project is yet to be developed about how Nichtenhauser defined the corpus of public health education films and how this related to his vision of what constituted a good film. Our interest is less in improving the quality of films than in Nichtenhauser's interest in assessing how people assessed the quality of films.

The Chapters

The chapters are divided into four parts that focus on different families of corpuses. The first, commercial contexts, explores corpuses produced by commercial organizations or individuals working within commercial cinema: film production companies, pharmaceutical companies, and Hollywood film directors. In these corpuses, the principle interest of the organization or individual is often not medicine or health. They turned to health films for a variety of reasons (perhaps as a source of additional income to help a struggling film company; perhaps as a means of promoting company products or image), and they ensured that techniques and practices from the commercial world (marketing techniques development by film companies and pharmaceutical corporations; filmmaking techniques from the entertainment film world) shaped the health film. The films in this section were thus hybrid creations, partly the product of the commissioning body, partly the product of the organization that made the film, partly the product of the directors and other members of the film production team. They thus straddle the boundaries between health film, advertising, and the commercial work of filmmakers. As such this corpus of health films is a very unstable entity, constantly blurring into other corpuses of films, many of which may have little to do with health.

David Cantor shows how American film producers turned to medical film, and he finds, unsurprisingly, that much of it had little to do with medical issues. The Eastern Film Corporation began life in 1915 as an entertainment film company that its founder, Frank Tichenor, hoped would rival the largest in the industry. There were good reasons for this hope. Tichenor had been a major figure in the entertainment film world since at least 1910; the company was well capitalized; it had perhaps the largest film studios in the country, located in Providence, Rhode Island; and some of the best-known actors in the film business. But it was not to be, and as Cantor details, as his hopes of a place in the entertainment film world began to crumble, Tichenor began looking for other revenue streams. Medical and health films were part of this strategy, but only one part. Tichenor also turned to other sponsored films, to advertising, and to efforts to create film libraries; he also continued trying to break into the commercial film world, first as producer and later as distributor. He was also a supporter of pioneer efforts in the early 1920s to mix film and sound. His efforts managed to keep Eastern alive until the late 1920s or early 1930s when the company—and Tichenor's other film ventures—folded. Cantor thus shows how medical and health film were part of a broader strategy of commercial survival. He also shows how for Tichenor these films blurred the boundaries between entertainment and education, theatrical and nontheatrical, and advertising and education. Tichenor saw the markets in medical film (films aimed at a medical audience) and health film (those aimed at the public) as very different and that different commercial strategies were needed to exploit them. So how to define the corpus of Eastern's health education films? The characteristics of the market distinguished this corpus from medical films but not from other markets such as for political, advertising, or social service films. Moreover, it shared with these later corpuses the central problem of shaping people's beliefs and behaviors. The corpus of health education films thus has leaky boundaries that bleed into corpuses of other types of film in terms of market characteristics and the central problem. Indeed, they may have blurred into others in other ways. Eastern's film libraries meant that film footage from medical or health films could be found in other types of film and vice versa. This library was a repository of stock footage that could be inserted into other films, either produced by Tichenor's companies or by other corporations that would pay for the footage.

Christian Bonah looks at another commercial corpus: that produced by the pharmaceutical company Bayer from the 1920s to the 1940s. Like Cantor, he argues, that one must take account of the historical actor's definition of film. Where Cantor highlights Tichenor's distinction between medical and health films, Bonah highlights the different ways in which the Bayer pharmaceutical company defined films produced by its in-house film unit, founded in 1934. As Bonah shows, Bayer saw its film production as part of a broader marketing strategy of image building that sought not only to promote Bayer products, such as aspirin, but also the corporation itself and its reputation as a trustworthy, science-based, and efficient manufacturer and supplier. To do this, the corporation produced a variety of different types of film, each targeted at different audiences and each with different goals. Indeed, Bayer divided its film production into several different types: (1) popular advertisement films, (2) scientific demonstration films, (3) Kulturfilm, (4) image-building films (*Wert-Werbungsfilm*), and finally (5) special films (films that aimed to increase the entertainment aspect of film events or to obtain access to audiences that otherwise would have been difficult to reach). Bonah shows how Bayer used this classification to target different audiences and to distinguish many of its promotional films from traditional advertising. These film types were distinct corpuses within the broader category of the company's industrial film corpus.

Bonah pays particular attention to a series of image-building films that Bayer produced between 1934 and 1943. Bayer's policy in regard to this type of film meant that the films generally avoided references to any Bayer product or to the company, except that Bayer was mentioned in the opening credits and at the end of the films. Thus, while these films were labeled as Bayer films, they did not promote its products or the company itself except as a sponsor of these films—much like the contemporaneous Shell film unit in the 1930s in the United Kingdom. As Bonah shows, such films do not easily fit film categories of industrial, educational, health film, advertising, or propaganda film (though some were produced under the National Socialist regime and by directors sympathetic to the Nazis), and they could contain elements of some or all. Indeed, these films could serve advertising, information, instruction, and education all at once, depending on the settings in which they were shown and the audiences before which they were screened, as much as they also served Bayer's intent in commissioning them, and the various aims of the filmmakers hired to make them. Thus, the chapter argues that these films not only promoted Bayer's goals but could also promote others as well, not all of which were in harmony with the intent of the sponsor. Finally, it should be noted that Bayer's films were not only part of a corpus of Bayer films, but also a corpus of other Bayer media productions. The unifying image across all these media was the Bayer Cross—a display of the corporation's name twice in form of a cross that could appear as an illumination strung between the factory chimneys of Bayer's industrial places, in a pharmacy advertisement in Latin America, an information leaflet in China, a film still in a 1934 Malaria reel, and stamped onto every tablet that left the factory. In incorporating this symbol into its production, Bayer used films as part of its broader goal of branding. It is at moments such as this that the corpus can extend beyond film to include many other media productions.

Finally, Vincent Lowy and David Cantor construct their corpus not from an institutional corpus—a film company or a drug manufacturer—but from the films of Hollywood directors who also made health education films and from health education and entertainment films that employ conversion narratives. Their corpuses are analytical and comparative in nature. Theirs is an account of the complex relations between commercial entertainment films and health films. The point has been made by other chapters in this section: Cantor's first piece looks at this porous boundary in the context of Frank Tichenor's business rationales for moving into health education and medical films production and distribution; Bonah shows how film techniques and approaches developed in the entertainment setting were applied in the industrially commissioned health film; Lowy and Cantor develop the latter point, looking at how conversion narratives employed in entertainments were applied (or not) to educational films.

Lowy's and Cantor's focus is the health education films of three Hollywood directors—Edgar Ulmer, John Huston, and John Ford. These three directors were part of a broader influx of Hollywood talent into educational, training, and propaganda filmmaking during the 1930s and 1940s that allowed the transfer of film techniques developed in Hollywood entertainment movies as part of broader efforts to mobilize support for and participation in public health programs. Much scholarly attention has focused on the efforts by government during the World War II to use Hollywood to mobilize for war and on how filmmakers—Huston and Ford among them—were recruited to make public health films as part of this broader wartime effort.[70] However, Lowy's and Cantor's chapter shows that while the influx of Hollywood talent might have expanded during the war, it also predated it, as when the director, Edgar Ulmer, already known for his "ethnic" films was hired in the 1930s by the National Tuberculosis Association to make a series of such films about tuberculosis—for African Americans, Native Americans, and Hispanics—as well as for white, nonethnic (in the view of the Association) audiences.[71]

Elsewhere, Cantor has argued that conversion narratives formed a key feature of cancer education films, and his collaboration with Lowy in this book expands the point to show that conversion narratives can be found in health education films on many other topics.[72] However, the focus on this one aspect of the health education film also reveals the complicated relations between health education films and entertainments. In the 1930s, the sorts of conversion narratives found in health education films were quite different from those found in many entertainment films of the same period. However, as both Hollywood and the health education film went to war in the 1940s, the conversions in both forms of film seem to have come much closer as both sought to mobilize the nation for war. The focus on three directors further complicates the picture. On the one hand, Ulmer's TB conversion narratives echoed that found in one of his entertainments, an exploitation movie on venereal disease, suggesting that the story of the divergence of conversion narratives in 1930s health educationals and entertainments did not apply universally. On the other hand, while both Ford and Huston deployed critiques of American society in their prewar entertainments, such critiques were largely absent from their wartime educationals and the conversion narratives they deployed, as they were from many entertainments. Such critiques did not fit well with efforts to mobilize and prepare Americans for war. Even Huston, who seems to have become disillusioned with some aspects of the war, was to produce an optimistic account of medicine's ability to turn psychologically wounded soldiers back into psychologically healthy civilians.

Part two of the book—Campaigns—addresses the films that were part of noncommercial campaigns. While Cantor's and Bonah's corpuses were campaigns in that they promoted the commercial objectives of the organizations that made or sponsored them, the corpuses in this section were sponsored, produced, screened, or distributed by a variety of health-related agencies, including anti-disease campaigns, local government, and national government. While these corpuses were not sponsored for commercial gain, they nevertheless were produced and disseminated to meet the goals of the agencies that sponsored them. Yet like the films in commercial corpuses, they were often hybrid creations. The agencies that sponsored them sometimes did so for a mix of reasons, which might include promoting public health but also the broader policy goals of local and national governments and the complex politics of disease agencies. They were also hybrids in the sense that while some were produced by the sponsoring agencies themselves, others relied on commercial or other agencies to make or distribute them, and films made for a public health purpose could also stray into the commercial theatrical arena where their meaning could change. And even those that made their own films had to rely on filmmakers—not always of the stature of an Ulmer, Ford, or Huston—to turn their policy goals into something that worked as a film, which could leave ample room for other interests and agendas to shape the movie. Finally, these films were also hybrids in the sense that they highlight the emergent distinctions between entertainment and nonentertainment, theatrical and nontheatrical, or commercial and noncommercial films. Public health films could fall into any of these categories, but increasingly they came to be defined as nonentertainment, nontheatrical, and noncommercial, while often drawing on techniques and practices from the entertainment, theatrical, and commercial film worlds.

Focusing on US venereal-disease movies produced in the 1910s, Miriam Posner's chapter explores the hostile worlds of sex and commerce in the United States and what happened when films originally intended for educational purposes entered the commercial sphere. Her focus is *The End of the Road* (1919) and the corpus of social hygiene films produced during the war. But as Posner notes, the corpus of films into which a film might fit can change. *The End of the Road* was originally produced as an educational film during the war as part of a broader effort to combat venereal disease and to regulate sexual activities of men in uniform and the women they encountered, at least outside of marriage and family. The film was originally shown in noncommercial settings: church halls, YWCAs, factories, and elsewhere. However, by the end of the war, a slightly different version of the movie was shown in commercial theaters, and then the trouble started. A film that had been uplifting in the educational setting had turned to smut, as Posner puts it, when it entered the commercial sector. It no longer belonged solely to the corpus of public health education films or even of commercial entertainment films. It had entered a corpus of exploitation films where concerns about the commercialization of cinema paralleled concerns about the commercialization of its subject matter, sex. Posner thus shows that commercial release of *End of the Road* was a key moment when the boundary between "educational" and "entertainment" films was drawn, and it led to the film studios recruiting Presbyterian elder Will H. Hays to rehabilitate the industry's image. Moreover, she also shows that by following one film, and its protean meanings, one can also beginning to raise questions highlighted by other authors in this volume about the problematic definition of corpuses of films. If one film within a corpus could change meaning so dramatically, then the corpus of which it was a part was also in danger of dissolving into others.

If Posner explores the boundaries between commercial and educational film in capitalist America, Alexandre Sumpf explores the boundaries between political ideology and the public health education film at the heart of Communism: the Soviet Union in the 1920s. His focus is the corpus of films produced by Russian and later Soviet anti-alcohol campaigns, a hybrid corpus, like so many others in this volume, that includes different genres or types of film. Sumpf highlights the porous boundary between films designed to promote the goals of public health and those designed to promote Soviet ideology—a corpus that could include a much broader range of films than those focused on alcohol. In Sumpf's account, anti-alcohol films were not only about promoting sobriety, but also about helping to create the "new man" who would build a Communist utopia. Yet the Soviet authorities had a mixed attitude toward alcohol, sometimes promoting alcohol reform, sometimes promoting the sale and consumption of vodka, which raised questions about the role of alcohol reform in promoting communism and the ability of anti-alcohol films to deliver such reform.

Sumpf also discusses the complex ways in which physicians were involved in these films: sometimes they were advisors, sometimes directors, sometimes sponsors. Whatever the role, they found themselves struggling to figure out how to mesh the public health goals of the film with the emergent visual language of the film medium and the developing political realities of the new Communist regime, and not always successfully—discussions of what constituted a Soviet film could work for physicians, but equally it could work against them. Even if they produced a film that somehow brought together the various agendas and skills and hopes of the new medium, it was not certain how audiences would respond. Their status as medical experts did not necessarily mean that they were accepted as film experts by audiences, while medical popularizers were not always accepted as medical experts by their professional peers; such were some of the complexities of medical expertise in film. Moreover, like Posner, Sumpf looks at what happens to films during distribution and screening in the immense country that was the Soviet Union, with a scattering of cities and rural populations in the vast tracts of land between. Sumpf shows how, in the cities, workers' committees could be difficult audiences to please, while other audiences could turn the rhetoric of Communism against the film. In one instance, a projectionist's suggestion that one of the members of Komsomol (the Soviet youth organization) in a rural village read the insert titles was rejected by the peasant audience on the grounds that on the tenth anniversary of the October

Revolution there should no longer be a single illiterate. Everyone could read the titles for themselves.

Elizabeth Lebas's focus is on the relationship between the public health film and municipal policy and politics. She explores municipal public health films in Britain between the wars, and in particular the corpuses of films produced by two left-leaning local councils, Bermondsey and Glasgow, each representing different strands of Labour Party politics. Once again the corpus of public health films blurs into others, notably the broader film corpus of these two municipalities. In Lebas's account, these municipal health films were distinctive in that, unlike other health films produced at the same time, they made citizenship and entitlement universal and introduced their audiences to an imagined future of everyday life in a new class(less) society, albeit sometimes defined in middle-class terms. Municipal health films allowed local councils to both distinguish themselves from national policy while at the same time sharing with national policy a goal of improving the health of the people. The level of observation of a corpus may thus be adjusted according to the analytical aims pursued; in this case it serves the national versus the local divide, reminding us that health missions and film production played out at many different levels in different ways.

Bermondsey and Glasgow turned to film for remarkably similar purposes, in part to promote public health, but also for other reasons. Some films were little more than promotional exercises, some were visual annual reports, others were commemorative, and yet others had a more didactic goal. Some were made locally, using local scenes and people, and so provided opportunities for local residents to star in or comment on themselves or others or the localities where they were shot. Production could thus include spectatorship directly as a vehicle of mobilization and concern. Hence, Lebas tells us not only much about why local authorities decided to make these films, but also how they were distributed and screened and the responses of local audiences. Municipal public health films, in Lebas's telling, were only in part about public health, not only for the local councils that sponsored and produced them, but also for their audiences. They were part of a broader history of local authority activism, their efforts to create local civic identities, and of audience responses to these efforts.

Part three of this volume moves beyond the nation and locality to explore the theme of international reorganization in public health films, especially after World War II. International organizations had turned to film much earlier: the Red Cross, the League of Nations, and others all produced, distributed, and screened films before the Second World War. Indeed, institutions such as the League of Nations, and later the United Nations, that sought to project a neutral voice that brought together nations with different interests and agendas, helped to construct the idea of documentary film as somehow neutral and above politics. As Zoë Druick argues, the League of Nations and the United Nations helped to turn (especially documentary) film into a particularly modern educational technology that balanced the perceived threats posed by modernity to traditional culture with a world increasingly mediated by information technology.[73] Indeed, in documentary film this mediation was central to the visibility and validation of traditional cultures. Representations of educational film as apolitical persisted into the postwar years, where their seeming neutrality helped to promote disparate values in the emergent Cold War, even if national governments sometimes attempted to turn international organizations into their tools. WHO, for example, was dominated by the Americans in the immediate postwar period.

Ursula von Keitz's contribution highlights the role of film in mediating political tensions in postwar Germany. It is an international story focused on one country that became two, in the four zones—British, French, American, and Soviet—of the occupying powers. In particular, her focus is on how the institutional structures of the film industry that predated Germany's wartime defeat continued to shape filmmaking in the defeated and occupied Germany, as did prewar styles of filmmaking. Her story is thus in part about how local filmmaking institutions and cultures are important to an understanding of film in international context.

In von Keitz's account, the four occupying powers first turned to film as a means of de-nazification. Film provided a means of confronting Germans with the horrors of Nazi racial policy, and the occupying powers regarded medicine as a particularly important area for reeducation, given the role of physicians in Nazi policies of sterilization, euthanasia programs and "scientific" experiments on prisoners and concentration camp inmates. But the occupying powers' policies began to separate out after 1946, when American occupation policy shifted from a predominantly punitive focus that emphasized collective guilt to a focus that was intended to highlight the commitment of that occupying power to the task of rebuilding a democratic political system in Germany. This, however, was a specifically American twist on democracy, one that the Soviets in particular did not share, and their policy shifted from support for a democratic system to the promotion of Communist ideology and pro-Soviet ideology. Both sides sought to include health films in this new focus to mobilize German support for their occupation and to prepare them for different political futures. Her corpus of films is thus not only about health but also about the transformation of Germany toward its postwar futures and how this was shaped by the different political agendas and resources of the occupying powers.

If Keitz emphasizes postwar changes, she also emphasizes continuity with prewar Germany. The availability of film production facilities after the war, for example, was based less on the postwar occupation than on those prewar facilities that survived, a factor that even affected the importation of foreign made films into Germany: films in English, French or Russian had to be dubbed into German, and prewar production facilities were turned to this purpose. Von Keitz shows that films released across the four sectors were often quite similar, in part because the major center of the filmmaking was in one sector (the Soviet sector). It was also the case that filmmakers themselves drew on older filmmaking traditions that sometimes seemed to undermine the message of the occupying powers, as when for example, antityphus films evoked Nazi tropes of Jews as lice. In focusing on one specific venereal disease film screened in all four

German occupied zones and sectors of Berlin, the chapter further explores the role of medical institutions in modeling gender relations and emotions. Thus, this chapter also highlights limits to the cultural hegemony of the occupying powers, for they did not always foresee the various meanings of the films they commissioned or permitted.

If von Keitz looks at how local conditions shaped international efforts to denazify Germany and build democratic institutions, Kirsten Ostherr's contribution focuses on the corpus of films sponsored by a transnational player, the World Health Organization (WHO), and how they sought to address many different audiences in different localities across the world. Her corpus, however, is not solely films produced by the WHO. It is rather the intersection of WHO films with a broader corpus of postwar animated films, as illuminated by one of the WHO's most successful, widely distributed films, the anti-alcohol production, *To Your Health* (1956). Ostherr argues that in common with many mid-century animators, the makers of *To Your Health* broke from the dominant Disney style, dropping the earlier reliance on circle and oval graphic formulas in favor of cartoon characters with a variety of sophisticated "modern" elements: abstract forms, sparse backgrounds, and cubist shapes and organic biomorphic forms reminiscent of Miró, Calder, and Noguchi. In Ostherr's telling, the abstraction of 1950s animation may have functioned as a powerful code for viewers that offered alternate conceptions of realism which allowed for a wider range of interpretations across national boundaries. Thus, although the central figure in this film is clearly white and male, and with an American accent, the visual style of *To Your Health* meant that he could change national identity with just a change of soundtrack. A different language or accent could turn a figure who was American or European in some versions into someone with a different national or regional characteristic. Such mutable figures, Ostherr suggests, were possible because of the nature of animation to the studios that adopted modernist forms. Whereas live action particularized, it was suggested, animation generalized and so made what it sought to represent universal. If international organizations helped to construct a view of documentary film as neutral and above politics, Ostherr's argument is that they also helped to construct a view of modernist animation as particularly suited to reaching diverse audiences.

Ostherr makes a further point, which is that an understanding of the WHO corpus provides a further refinement of this argument about the relationship of international organizations to animation. In her account, there was no master plan behind the WHO film corpus, not even a set of clearly defined goals. It came together in a more haphazard way and sought to address a mix of agendas and audiences. Sometimes films in the corpus such as *To Your Health* addressed issues of broad concern that traveled well; others addressed local issues that did not travel so well. Some were documentaries; others were animated. In Ostherr's story, audiences would likely have responded differently to *To Your Health* had it been a documentary rather than an animated production, and even among animated films none was as successful as *To Your Health.* Her point, however, is that the success of this film made it a model for the impact a health film could have, an ideal that shaped decisions large and small concerning future WHO film productions. From this perspective, she suggests, the study of any film corpus can be greatly enhanced by close examination of an exemplary film that demonstrates the ideals to which the total corpus aspired, even if many productions fell short of such ideals.

The fourth and final part of the book turns to questions of how audiences might be constructed by historical actors and by historians themselves. Our goal is here, in part, to start to address what audiences, and those who study them, define as corpuses, and how seemingly well-defined corpuses can lose some of their characteristics when we view how audiences are themselves imagined or constructed. Anja Laukötter's contribution returns us to the social hygiene corpus examined earlier by Miriam Posner. However, where Posner situates *End of the Road* within the overlapping corpuses of exploitation and educational social hygiene films, Laukötter looks at it within the context of corpuses constructed for the purposes of audience research on educational film. In this case, the corpus was put together by the psychologists John B. Watson and Karl S. Lashley, who were hired to explore how health education films affected audiences, the first time psychologists had been brought in to address this issue. In 1919 Watson was given a $6,600 grant by the US Interdepartmental Social Hygiene Board to examine the educational effects of a motion picture campaign against venereal diseases (VD). A central part of this research involved selecting suitable films for study from a self-compiled corpus of social hygiene films. In the end they chose *End of the Road* and *Fit to Win*, films that Watson and Lashley hoped would not only allow them to address educator's concerns about the value of film as an educational technology but also their own professional goals. An established academic psychologist with a full professorship at Johns Hopkins, Watson saw in this research an opportunity to extend psychology's reach to include the fields of marketing, education, and advertising. These films, and the corpus from which they derived, thus served a double purpose of evaluating social hygiene films and of expanding the scope of experimental psychology. More generally, Laukötter's chapter also suggests that the creation of a corpus of films does not necessarily predetermine how it may be studied. A corpus may be shaped by analytical aims or historical contingencies, but it can also be a field on which to apply a specific set of questions.

Timothy Boon's contribution ends the book on a methodological note, exploring how historians might approach the question of audiences' responses to health education films—his focus is the corpus of health education films in interwar Britain, which he uses to argue for greater scholarly focus on what films meant for audiences as much as what it meant for producers, sponsors, filmmakers, or even psychologists studying audience response. In particular, Boon uses the "moral tale" genre (fictional stories with moral narratives presented as entertainment films) produced and promoted by the British Social Hygiene Council to describe two approaches that scholars might take to the study of audiences understood as "historical social audience" for films. In a first step the chapter discusses the "truffle hunter" perspective that focuses on context, numbers, and sociological approaches to cinema in Britain and the possibilities of oral history. In a second step, the chapter introduces the "parachutist" perspective, discussing several approaches and conceptions provided by film studies to identify patterns or the ideal or typical spectator, before the chapter closes with an attempt to synthesize these different approaches, presented as thesis and antithesis.

Boon's approach highlights the question of how historians construct their corpuses. As with many other authors in this volume, his corpus is partly a product of an institution, and like others in this book, this institutional corpus overlaps, like a Venn diagram, with other ways of grouping the film. One of the points of this book is that films rarely fall within one corpus but often belong to many different corpuses, and that it can be fruitful to explore these different corpuses and the tensions between them. But in focusing on methodological issues, Boon also highlights the constructed nature of these corpuses. The films that historians use are part of many different corpuses—the corpuses of the commercial companies that made them, of the agencies that sponsored them, of the directors who made them, of the scholars who studied them, as well as the audiences that viewed them. They are also part of the corpuses of the libraries and archives that collect them and of the historians who study and (re)construct them. By exploring public health films as part of all these corpuses, we can gain a richer knowledge of this form of film and how these corpuses have shaped our own understanding of film as a public education tool.

Notes

1. For surveys of the historiography of medicine and public health in film, see Timothy Boon, "Medical Films and Television: Alternative Paths to the Cultures of Biomedicine," in *The Oxford Handbook of the History of Medicine*, ed. Mark Jackson (Oxford: Oxford University Press, 2011), 617–33; Susan E. Lederer and Naomi Rogers, "Media," in *Medicine in the Twentieth Century*, ed. Roger Cooter and John Pickstone (Amsterdam: Harwood Academic Publishers, 2000), 487–502; Christian Bonah and Anja Laukötter, "Moving Pictures and Medicine in the First Half of the 20th Century: Some Notes on International Historical Developments and the Potential of Medical Film Research," *Gesnerus* 66 (2009): 121–45; and Christian Bonah and Anja Laukötter, eds., "Screening Sex Hygiene Films in the first Half of the 20th Century," special issue, *Gesnerus* 72, no. 1 (2015).

2. See, for example, David Cantor, "Uncertain Enthusiasm: The American Cancer Society, Public Education, and the Problems of the Movie, 1921–1960," *Bulletin of the History of Medicine* 81 (2007): 39–69. More generally on early twentieth-century anxieties about cinema, see Lee Grieveson, *Policing Cinema: Movies and Censorship in Early-Twentieth Century America* (Berkeley: University of California Press, 2004).

3. Health education films also played a role in other countries and regions—including Canada, India, and Latin America—not discussed in this collection. We would have

loved to have taken a more global perspective on health education films beyond North America and Europe, but it was not possible. Our hope is that the approaches set out here will be applied to public health education films produced elsewhere.

4. Utility film may be defined as documentary film produced under contract from industrial, corporate, teaching, or educational bodies. These films were produced under commission as purpose-oriented audio-visual communication tools with clearly established objectives addressed to specific audiences. As such, utility films are primarily neither art works nor commercial entities but media tools guiding public opinion that accomplish their job when messages are received by specified spectators whose behavior is influenced according to commissioners' interests. Vinzenz Hediger and Patrick Vonderau, eds., *Films That Work: Industrial Film and the Productivity of Media* (Amsterdam: Amsterdam University Press, 2009), esp. "Introduction," 10; and Yvonne Zimmermann, "'What Hollywood Is to America, the Corporate Film Is to Switzerland': Remarks on Industrial Film as Utility Film," in Hediger and Vonderau, *Films That Work*, 101–17. See also the earlier, slightly different German version of *Films That Work*: Vinzenz Hediger and Patrick Vonderau, eds., *Filmische Mittel, industrielle Zwecke: Das Werk des Industriefilms* (Berlin: Vorwerk 8, 2007). Two special issues of the periodical *AV Montage* were dedicated to "utility film" in 2005 and 2006: *Montage AV Zeitschrift für Theorie & Geschichte audiovisueller Kommunikation*, special issues, *Gebrauchsfilm* 14, no. 2 (2005), and 15, no. 1 (2006). See especially Vinzenz Hediger, "'Dann sind Bilder also nichts!' Vorüberlegungen zur Konstitution des Forschundsfeldes 'Gebrauchsfilm,'" *Montage AV* 14, no. 2 (2005): 11–22. See as well the annotated international bibliography, Anna Heymer and Patrick Vonderau, "Industrial Films: An Analytical Bibliography," in Hediger and Vonderau, *Films That Work*, 404–61; Yvonne Zimmermann, *Schaufenster Schweiz: Dokumentarische Gebrauchsfilme 1896–1964* (Zürich: Limmat Verlag, 2011); and Charles R. Acland and Haidee Wasson, eds., *Useful Cinema* (Durham, NC: Duke University Press, 2011).

5. Thomas Elsaesser, "Archives and Archaeologies: The Place of Non-fiction Film in Contemporary Media," in Hediger and Vonderau, *Films That Work*, 19–34.

6. Patrick Vonderau, "Vernacular Archiving: An Interview with Rick Prelinger," in Hediger and Vonderau, *Films That Work*, 51–61; and Rick Prelinger, *The Field Guide to Sponsored Films* (San Francisco: National Film Preservation Foundation, 2006). See also a description on Rick Prelinger's website, http://www.prelinger.com (accessed May 9, 2017).

7. Annette Melville and Scott Simmon, *Film Preservation 1993: A Study of the Current State of American Film Preservation: Report of the Librarian of Congress* (Washington, DC: NFPB/LOC, 1993), https://www.loc.gov/programs/national-film-preservation-board/preservation-research/film-preservation-study/current-state-of-american-film-preservation-study/.

8. See, for example, The Prelinger Archives, on the Internet Archive, accessed September 6, 2017, https://archive.org/details/prelinger; US National Library of Medicine (NLM), "Historical Audiovisuals Program," accessed September 6, 2017, http://www.nlm.nih.gov/hmd/collections/films; and the Wellcome Library, "Moving Image and Sound Collection," accessed September 6, 2017, https://wellcomelibrary.org/collections/about-the-collections/moving-image-and-sound-collection/. For an example of how film scholarship and film preservation might go hand

in hand, see David Cantor, *The Reward of Courage (1921): A Rediscovered Cancer Film of the Silent Era* (Bethesda, MD: National Library of Medicine, 2013).

9. Lester D. Friedman, ed., *Cultural Sutures: Medicine, Media and Morals* (Durham, NC: Duke University Press, 2004); Graeme Harper and Andrew Moor, eds., *Signs of Life: Medicine and Cinema* (London: Wallflower Press, 2005); Leslie J. Reagan, Nancy Tomes, and Paula A. Treichler, eds., *Medicine's Moving Pictures: Medicine, Health, and Bodies in American Film and Television* (Rochester, NY: University of Rochester Press, 2007); Ludmilla Jordanova, "Medicine and Visual Culture," *Social History of Medicine* 3 (1990): 89–99; Marcus Krause and Nicolas Pethes, eds., *Mr. Münsterberg und Dr. Hyde: Zur Filmgeschichte des Menschenexperiments* (Bielefeld, Germany: Transcript, 2007); and Ramón Reichert, *Im Kino der Humanwissenschaften: Studien zur Medialisierung des wissenschaftlichen Wissens* (Bielefeld, Germany: Transcript, 2007).

10. Zoë Druick, *Projecting Canada: Government Policy and Documentary Film at the National Film Board of Canada* (Montreal: McGill-Queen's University Press, 2007); and Tim Boon, *Films of Fact: A History of Science in Documentary Films and Television* (London: Wallflower Press, 2008).

11. Vinzenz Hediger and Patrick Vonderau, "Record, Rhetoric, Rationalization," in Hediger and Vonderau, *Films That Work*, 35–49, 37; and Zimmermann, "'What Hollywood Is to America,'" 102–4.

12. For a synthesis on comparative history approaches, see Marc Bloch, "Pour une histoire comparée des sociétés européennes," *Revue de Synthèse Historique* 46 (1928): 15–50; Raymond Grew, "On the Current State of Comparative Studies," in *Marc Bloch aujourd'hui: Histoire comparée et sciences sociales*, ed. Hartmut Atsma and André Burgière (Paris: Editions de l'Ecole des hautes études en sciences sociales, 1990), 323–34; and Jürgen Kocka, "Comparative Historical Research: German Examples," *International Review of Social History* 38 (1993): 369–79.

13. In 2006 Paul Theerman, Michael Sappol, and David Cantor at the US National Library of Medicine (NLM) proposed the creation of a searchable online database census of historical medical films, which would collect in one place information on production, content, and location and which would be updateable. The idea was that this census would include both films that had survived and the many more that had not. A prototype database was developed in 2007, but the library decided not to develop a full-scale database. In addition, an effort to create a DVD series based on the NLM's film collections foundered after a prototype was developed. A website, *Medical Movies on the Web*, was launched in 2013, superceding plans for the DVD series.

14. At the same time as the NLM began its plans for a database, Christian Bonah, Joël Danet, Anja Laukötter, and Vincent Lowy started a related exercise in France. They not only sought to develop a census of French films, but also to collect, digitize, describe, and contextualize these films. This work provided the basis of MedFilm, a research and teaching online database of French medical and health education film that has been developed since 2010 with financial support from the French National Research Agency (ANR) and based at the University of Strasbourg: http://www.medfilm.unistra.fr. In 2017 the database included 450 films and their descriptions as well as related materials such as contemporary film reviews, present-day scholarly research materials (including research papers and master's theses), teaching curricula, and archival sources related to the films. Conceived as a Wikimedia, the database is collaborative in nature and is moderated through editorial overview and fact-checking

or verification of content. The latter has avoided the definitional/boundary problems by taking a pragmatic approach. It included any rescued and available film that might loosely be defined as health or medical education: they can be part of health campaigns or of school and training programs as well as nonentertainment medical, scientific, or documentary subject films.

15. *The Story of Wendy Hill* (Produced by Warner News Inc.; Presented by Federal Security Agency, Public Health Service and the American Diabetes Association, 1949).

16. On conversion narratives in health education films, see David Cantor, "Choosing to Live: Cancer Education, Movies, and the Conversion Narrative in America, 1921–1960," *Literature and Medicine* 28 (2009): 278–332.

17. See, for example, the traffic accident in the cancer film *A Fortunate Accident* (1925) discussed in David Cantor, "Uncertain Enthusiasm: The American Cancer Society, Public Education, and the Problems of the Movie, 1921–1960," *Bulletin of the History of Medicine* 81 (2007): 39–69, 46.

18. "Sneeze" (United States: Edison Manufacturing Co., 1894), Library of Congress, http://www.loc.gov/item/00694192; "Sandow" (United States: Edison Manufacturing Co., 1894), Library of Congress, http://www.loc.gov/item/00694298; "A Morning Bath" (United States: Edison Manufacturing Co., 1896), Library of Congress, http://www.loc.gov/item/00694249; "A Morning Alarm" (United States: Edison Manufacturing Co., 1896), Library of Congress, http://www.loc.gov/item/00694248; "US Troops and Red Cross in the Trenches before Caloocan" (United States: Edison Manufacturing Co., 1899), Library of Congress, http://www.loc.gov/item/98501181; "Fun in Camp" (United States: Edison Manufacturing Co., 1899), Library of Congress, http://www.loc.gov/item/00694212; "Love and War" (United States: Edison Manufacturing Co., 1899), Library of Congress, http://www.loc.gov/item/98501279; "Red Cross Ambulance on Battlefield" (United States: Edison Manufacturing Co., 1900), Library of Congress, http://www.loc.gov/item/00694286; and "Life Rescue at Long Branch" (United States: Edison Manufacturing Co., 1901), Library of Congress, http://www.loc.gov/item/00694235.

19. The well-documented case of Eugène Doyen's surgical films (produced from 1898 onward) illustrates the point. To counteract accusations of self-publicity, the surgeon filed a legal suit against his film operator, Parnaland, for screening these motion pictures in fairs and barracks. Thierry Lefebvre, *La chair et le celluloïd: Le cinéma chirurgical du docteur Doyen* (Brionne, France: Jean Doyen Editeur, 2004).

20. Tom Gunning, "The Cinema of Attraction: Early Film, Its Spectator and the AvantGarde," *Wide Angle* 8, nos. 3–4 (Fall 1986): 63–70. A revised version of Gunning's article was published as Tom Gunning, "The Cinema of Attractions: Early Film, Its Spectator and the Avant-Garde," in *Early Cinema: Space, Frame, Narrative*, ed. Thomas Elsaesser and Adam Barker (London: BFI Publications, 1990), 56–63. Other historians have extended Gunning's efforts to open up the history of early cinema in a way that does not make it a simple prelude to later forms of film. See Thierry Lefebvre, "Images du réel: La non-fiction en France (1890–1930)," special issue, *1895 Revue d'Histoire du Cinéma* 18 (1995); Daan Hertogs and Nico DeKlerk, *Uncharted Territory: Essays on Early Nonfiction* (Amsterdam: Stichtung Nederlands Filmmuseum, 1997); Laurent Mannoni, *The Great Art of Light and Shadow: Archaeology of the Cinema* (Exeter, UK: Exeter University Press, 2000); Virgilio Tosi, *Cinema before*

Cinema: The Origins of Scientific Cinematography (London: British Universities Film and Video Council, 2005); Richard Abel ed., *The Encyclopedia of Early Cinema* (New York: Routledge, 2005); Paula Amad, *Counter-Archive: Film, the Everyday, and Albert Kahn's Archives de la Planète* (New York: Columbia University Press, 2010); Matthew Solomon, *Disappearing Tricks: Silent Film, Houdini, and the New Magic of the Twentieth Century* (Champaign: University of Illinois Press, 2010); Kristin Whissel, *Picturing American Modernity: Traffic, Technology, and Silent Cinema* (Durham, NC: Duke University Press, 2010); Luke McKernan *Charles Urban: Pioneering the Non-fiction Film in Britain and America, 1897–1925* (Exeter, UK: Exeter University Press, 2013); Jennifer Peterson, *Education in the School of Dreams: Travelogues and Early Nonfiction Film* (Durham, NC: Duke University Press, 2013); Oliver Gaycken *Devices of Curiosity: Early Cinema & Popular Science* (New York: Oxford University Press, 2015); and Scott Curtis, *Managing Modernity: Art, Science, and Early Cinema in Germany* (New York: Columbia University Press, 2015).

21. Charles Musser, "Rethinking Early Cinema: Cinema of Attractions and Narrativity," in *The Cinema of Attractions Reloaded*, ed. Wanda Strauven (Amsterdam: Amsterdam University Press, 2006), 389–416; and Charles Musser, *The Emergence of Cinema: The American Screen to 1907* (Berkeley: University of California Press, 1990).

22. Gaycken, *Devices of Curiosity*, 15–53.

23. Tom Gunning, "From the Opium Den to the Theatre of Morality: Moral Discourse and the Film Process in Early American Cinema," in *The Silent Cinema Reader*, ed. Lee Grieveson and Peter Krämer (London: Routledge, 2004), 145–54; Lee Grieveson, "'A Kind of Recreative School for the Whole Family': Making Cinema Respectable, 1907–09," *Screen* 42 (2001): 64–76; and Tom Gunning, *D. W. Griffith and the Origins of American Narrative Film: The Early Years at Biograph* (Urbana: University of Illinois Press, 1991).

24. Gunning, "From the Opium Den"; Grieveson, "'A Kind of Recreative School.'"

25. Gunning, *D. W. Griffith*, 6. On melodrama, see Gaycken, *Devices of Curiosity*, 158–80.

26. Cantor, "Choosing to Live."

27. For example, the series of antituberculosis films produced at the end of the 1930s by Edgar Ulmer for the National Tuberculosis Association: Devin Orgeron, "Spreading the Word: Race, Religion, and the Rhetoric of Contagion in Edgar G. Ulmer's TB Films," in *Learning with the Lights Off: Educational Film in the United States*, ed. Devin Orgeron, Marsha Orgeron, and Dan Streible (New York: Oxford University Press, 2012), 295–315; and Christian Bonah and Vincent Lowy, "Lorsque le regard l'emporte sur le message: Les courts-métrages de lutte contre la tuberculose d'Edgar G. Ulmer, *Alliage* 71 (Winter 2012–13): 46–56. More generally, Cantor, "Choosing to Live."

28. Anja Laukötter, "Listen and Watch: The Practice of Lecturing a Film and the Epistemological Status of Sex Education Films in Germany," *Gesnerus* 1 (2015): 56–76.

29. Laukötter, "Listen and Watch." See also Richard Abel, "The Cinema of Attractions in France, 1896–1904," in *The Silent Cinema Reader*, ed. Lee Grieveson and Peter Krämer (London: Routledge, 2004), 63–75.

30. An example is *Reborn to Life* (1916), commissioned by the Maria Pavlovna Committee for War Veterans Assistance.

31. Elizabeth Toon, "'Cancer as the General Population Knows It': Knowledge, Fear, and Lay Education in 1950s Britain," *Bulletin of the History of Medicine* 81 (2007): 116–38; and Virginia Berridge, "Medicine and the Public: The 1962 Report of the Royal College of Physicians and the New Public Health," *Bulletin of the History of Medicine* 81 (2007): 286–311.

32. Stephen Snelders, Frans J. Meijman, and Toine Pieters, "Cancer Health Communication in the Netherlands 1910–1950: Paternalism or Popularization?," *Medizinhistorisches Journal* 41 (2006): 271–89.

33. David Cantor, "Cancer Control and Prevention in the Twentieth Century," *Bulletin of the History of Medicine* 81 (2007): 1–38, esp. 9–10.

34. Bonah and Laukötter, "Moving Pictures and Medicine."

35. Louis L. Thurstone, "What Is an Education Movie," *Visual Education* 1 (April 1920): 25. Quoted in Devin Orgeron, Marsha Orgeron, and Dan Streible, "A History of Learning With the Lights Off," in *Learning with the Lights Off,* by Devin Orgeron, Marsha Orgeron, and David Streible, 16.

36. On film as a form of virtual witnessing, see David A Kirby, *Lab Coats in Hollywood: Science, Scientists, and Cinema* (Cambridge, MA: MIT Press, 2011), 21–40.

37. Gaycken, *Devices of Curiosity,* 15–53.

38. Lee Grieveson, "Cinema Studies and the Conduct of Conduct," in *Inventing Film Studies,* ed. Lee Grieveson and Haidee Wasson (Durham, NC: Duke University Press, 2008), 3–37; and Hugo Münsterberg, *The Photoplay: A Psychological Study* (New York: D. Appleton, 1916).

39. Anja Laukötter, "How Films Entered the Classroom: The Sciences and the Emotional Education of Youth through Health Education Films in the United States and Germany, 1910–1930," *Osiris* 31 (2016): 181–200.

40. "The Red Cross Seal," 1910; "The Awakening of John Bond," 1911; "Hope: A Red Cross Seal Story," 1912; "The Price of Human Lives," 1913; "The Temple of Moloch," 1914 (see the film on the Internet Archive at https://archive.org/details/temple_of_moloch, accessed September 6, 2017); "The Lone Game," 1914 (see "The Lone Game, A Red Cross Seal Drama (1915)—Edward C. Taylor | Thomas Edison," YouTube video, posted by Change Before Going Productions, August 26, 2014, https://www.youtube.com/watch?v=AJgkMjE-zbg).

41. Nancy Tomes, *The Gospel of Germs: Men, Women and the Microbe in American Life* (Cambridge, MA: Harvard University Press, 1998), 113–34.

42. Bonah and Laukötter, "Moving Pictures and Medicine."

43. On the Edison films, see Martin S. Pernick, "Thomas Edison's Tuberculosis Films: Mass Media and Health Propaganda," *The Hastings Center Report* 8, no. 3 (June 1978): 21–27; Martin S. Pernick, "More than Illustrations: Early Twentieth-Century Health Films as Contributors to the Histories of Medicine and of Motion Pictures," in Reagan, Tomes, and Treichler, *Medicine's Moving Pictures,* 19–35; and Miriam Posner, "Communicating Disease: Tuberculosis, Narrative, and Social Order in Thomas Edison's Red Cross Seal Films," in *Learning with the Lights Off,* by Devin Orgeron, Marsha Orgeron, and Dan Streible (New York: Oxford University Press, 2012), 90–106. More generally, on Edison and educational film see Oliver Gaycken, "The School of the Future or Ganod's Physics? Edison's Foray into Educational Cinema," in *Beyond the Screen: Institutions, Networks and Publics of Early Cinema,* ed. Marta Braun, Charlie Keil, Rob King, Paul Moore, and Louis Pelletier (New Barnet, UK: John

Libbey, 2012), 143–52; and Amanda R. Keeler, "John Collier, Thomas Edison and the Educational Promotion of Moving Pictures," in Braun, Keil, King, Moore, and Pelletier, *Beyond the Screen*, 117–25.

44. Posner, "Communicating Disease." Pernick. "Thomas Edison's Tuberculosis Films."

45. "The Moving Picture and the National Character," *American Review of Reviews* 42 (1910): 315–20, 317.

46. Grieveson, *Policing Cinema.*

47. For an exception, see Man Alive!, which crossed the boundary between theatrical and nontheatrical production. See David Cantor, *Man Alive!* (1952): *Cartoon Fun with Cancer, Cars and Companionate Marriage in Suburban America* (Bethesda, MD: National Library of Medicine, 2014).

48. For developments in Europe, see Christian Bonah and Anja Laukötter, "Screening Diseases: Sex Educations Films in Germany and France in the First Half of the 20th Century," special issue, *Gesnerus* 72, no. 1 (2015). For an overview see Bonah and Laukötter, "Moving Pictures and Medicine."

49. See the discussion of the Swiss film *Women's Joy—Women's Misery*, below.

50. Kirsten Ostherr, *Medical Visions: Producing the Patient through Film, Television and Imaging Technologies* (New York: Oxford University Press, 2012).

51. Lefebvre, *La chair et le celluloïd.*

52. As Leslie Reagan has noted in the case of cancer education films, the messages could be quite different. Leslie J. Reagan, "Projecting Breast Cancer: Self-Examination Films and the Making of a New Cultural Practice," in Reagan, Tomes, and Treichler, *Medicine's Moving Pictures*, 163–95.

53. On the Canti film, see Duncan Wilson, *Tissue Culture in Science and Society: The Public Life of a Biological Technique in Twentieth Century Britain* (Basingstoke, UK: Macmillan Palgrave, 2011); David Cantor, "The Definition of Radiobiology: The Medical Research Council's Support for Research into the Biological Effects of Radiation in Britain, 1919–1939" (PhD diss., University of Lancaster, 1987); and Gaycken, *Devices of Curiosity*. For other films about cells see Hannah Landecker, "Microcinematography and the History of Science and Film," *Isis* 97 (2006): 121–32; Christopher Kelty and Hannah Landecker, "A Theory of Animation: Cells, L-Systems, and Film," *Grey Room* 17 (2004): 30–63; Hannah Landecker, "The Lewis Films: Tissue Culture and 'Living Anatomy,' 1919–1940," in *Centennial History of the Carnegie Institute*, vol. 5, *Department of Embryology*, ed. Jane Maienschein, Marie Glitz, and Garland Allan (Cambridge: Cambridge University Press, 2004), 117–44; Hannah Landecker, "Seeing Things: From Microcinematography to Live Cell Imaging," *Nature Methods* 6 (2009): 707–9; Hannah Landecker, "Cellular Features: Microcinematography and Early Film Theory," *Critical Inquiry* 31 (2005): 903–37; Hannah Landecker, "The Life of Movement: From Microcinematography to Live-Cell Imaging," *Journal of Visual Culture* 11 (2012): 378–99; and Hannah Landecker, "Creeping, Drinking, Dying: The Cinematic Portal and the Microscopic World of the Twentieth Century Cell," *Science in Context* 24 (2011): 381–416.

54. Christian Bonah and Alexis Zimmer, "Le calvaire du *Steinach Film*" (1922/23). "Représentations du médecin dans le film de recherche et d'enseignement médical," *Sociétés & Représentations* 28 (2009): 87–106. Rainer Herrn and Christine N. Brinckmann, "Rats and Men: Rejuvenation and the Steinach Film," in *Not Straight*

from Germany: Sexual Publics and Sexual Citizenship since Magnus Hirschfeld, ed. Michael Thomas Taylor, Annette F. Timm and Rainer Herrn (Ann Arbor: University Michigan Press, 2017 (forthcoming).

55. Peter Baechlin and Maurice Muller-Strauss, eds., *Newsreels across the World* (Paris: Unesco, 1952); Raymond Fielding, *The American Newsreel 1911–1967* (Norman: University of Oklahoma Press, 1972); Roger Smither and Wolfgang Klaue, eds., *Newsreels in Film Archives: A Survey Based on the FIAF Symposium* (Wiltshire, UK: Flicks Books, 1996); and Roel Vande Winkel, "Newsreel Series: World Overview," in *Encyclopedia of the Documentary Film*, ed., Ian Aitken (New York: Routledge, 2006), 985–91.

56. Many scenes of the German film *Geissel der Menschheit* (1926) were reused in the widely shown Kulturfilm *Falsche Scham* (1925–26).

57. Barnett Addis, producer and director, *Nurse-patient Interaction* (Los Angeles: Behavioral Sciences Media Laboratory, Neuropsychiatric Institute, UCLA Center for the Health Sciences, 1976).

58. For the complicated production history of the film, see François Albera, "Un destin mouvementé: *Frauennot-Frauenglück*," in *Cinéma suisse muet: Lumières et ombres*, ed. Rémy Pithon (Lausanne, Switzerland: Antipodes et Cinémathèque Suisse de Lausanne, 2002), 73–84; and Ursula von Keitz, *Im Schatten des Gesetzes: Schwangerschaftskonflikt und Reproduktion im deutschsprachigen Film 1918 bis 1933* (Marburg, Germany: Schüren, 2005).

59. Russia depenalized abortion in 1920. Debates stirred by the Communist and Socialist parties in Germany led in July 1920 to a first proposal to parliament to reform §218 of criminal law depenalizing abortion, which remained a criminal act but without penal consequences. Between 1920 and 1932, nineteen parliament propositions were filed to reform or abandon criminal prosecution for abortion.

60. The four profiles include an undesired pregnancy in a poor working-class family environment with four children already; the case of a seduced and abandoned naïve working-class woman; a pleasure-seeking, hedonist bourgeois female; and an unmarried future mother after a workplace accident of her fiancé.

61. The film title changes from country to country: Switzerland Frauennot—Frauenglück / Misères des femmes—Joies des femmes/Miseria e felicità delle donne; Germany: Frauennot—Frauenglück (German Censored); France: L'appel de la vie; England: Misery and Fortune of Women; USA: Women's Misery—Women's Happiness; Brazil: Miséria e Fortuna de uma Mulher.

62. Adolf Nichtenhauser, "A History of Motion Pictures in Medicine" (unpublished manuscript, ca. 1950), Adolf Nichtenhauser History of Motion Pictures in Medicine Collection, MS C 380, Archives and Modern Manuscripts Program, History of Medicine Division, National Library of Medicine, Bethesda, MD.

63. For example, Kirsten Ostherr, *Cinematic Prophylaxis: Globalization and Contagion in the Discourse of World Health* (Durham, NC: Duke University Press, 2006); Lisa Cartwright, *Screening the Body: Tracing Medicine's Visual Culture* (Minneapolis: University of Minnesota Press, 1995); and John Parascandola, "Syphilis at the Cinema: Medicine and Morals in VD Films of the U.S. Public Health Service in World War II," in Reagan, Tomes, and Treichler, *Medicine's Moving Pictures*, 71–92.

64. In some countries, the government took the lead in producing and sponsoring such films, while in others it was private organizations (commercial and voluntary), in others individual physicians and public health officials, among others. And

the mix of public, private, and individual varied over time in each country, so that sometimes governments dominate, and at others commercial organizations, philanthropic, or medical/public health ones.

65. Nichtenhauser, "A History of Motion Pictures in Medicine," 2:136.

66. Ibid., 3:351–54.

67. Ibid., 4:1–25.

68. Adolf Nichtenhauser Medical Film Materials, 1933–55, Archives and Modern Manuscripts Program, History of Medicine Division, National Library of Medicine.

69. Nichtenhauser, "A History of Motion Pictures in Medicine," 4:298.

70. Marianne Fedunkiw, "Malaria Films: Motion Pictures as a Public Health Tool," *American Journal of Public Health* 93 (2003): 1046–57; and Michael Sappol, "The Public Health Film Goes to War," ed. Paul Theerman and David Cantor, US National Library of Medicine, first published January 31, 2011, http://www.nlm.nih.gov/hmd/digicolls/phfgtw/.

71. Bonah and Lowy, "Lorsque le regard l'emporte sur le message," 46–56; Noah Isenberg, *Edgar G. Ulmer: A Filmmaker at the Margins* (Berkeley: University of California Press, 2014); and Orgeron, "Spreading the Word."

72. Cantor, "Choosing to Live."

73. Zoë Druick, "'Reaching the Multimillions': Liberal Internationalism and the Establishment of Documentary Film," in *Inventing Film Studies*, ed. Lee Grieveson and Haidee Wasson (Durham, NC: Duke University Press, 2008), 66–92. See also Richard Maltby, "The Cinema and the League of Nations," in *"Film Europe" and "Film America": Cinema, Commerce and Cultural Exchange, 1920–1939*, ed. Andrew Higson and Richard Maltby (Exeter, UK: University of Exeter Press, 1999), 82–106.

Part One

Commercial Contexts

Chapter One

Between Movies, Markets, and Medicine

The Eastern Film Corporation, Frank A. Tichenor, and Medical and Health Films in the 1920s

DAVID CANTOR

The Eastern Film Corporation may not be the most readily recognized name in medical history. Incorporated in 1915, it began life making feature films and comedies, and for a while it seemed to rival some of the largest film production companies in the business. Yet this early promise faded, and during the late 1910s and 1920s it shifted focus to concentrate on industrials and educationals, emerging in the 1920s as a major producer and distributor of technical movies for medical and dental audiences and of health and safety movies for the public. But its life was short. By the end of the 1920s the company was in trouble, and it seems to have folded early in the following decade.

Hitherto, historians of medicine have paid little attention to the commercial context in which early twentieth-century medical and health movies were made and distributed.[1] Yet in the late 1910s and early 1920s many new companies flooded into the field, with perhaps forty-six firms making and distributing films in the United States by the end of the 1920s, all jostling for market share.[2] Eastern—headed by its manager and president, Frank A. Tichenor (1882–1950)[3]—was one of the companies that jumped on the bandwagon, and it provides an opportunity to explore why commercial film companies came to be interested in medical and public health education films in the years after

World War I and what happened to them as them as the economy dipped in the late 1920s and early 1930s.

Commercial companies involved in medical and health films fall along a spectrum in the 1920s. Some (such as Visugraph,[4] the Coronet Film Corporation,[5] and the Carter Film Company) specialized almost entirely in educationals and industrials. Others (such as Edison, Bray, Pathé, Eastman Kodak, or the General Film Company)[6] were primarily interested in the production or distribution of entertainment films but created departments specializing in sponsored or didactic movies within the larger organization. Others straddled the divide between the two, sometimes tending toward entertainment, sometimes toward education, the balance shifting one way or another within each business over time and differing from company to company.[7] Eastern falls into this shifting, in-between category. It started as with a focus on theatricals and, despite hopes of remaining a producer or distributor of features and comedies, it shifted over time to educationals and industrials. Its story thus provides a window onto why entertainment companies moved into educationals and industrials (including medical and health education films) at a time when the latter were, on the one hand, increasingly being marginalized by the theatrical film exhibitors and, on the other hand, increasingly being promoted (by some advocates) as quite distinct from entertainment films.

If this chapter is a case study of why film companies came to be interested in medical and public health films, it is also a case study of why film entrepreneurs such as Tichenor came to be interested in these types of film.[8] The historian of "nontheatrical" film, Edwin Krows—an admirer and one-time employee of Tichenor—claims that Tichenor was a crucial figure in the mass production and distribution of medical and surgical films.[9] But if medicine and health were important to his business interests, they were only one part. Until the late 1910s, he seems to have had little interest in medical or health movies, and he only became interested in them as part of a broader effort to diversify his own business interests as Eastern got into difficulties. Furthermore, although Tichenor had been involved with Eastern from the start, it was never his sole business interest. Between 1910 and 1930, he founded many different film companies and often ran more than one at the same time. Eastern had to share his attentions with his other business interests, and by the end of the 1920s and early 1930s he had abandoned the company, as he also abandoned his interest in making and distributing movies about medicine and health.

Tichenor had once been at the center of the entertainment film industry, a colleague of many of the leading filmmakers of the early twentieth century. But by the 1930s, all his dreams in this area had come to nothing. Instead he moved into politics, publishing, and the problems of the airplane industry. Medicine was thus doubly marginalized within Eastern; it was only one part of Eastern's interest in film, and Eastern itself was only one part of Tichenor's business interests.

This last comment draws attention to two final points that this essay seeks to highlight. The first concerns the problematic place of medicine and health in the story of medical and health films, at least from a commercial perspective. Medicine and health were never the center of Eastern's or Tichenor's interests, and their turns to medical and health films were as much the result of their failures in feature and comedy film production as it was to do with any specific interest in medicine or health. Moreover, when Eastern and Tichenor did get interested in making medical and health movies, it was only part of a broader strategy of cultivating new markets in film after the war. As their efforts to produce entertainment films failed, Eastern and Tichenor diversified into film distribution, new film technologies such as sound, and a variety of different types of "special interest" or "purpose" films, including medical and health movies. Medical and health movies were thus part of a broader effort to reinvent the company and to diversify Tichenor's business interests, but they were not their complete stories.

The second point concerns the corpus of health education films produced and distributed by Eastern. In some ways, Tichenor saw this as a discrete corpus, since the market in health education films could be distinguished from other related markets such as for films targeted at a professional medical audience. Yet in general it was a corpus that was always in danger of dissolving into others. The key problem of the public health movie—that of shaping people's beliefs and behaviors—was the same as for many other forms of sponsored motion pictures such as advertising, political, and social service films. Its subject matter—health, illness, and healing—blurred into other subjects such as accident prevention, fire prevention, and industrial safety also made and distributed by Eastern. And while its market could be distinguished from that for medical films, the two markets overlapped in places, and the market in health education films was not dissimilar to others such as advertising or political films. Eastern's corpus of public health films was thus an unstable corpus from a commercial point of view, always at risk of vanishing into other corpuses—films that shaped people's behaviors, corpuses of films of other related subject matter, and films that required similar business approaches. It was also part of a corpus of films that were intended to solve the commercial problems that Eastern faced from the late 1910s onward; they were made by the same filmmakers who would at other times make other sponsored films for Eastern, and Tichenor hoped that these films would help to blur other boundaries as between educational and entertainment, theatrical and nontheatrical. A focus on the commercial aspects of the public health film thus raises questions about the identity of the public health film and the corpuses in which it should be included.

From Features and Comedies . . .

In order to understand why Eastern turned to medical and other sponsored films, it is first necessary to explore Tichenor's involvement in the entertainment film world. Tichenor's story is the tale of someone who would come to be central to this world in the 1910s, working alongside some of the biggest names in the business, but who by the 1920s was an increasingly marginal figure. The Eastern Film Corporation was central to this transition, for while it began in 1915 amid high hopes that it could compete with the major entertainment film companies, by the late 1910s such hopes had disappeared, and Tichenor began to focus its activities on sponsored films, including public health education films. The careers of many of Tichenor's former business associates—including Cecil B. De Mille and Samuel Goldwyn—are well documented, but there is very little on the careers of men like Tichenor, who struggled to produce entertainment films and who moved into sponsored films to keep their businesses (and their hopes of maintaining a foothold in the entertainment world) alive.

Born in Gethsemane, Kentucky, Tichenor was educated at Villanova College (1895–1901)[10] He moved to New York and got involved in the motion picture business in around 1909.[11] Within a few years, Tichenor was, as one report claimed, "known personally to practically every motion picture manufacturer and exhibitor in the United States by reason of his former business connections,"[12] and he was "one of the most esteemed members of the Screen club [founded 1912], the New York organization of photoplayers and photoplay producers."[13]

Tichenor's rise to prominence in the film world began in 1910, when he helped to found the Manhattan Slide Company, later the Manhattan Slide and Film Company (see table 1.1).[14] This was followed in 1913 by his appointment as chairman of the Third Annual Convention and First International Exhibition of the Motion Picture Art held at the Grand Central Palace, New York, July 7–12, 1913.[15] A bundle of inexhaustible energy, according to most reports, Tichenor was widely credited with the success of the exhibition. He made the cover of *Moving Picture News*, and his caricature graced the New York *Evening World*. His new prominence opened up new opportunities, and shortly after the exhibition ended, he joined the Jesse L. Lasky Feature Motion Picture Company, founded in the summer of 1913 by Lasky (a prominent vaudeville impresario), Samuel Goldfish (later Goldwyn), and Cecil B. De Mille. Tichenor joined the company as general sales manager, assisting Goldfish and Lasky in New York selling films, while De Mille traveled west to make movies.[16]

But Tichenor did not stay long with Lasky. Ambitious to run his own film production company, a year later in April 1914 he started up Photo-Play Productions, headquartered in the recently opened Candler Building at 220 West Forty-Second Street, New York, at the center of the city's entertainment district, where his main role was to be behind the scenes, as was to be the case in all his future film companies.[17] Lasky's business model had involved making feature length theatrical films with theater stars duplicating their stage roles on screen; Photo-Play Productions' model was much the same.[18] Its first movie, *The Littlest Rebel* (1914), was based on Edward Peple's 1911 Civil War play of the same name, which had recently been staged, starring the brothers Dustin and William Farnum.[19]

Photo-Play Productions collapsed in early 1915 after falling out with its main financial backer.[20] And it was in this context that the Eastern Film Corporation

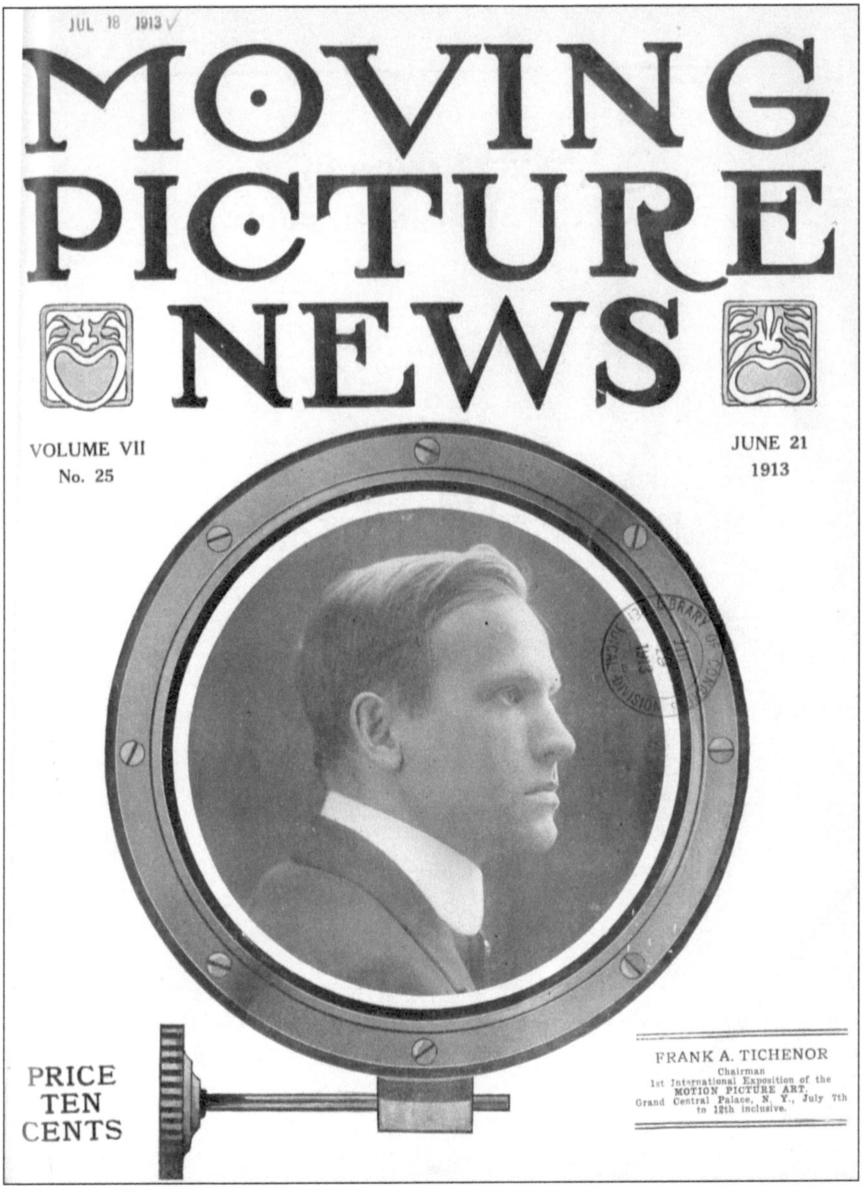

Figure 1.1a. Frank A. Tichenor on the cover of the *Moving Picture News*, June 21, 1913.

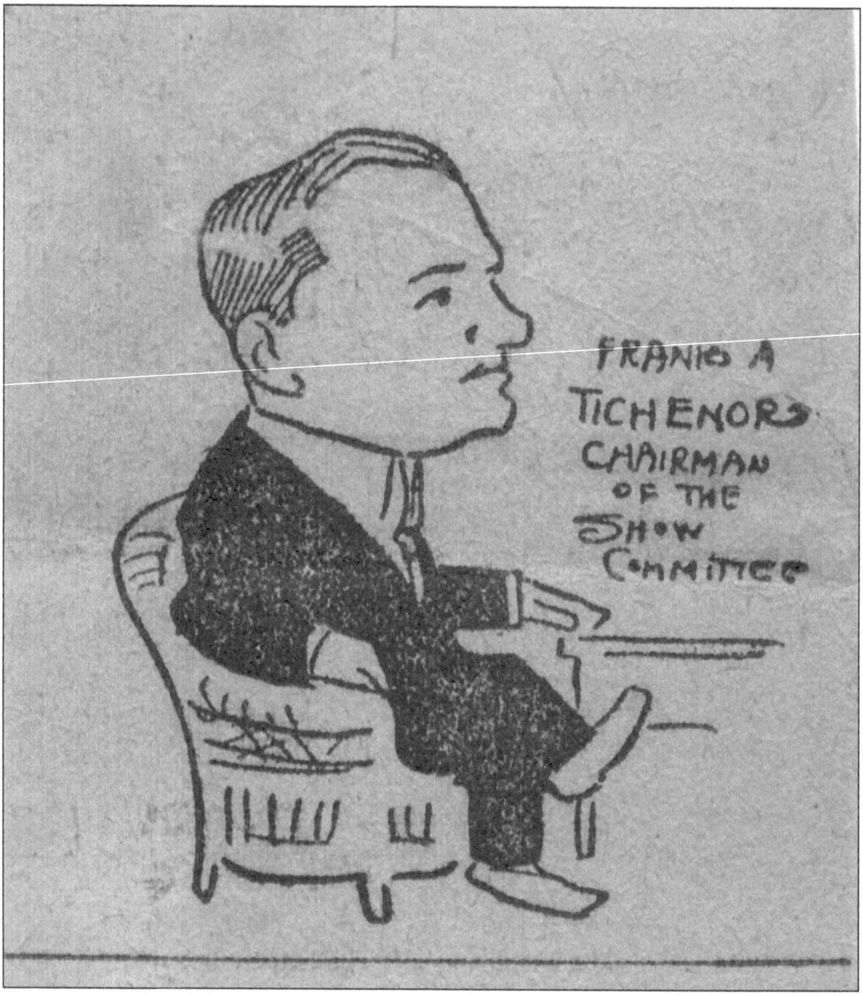

Figure 1.1b. Tichenor caricatured in a clipping from the *Evening World* (New York), July 8, 1913.

came into being, a few months after the demise of Photo-Play. By this stage, Tichenor had found another financial backer in Frederick Peck (1868–1947), a banker and one of the richest men in New England, with whom he had forged a close business relationship during troubles at the General Film Company, which threatened their financial investments in the film distribution company. Tichenor would eventually become general manager and vice-president of General.[21]

In December 1914, Peck, fellow Rhode Island businessman, Benjamin L. Cook, and the stage director turned film producer, Elwood F. Bostwick filed an

Table 1.1. Frank A Tichenor's involvement in film

Dates	Company	Position(s)
1910–c. 1913	Manhattan Slide (and Film) Company	Codirector
1913	Motion picture exhibition and convention at Grand Central Palace, New York	Chairman
1910s–1919	General Film Company	General manager; then president
1913–c. 1914	Jesse L. Lasky Feature Motion Picture Company	General sales manager
c.1914–c. 1915	Photo-Productions Company, Inc.	General manager
1915–1930s	Eastern Film Corporation	Manager; then president
1916–1920s	Amber Star Films Corporation	
1916[?]–1917	Vim Comedy Company	
1917–1930s	Jaxon Film Corporation	
1919–1920s[?]	Photoproducts Export Company	
1920s	DeForest Phonofilm Company	
1928–[?]	General Talking Picture Company	General manager and treasurer
1936		Mayor LaGuardia's mediator in a dispute with theatre exhibitors

agreement to form the Eastern Film Corporation, with the capital stock of one hundred thousand dollars. Eastern was formally incorporated in August 1915, with Peck as president, Cook as vice-president, Bostwick as general manager, and Walter Young—a business associate of Peck's—as treasurer. Tichenor's connections to Eastern in its early days are unclear. He is not mentioned in the articles of incorporation or in the early publicity for the organization. Arthur Krows suggests he joined Peck as a silent partner. Eastern took over Photo-Play Productions' New York offices at the Candler Building, which were to serve all of Tichenor's future film companies and to prove a valuable location for Tichenor's business dealings.[22]

Eastern was an altogether different and larger venture than Photo-Play Productions. Backed by Peck's "unlimited capital, brains, and shrewd business perception,"[23] the company sought to release each week two or three comedies ("high grade," not "slapstick,"[24] according to an Eastern advertisement) in addition to two three-, four-, five-, or six-part features under the "Pelican" brand.[25] Eastern appointed the former actor turned screenwriter, Mary Murillo, as the editor of the scenario department and advertised that it was in the market for two-part comedy stories and strong high-class four-to-six part feature films.[26]

At first Eastern seemed set to rival other commercial film companies. Its movie studios, laboratory, and offices in Providence were, according to one report, larger than any film plant in the country.[27] With "facilities of the finest kind"[28] and Peck's seemingly bottomless pockets, the company attracted "a roster of international stage and screen favorites."[29] Among these "favorites" were the actor, director, and producer George Lessey,[30] the former vaudeville performer and journalist, Lambert Hillyer,[31] the comedian, George Bunny, actress Helen Lowell, and cinematographer Frank M Blount. Its screenwriters included a young playwright, Eugene O'Neill.[32]

The first films were released in 1915, including two adaptations of Joseph C. Lincoln's sea stories, *Cap'n Eri* and *Partners of the Tide.*[33] Large crowds came to watch the filming of these movies, attracted by the stars and the spectacular set pieces. Lessey burned a $500 specially erected house to the ground for *Cap'n Eri*,[34] and Hillyer dynamited a $3,000 fishing schooner, *Conquest*, captained by a Charlie Chaplin (no relation to the actor, but apparently an admirer) for *Partners of the Tide.*[35] In the case of *Cap'n Eri* things got out of hand, and Lessey had to create a temporary emergency hospital when some people were injured by burning embers and overcome by excitement.[36]

But the early promise soon faded. Production stopped in the fall of 1915 due, according to historian Kathleen Karr, to mismanagement of company funds.[37] Elwood F. Bostwick resigned as general manager in October 1915.[38] Soon after, Lessey abandoned Eastern and returned to Universal.[39] Hillyer also moved on, eventually to Paramount, where he directed William S. Hart in his first starring role, in the Western *The Narrow Trail* (1917). Blount also ended up at Paramount, where he filmed the escapologist, Harry Houdini, in the *Grim Game* (1919), while Murillo left in 1915 to work for Fox films, where she became chief screenwriter in 1916.[40] Another screenwriter—Beta Brueil—later became head screenwriter with Vitagraph.[41]

Against this backdrop, the company began to produce a different class of movie. In January 1916, one disappointed screenwriter reported that Eastern now only wanted one- and two-reel scenarios, "and that the paramount requirements are that these be cheap and easy of production."[42] In April it was announced that the studio would release its films through a merger office in the summer.[43]

As Eastern got into trouble, Tichenor sought to diversify his film interests. On August 11, 1916, he (and business partners Herbert S. Tillinghast and George F. Maguire) filed an agreement to form the Amber Star Films Corporation with the capital stock of $5,000—Tillinghast was its first president, Walter F. Young its secretary-treasurer, with Peck was a major stockholder.[44] But no sooner had it started than this new company, like many previous Tichenor ventures, got into trouble. This time the problem came about because of Amber Star's involvement with the Vim Comedy Company, founded in late 1915 by Louis Burstein and Mark Dintenfass, with studios in New Jersey and Jacksonville, Florida, best known for comedy film series such as "Pokes and Jabs" (starring Bob Burns as Pokes and Walter Stull as Jabs) and the "Plump and Runt" series (starring Oliver Hardy as Plump and Billy Ruge as Runt).[45]

The problems started when Oliver Hardy claimed that Burstein and Dintenfass were stealing money from the Vim payroll. The allegations prompted an immediate reaction from Tichenor and Peck at Amber Star. Peck refused to pay the salaries, and Tichenor demanded answers from Burstein and Dintenfass and threatened to go to court. Burstein telegrammed Dintenfass in October 1916 suggesting that they be prepared to "grab the pictures,"[46] that is, cut their losses and make off with any films they could. But Dintenfass urged caution, not to "break contracts yet"[47] and to adjust things amicably with Tichenor so as not to jeopardize the business. Then, between October and December 1916, Tichenor, Peck, and Young removed Dintenfass from the presidency of Amber Star.[48] Dintenfass went to court arguing that Tichenor, Peck, and Young had done this illegally.[49] Dintenfass eventually abandoned his court case, and Vim ceased production in 1917. Tichenor traveled to Florida to reorganize the business.[50]

In January 1917 a new company, the Jaxon Film Corporation, was incorporated.[51] It took over the extensive Vim studios in Florida.[52] By March, Jaxon's first feature film was in production: *Strife*, directed by Lambert Hillyer, briefly returned to Tichenor's fold.[53] Billy Ruge stayed on with Jaxon, starring in a new comedy series without Hardy (Sparkle Comedies), while Burns and Stull continued the Pokes and Jabs series with Jaxon.[54]

Tichenor thus began with interests in both the production and distribution of Jaxon films. However, Jaxon does not appear to have been very active in film production after 1921, though it was still listed at Tichenor's New York address in 1933.[55] Amber Star appears to have established an office in Jacksonville but was listed as out of business at that address by 1921.[56]

So after a brief foray into the troubled waters to the Jacksonville film industry, Tichenor was back with Eastern in Providence.[57] However, his problems did not end there. On August 23, 1917, Eastern's Rhode Island Studios were partially destroyed by fire with estimated losses of $75,000–$100,000.[58] The fire forced a scaled-down operation and accelerated an existing trend in which Eastern moved away from producing entertainment films. The problems of coal rationing in the winter of 1918–19 cannot have helped. It forced many film companies to close their East Coast studios and consolidate operations on the West Coast.[59] This option was not available to Eastern, which had no West Coast facilities, and it was struggling after 1917.

None of this is to say that Eastern or Tichenor gave up on producing features and comedies. On the contrary, Tichenor seems to have taken advantage of the postwar boom in studio building in the New York area to revive Eastern's fortunes in this field.[60] An advertisement published in 1920 noted that Eastern was

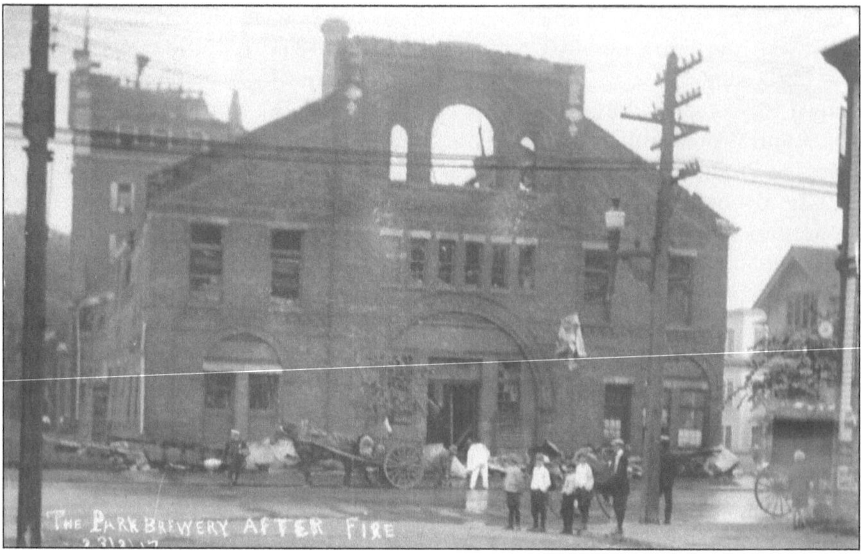

Figure 1.2. Park Brewery after the fire of 1917. Founded, in 1899, the Park Brew Company closed in 1913 and its buildings were taken over by Eastern. Courtesy of Gregory Theberge.

in the market for "all kinds of serials and comedies,"[61] and it worked on at least one feature in the early to mid 1920s—*Beyond the Great Wall* (1921), directed by Arch Heath and written and produced by Charles Beahan.[62]

In addition, Eastern and Tichenor also had a continuing interest in film distribution. Tichenor resigned as general manager and vice-president of the General Film Company in 1919, when the company also folded.[63] Left without a way of distributing Jaxon and Eastern theatricals (except though the independent exchanges; sometimes a risky business), in 1919 he founded the Photo Products Export Company, which distributed older movies from these companies and reedited versions of earlier feature films released by George Kleine and Thomas Edison.[64] In 1921 Tichenor secured rights to *The Rubaiyat of Omar Khayyam.*[65] Starring Ramon Novarro as Ben Ali, filming of the *Rubaiyat* started in June 1921, but after a falling out between the director and his impresario partner, the movie was unable to find a distributor. It lay in a vault until 1925, when it was released as *A Lover's Oath* to take advantage of the publicity for another Novarro film, *Ben Hur* (1925). Even so the film was not a success, and with bad reviews and poor box office receipts, it quickly disappeared.[66]

The fate of the Photo Products Export Company is unknown, but later in the 1920s Tichenor tried to establish Eastern itself as a distributor of nontheatricals and of foreign theatrical films. He had some luck with the former when he took over some of the films of the defunct Clinical Film Company (fl. 1915–17), but his efforts to distribute theatrical films for the French company Albatros in the

United States seem to have been stymied. He told the French company that this was in part because French films were often not to American tastes and because the French government's attempts to restrict the showing of foreign films undermined the efforts of French filmmakers to export to the United States.[67]

Tichenor also branched out in new directions. During the 1920s, he acquired a large film library in Eastern's name.[68] According to a 1927 advertisement, this library was one of the largest in the country, comprising some 40 million feet of film, protected in fireproof vaults. It included stock footage on an immense variety of subjects. Tichenor loaned some of these films out for profit, donated them for charitable purposes, rereleased edited versions of others, and plundered the vault for stock footage for Eastern's growing range of sponsored films. In its 1927 advertisement, Eastern cited the example of a food supplier that sold a range of thirty-two spices. Eastern found footage of thirty of these spices in the vault—growing and harvesting, "rich in atmosphere"—which it wove into a film "packed with interest and loaded with sales dynamite."[69]

Finally, in the 1920s Tichenor joined with the inventor Lee De Forest in promoting Phonofilm, an early sound-on-film technique, which recorded synchronized sound directly onto film.[70] According to Krows, Tichenor became the general manager and treasurer of the General Talking Picture Corporation founded in 1928 by De Forest to handle equipment distribution, with the financial backing of the New York City–based South African theatrical magnate, M. A. Schlesinger.[71] In addition, Tichenor's Simplex Projection Room at the 220 West Forty-Second Street address was outfitted for private demonstrations of De Forest's Phonofilm, which also had sublet offices in Tichenor's suites in the Candler Building.[72]

To Industrials and Educationals . . .

It should be clear by now that neither Tichenor nor Eastern had much interest in medical or health films before the 1920s. Indeed, with the exception of a Beta Brueil feature *Daisies* (a story about a doctor, released ca. 1915), they had almost no interest in these subjects. All this changed around 1919 or 1920, when Eastern produced its first medical and health films—sponsored films, not features. Tichenor quickly became an enthusiast for these sorts of film, but then he was also an enthusiast for many other types of sponsored movie. In his view, sponsored movies—of all types, including medical and health films—offered a solution to the problems that Eastern faced in the late 1910s and early 1920s. They provided the possibility of a return on the investment in the studios in Rhode Island and elsewhere. They built upon the skills that Eastern had already developed in producing features and comedies. And they shared a similar function, that of changing or reinforcing people's behaviors or ideas. Before I can set out how Eastern imagined the specific markets in medicine and health, then I need to set out how and why it became interested in the broader category of sponsored movies and how medical and health films fit into this category.

Tichenor himself claimed that he was first alerted to the possibility of sponsored films in 1910 when he received a letter from Cuba inquiring about the purchase of a "spanking machine" that had featured in a slapstick comedy he had produced.[73] Whatever the truth of such a recollection, Tichenor soon had a business in industrials, newsreels, political campaign, and educational movies, many produced by the Manhattan Slide (and Film) Company.[74] By 1913 he seems to have gained a reputation as someone with an expertise in this field, consulted by industry groups on the use of motion pictures to reach a mass audience.[75]

Tichenor's interest in what he called "special interest" or "purpose" movies—was further developed in 1915 when Eastern produced newsreels for local use in Providence, supplied educational, religious, and comedy films to the Rhode Island state prison, considered producing a film on the care of babies in Providence for baby week, and filmed the results of a major fire in Fall River, Massachusetts, under Tichenor's direction.[76] But between 1915 and 1920, these activities were subsidiary to Tichenor's and Eastern's interests in features and comedies.

All this changed in the late 1910s, as Tichenor's efforts to produce and distribute features and comedies were increasingly frustrated and pressures mounted to get a return on the huge investment in studios and equipment.[77] Eastern had acquired the Jacksonville plant (at least until its disposal in 1917), a small studio in the 220 West Forty-Second Street building, and the large studio in Providence, Rhode Island. All three were expensively equipped, and as commercial filmmaking began to fade, much of the equipment lay idle. The Rhode Island studio was a particular concern with its indoor and outdoor stages, well-filled scene docks and property rooms, lighting equipment, paint frames, and processing laboratories.[78] After 1915 Eastern sought to rent the facilities out to other production companies, but the promise of income from these sources remained uncertain, and after the 1917 fire it was difficult to lease the charred remains.[79] Employees—those who remained after the losses of 1915–16—were worried about their jobs and looking elsewhere for work.

Contemporary commentators highlighted a growing enthusiasm for industrials and educationals—including medical and health films—after the war. In Eastern's case, at least part of the impetus behind this enthusiasm was financial and commercial pressures of the sort that Tichenor faced. While Tichenor encountered unique problems with Eastern, the pressures that he faced in obtaining a return on investments and keeping employees on the payroll were not limited to his company. In such circumstances, film entrepreneurs began to look to new ventures to expand or stabilize their companies, to keep their investors happy, their cameras rolling, and their workers in place. Thus, businessmen like Tichenor worked feverishly behind the scenes trying to persuade potential sponsors that movies could promote their messages. But many would-be clients were cautious. There were, after all, many alternative, and often cheaper, ways of getting a message across, and educators and advertisers were not always convinced that movies were the best way to do it.

Tichenor himself became an eloquent advocate for movies as tools of advertising and education. To advertisers and businesses, he promoted films as "trade getters" that promoted American industry at home and abroad more effectively than any other medium.[80] To educators and politicians, he promoted films as equally effective in "selling" ideas and changing behaviors, including the ideas and behaviors that medical and public health sponsors wanted to promote or change. Indeed, there was, in his view, very little difference between a movie that sold commercial products and one that "sold" ideas or practices such as going to the doctor. At root, both involved changing or reinforcing peoples' behaviors, and in his view, movies were a powerful, perhaps the most powerful, way of doing this because of their unparalleled capacity to transmit vast amounts of information and to reach audiences that other media could not reach. "No other way," he enthused in 1926,[81] "ever has been devised by man by means of which so many ideas could be so rapidly and so graphically presented to the human mind." "One picture is worth a thousand words,"[82] he claimed, adopting the phrase popular among advertisers in the 1920s. In addition, in the case of public education films, he often recommended that films include a human interest story: this combination of visuals and narrative, he felt, worked best for popular audiences, as it did for the audiences of some professional training films, political campaign movies, and commercial advertisements. In other types of films—such as scientific or medical films—human interest narratives were less important.

In such ways, Tichenor sought to cultivate a market for sponsored films by trying to persuade potential sponsors that movies were a unique and immensely powerful way of selling ideas and behaviors. He also sought to find a place for Eastern within this market. "If your sales program requires a change of habit to bring success," a 1927 advertisement suggested, "or if the permanence of your business demands that no change of habit take place, you are urged to consult Eastern to find out how motion pictures can serve you."[83] Repeatedly, he highlighted the company's long experience in the film world, its skilled staff, and its comprehensive facilities.[84] As a 1924 advertisement put it,

> We maintain a very complete motion picture plant. It comprises cameras and cameramen, scenario writers, casting director, a staff of actors and actresses of ability, complete studios, developing and laboratory equipment, a title shop, etc. We can produce in our own plant a complete motion picture from the scenario to the finished print. We can send cameramen anywhere on the land, in the air or under the sea to secure a motion picture of anything that can be photographed with standard or slow motion cameras.[85]

Yet it was often a difficult task to persuade would-be clients to hire Eastern for their films. In the first place, Tichenor's salesmanship was hampered by growing concerns about the poor quality of films produced by the numerous companies jumping on the bandwagon of the sponsored film after the war. Critics claimed that many were recycled old commercial films that had been junked and reworked into films of dubious educational value.[86] The problem for Tichenor was that this trend threatened to undermine the market in sponsored films. The best companies in the field were likely to be tainted by the worst, while the hype around film threatened to harm the market in the long term by generating unrealistic expectations that were bound to be disappointed. In 1918 Evart G. and Mary Swain Routzahn of the progressive Sage Foundation cautioned against extravagant claims made for the value of movies to education and lamented the lack of films that met even basic standards for educational or propaganda purposes.[87]

In the second place, Tichenor's efforts to persuade would-be clients to hire Eastern were also stymied by growing concerns that sponsored films were difficult to distribute.[88] In 1923–24, Tichenor sought to counter such problems by reinventing Eastern as a distributor of sponsored movies; this shortly after his other company—the Photo Products Export Company—began distributing theatrical films. He also constantly talked up the potential for well-made films to get distribution, including theatrical distribution. In Tichenor's view, the best sponsored films found their way into the entertainment theaters as part of an evening's entertainment, and despite the naysayers, exhibitors—even in the 1920s—would pay good prices to insert such a film into a show. In 1926 he told the story of how one movie obtained theatrical release because of its entertainment and visual impact, a motion picture advertising fur coats for women in which he had been involved. People were willing to pay for it, he claimed, because of its high quality.[89]

In the third place, Tichenor's efforts to persuade would-be clients to hire Eastern were also challenged by concerns about the difficulties of reaching audiences of differing intellectual and emotional capacities. Eastern had long argued that movies were ideal for reaching audiences that other media could not. "It is stated that men who cannot read or write," one newspaper report on Eastern's 1915 gift of educational, religious, and comedy films to the Rhode Island State Prison noted, "can secure much knowledge from educational films such as those showing how automobiles are made or picturing the making of shoes."[90] But the Tichenor employee, Arthur Krows, also worried that variations in the intellectual level of the audience placed restrictions on the appeal of films. In Krows's view, the intelligence of the average moviegoer was that of a fourteen-year-old child, which made it impossible to produce educational films with any pretense of sophistication. "The lowest intellectual level" governed "the character of the appeal to be made."[91] Krows proposed to make different movies that fitted the different intellectual needs of audiences, but this was an expensive option for many sponsors.

Of equal concern was the possibility that films might produce unwanted emotional responses in an audience, or vulnerable sections of it, that would work against the goals of the sponsor. Tichenor often argued that the emotional impact of movies was a valuable tool in changing public behaviors. However, while many sponsors hoped for such an outcome, they also came to worry that audiences tended to react in unpredictable ways. For example, many medical, public health, and insurance sponsors wanted to use fear as a stimulus to get people to take actions that would prevent disease, promote public health, and avert accidents. But fear could also paralyze people into inaction or send them in a different (unapproved) direction, and it was often difficult to figure out how an audience might respond.[92]

Given all these concerns, Tichenor spent much of his time reassuring potential sponsors that their money would be well spent and that Eastern was the best company to ensure that movies fulfilled the goals of their sponsors. To this end, he often presented potential clients with a risk-free incentive for going with Eastern. According to Krows, this involved offering rock-bottom prices and frequently allowing clients as much as a year in which to pay.[93] Indeed, Krows heard Tichenor tell prospective customers that if they didn't like their subjects on first screen examination, they wouldn't have to pay at all. "If you do authorize work," one advertisement noted in 1926,[94] "you are not asked for any payment until we have finished and you have approved what we have done."

Such a business strategy was not without its dangers in that it placed much of the financial risk on the company rather than the client. It was always possible that the client would refuse to pay, protest dissatisfaction, or demand expensive changes, so that Eastern would be left with all the costs and insufficient return. Krows claimed that there were plenty of social service organizations, experienced in the art of begging, ready to take extreme advantage of Tichenor's offer.[95] A company could go under in such circumstances, if it was not sufficiently capitalized or did not understand the business of filmmaking. As regards capitalization, Peck's seemingly bottomless pockets provided a cushion against what were in effect loans to clients against future returns. As regards the business of filmmaking, Tichenor's long experience in the film industry now came into play. Eastern's survival in the early 1920s, Krows suggests, was due in part to the fact that Tichenor knew the business of production in amazing detail and knew where the cuts could be made. Indeed, he suggests that many film companies without this knowledge got into trouble.

. . . and the Markets in Medical and Health Movies

As the above discussion suggests, Eastern's interest in medical and health films was part of a broader shift toward sponsored movies, itself part of a broader effort to diversify Eastern's and Tichenor's interests in film and other media. They were important to these processes, but probably no more important than any other area of their film work. My story, so far, has thus focused on what medical and health films shared with Eastern's other sponsored films, for what made them attractive to Tichenor were the synergies between these films and those on other subjects. Together with other sponsored films, they helped to solve the commercial and financial problems that Tichenor faced in the 1910s. Moreover, the core problem of a medical or health film was much the same as that of other sponsored films. They were intended to change or reinforce behaviors and practices, and the ways in which Eastern approached this problem in the case of medical and health films were similar to the ways in which they approached other films that sought to change behaviors of other groups: medical films overlapped with science education films; health films overlapped with films targeted at consumers of fur coats, voters, automobile drivers, or people who came in contact with explosives. In the latter cases, Tichenor claimed to make films that told (often, human interest) stories that were visually exciting and that, when shown in an appropriate setting, worked with a variety of different audiences. To do this well, he argued, one needed a company like Eastern with long experience in the film industry.

But if medical and health films shared much with other types of film, Tichenor regarded the markets in these sorts of films as quite distinct. The market in medical education movies, he believed, was poorly developed in terms of production and distribution, and (despite appearances of enthusiasm) medical schools and physicians were often reluctant to use film in medical training and education. By contrast, the market in health education films was relatively well developed and was expanding rapidly. Thus, his strategies for dealing with each were quite different. In the case of the former, he tended to encourage the market in medical education films as a prelude to finding a place for Eastern within that market. In the case of the latter, he tended to differentiate Eastern within the established market of public health education movies. I write of tendencies here, for Tichenor never adopted one in place of the other. The two strategies coexisted for both types of film, each blurring into the other, but one or the other dominating.

Tichenor became interested in the first of these markets—that of medical and dental training films—in about 1917, when he became associated with the Clinical Film Company of New York, which produced surgical and dental films; the company established a library of teaching films which it rented out to societies and colleges.[96] The company was founded in about 1915 amid growing interest in the possibilities of medical film among physicians, but by 1917 it was in trouble and went out of business. Harry J. Elkan—the former manager of the industrial film department at Pathé—purchased its film stock with the aim of distributing clinical films, and he rented office space, storage and projection facilities from Tichenor at his 220 West Forty-Second Street address. Elkan's plan did not work out, and after a few years he gave up this space, in part, Krows claims, because the distribution of medical films was quite disorganized.[97] Tichenor seems to have acquired the film stock in the early 1920s.

Despite the problems faced by Elkan and the Clinical Film Company, Tichenor remained optimistic that a new market was emerging for medical film in the 1920s. The first audio-visual departments began to appear in medical schools during that decade, and the new interest in medical movies was signified by the creation in 1920 of the Society for Cinematographic Instruction in Medicine and Surgery (SCIMS) along with its journal, the *Bulletin of the Society for Cinematographic Instruction in Medicine and Surgery*.[98] The problem for Tichenor was that these developments were accompanied by a tendency among physicians to blame commercial film companies for some of the problems of the field. According to James S. Edlin, the president of SCIMS, "the principal factor which has hindered the profession in this country from accomplishing more in this direction lies in one big obstacle—*the cost.*"[99] In his view, commercial companies were often to blame. Edlin claimed that while professional motion picture producers charged $1.50–$3.00 a foot for film production, technicians at his own Society charged only 25¢ a foot.

In an effort to distance Eastern from the criticism of overcharging, Tichenor offered physicians a loss-leading "philanthropy." This was not the first time that Eastern had deployed philanthropic gifts to cultivate a market in educational film: recall the gift of films to the Rhode Island Prison. In this case, Tichenor not only provided free gifts of medical films for screening; he also helped in the production of such pictures. Specifically, Eastern's philanthropy involved assisting the surgeon and medical film pioneer, Joseph Franklin Montague, to produce a series of surgical films. Montague was to become an articulate spokesman for medical film, for Eastern, and more generally for the commercialization of the field. It was he who described Eastern's involvement as "philanthropy."[100]

Montague had been interested in medical film long before his association with Tichenor. According to Adolf Nichtenhauser, he began filming rectal cases at the Bellevue Hospital Medical College Clinic in New York in 1916; he later filmed surgical operations and added animation to them to clarify both operative principles and anatomical, physiological, and pathological details.[101] But Montague had limited resources at Bellevue to make the sorts of films that he wanted, and at some point—probably 1919 or 1920—he came to collaborate with Tichenor. The arrangement was that Tichenor made Eastern's production facilities available to Montague and provided production assistance—including that of the former cartoonist turned film director Arch B. Heath.[102] Krows claims that by the time the collaboration with Eastern ended, Montague had produced about sixty films, including a six-reel film showing the dissection of the entire body.[103]

At first Tichenor's gamble seems to have paid off. Montague's films were widely praised, and Montague himself became "one of the most enthusiastic advocates of the efficacy of motion pictures in medical and public health education."[104] Montague saw film as both a quintessentially modern way of educating physicians and (paradoxically) as a technology that would allow medicine to move beyond the modern age. In his view, the modern age was characterized by a focus on diseases rather than patients, but it was a dying age. Patients in the 1920s, he claimed, were much better educated than in the past. They objected to being an interesting case of a disease. They were sick men and women who wanted to be healthy. A new age was beginning to emerge, he argued, the era of the patient. Motion pictures could help to usher in this new age by shortening and enlivening medical training, which would allow a rehumanization of medicine and a new focus on the patient.

Film for Montague was thus part of a much broader effort at medical reform. Not only would it challenge the focus on diseases rather than patients, it would also reduce the need for vivisection in medical training and undermine the growing dominance of the specialist in medicine. In his view, specialists were part of the problem of modern medicine: they tended to classify patients according to their own narrow specialist viewpoints and so failed to understand the patient as a whole. In the new age of the patient envisaged by Montague, the specialist was to be reduced to a narrow technical expert, answerable to general practitioners (or their successors) and to patients. General practitioners, he claimed, were best suited to the new age of the patient. They knew them as individuals, their families and friends, their economic and social circumstances. They brought them into the world and saw them through childhood ailments, marriage, the birth of children, and into old age. In short, they understood the patient as a whole person, not as an interesting example of a particular disease. Of all physicians, they were best placed to determine what types of specialist care a patient needed.

Such themes were common in the discourse of interwar clinical holism.[105] They allowed generalists to claim authority over specialists and the laboratory by asserting the primacy of knowledge gained in the doctor's office, face-to-face with patients. At the same time, Montague argued, general practitioners had to recognize the limits of their own knowledge and skill, when to hand patients over to specialists, and what sorts of specialists to hand them on to. In the case of his own specialty of proctology, for example, Montague was critical of general practitioners who, out of ignorance, treated rectal diseases by "skillful neglect."[106] His goal was to reform proctological care by distancing the specialty from charlatans and by improving medical training in proctology, both for specialists and general physicians. Medical films had a key role in this reform. They allowed training to be tailored to the needs of students. Students could learn at their own pace, reviewing films as many times as they wished. They also gained a clearer view of surgical procedures and human anatomy than traditional demonstrations allowed. The next generation of textbooks for physicians, he claimed, would be made of celluloid, not paper.

Montague was quick not only to set out a golden future for medical film, but also to diagnose problems that might impede its beginnings. In the first place, he worried that the value of the medical motion picture to medical reform might be subverted. There was always the possibility of a monopoly of medical films by physicians who, by virtue of superior capital and organization, "further augment the inferiority complex which they now . . . wish upon the small town and city surgeon."[107] His solution was to produce film based on accepted and recognized medical books selected by medical demand. In this way, those books that were filmed would be those which the medical public most requested.

In the second place, Montague also worried that a major hindrance to the development of film as a tool of training was a lack of funds. Making films was expensive, and medical schools, conservative in outlook, were generally unwilling to fund them. Nor were physicians generally able or willing to help. Medical men, he claimed, were not rich and were often unprogressive in outlook, and so motion pictures had received little support. It was in this context that he mentioned Eastern. Writing in a 1926 volume edited by Tichenor, he noted that "to date the only successful series of motion picture films on surgical subjects has been that of my own and this has been produced through the philanthropy of the Eastern Film Corporation of New York."[108]

Montague's comments were important to Tichenor because they helped to challenge continuing dissatisfaction among physicians about how films were made and worked.[109] Not only were films expensive, critics noted, but operative films were often too short so that the technique could not be shown in full and the observer gained the false impression that they were not difficult to undertake; there was little emphasis on the disadvantages of surgery. Also, some films were less about education than self-advertising—before and after films in plastic surgery were often little more than promotional films, with the "after" being retouched. Montague's comments provided answers to all these criticisms. As importantly, for Tichenor they also helped to counter the possibility of commercial competition from George Eastman of Eastman Kodak. Nichtenhauser notes that Eastman had joined with the American College of Surgeons in around 1925 to stimulate the use of film in medical and surgical teaching.[110] The details of this initiative are not important here, but it is clear that they tended to bypass Eastern, and Montague offered some hope that Eastern could beat the competition from Eastman.[111]

But Montague was an unreliable ally. His own partnership with Eastern probably ended around 1925, when the last of his rectal films was complete. In 1927, the year after his favorable mention of Eastern, Montague proposed the creation of a Medical Film Foundation endowed not by Eastern but by the rival Eastman to "save us [the medical profession] from the distressing spectacle of unscientific 'scientific' films."[112] Montague's concern was that too many medical men were producing films themselves but without knowing how to make *good* films, and he saw businessmen such as Eastman as a solution to this problem. Under Eastman's leadership, Montague claimed, the Foundation would be assured of the highest technical excellence of the film produced. It would also "remedy a notorious defect in many enterprises run by the medical profession":[113] it would eliminate professional rivalries between medical men and ensure an adequate and proper supply of medical films and the continued freedom of the medical press. To Montague, it would also help to guarantee the availability of material that had been thoroughly appraised beforehand by the profession. He also hoped that the Foundation would help to increase the sales of books that were chosen for filming.

With Montague's desertion, Eastern began to abandon medical film production, focusing instead on film distribution. It had started distributing medical films in around 1924, when it distributed some old Clinical Film Company dental training movies: recall that Tichenor acquired the company's film stock around the time that Elkan had left the business. With its efforts to produce medical films beginning to fail, Clinical's film stock took on new importance as a source of revenue, albeit a short-lived one. A 1925 report suggests that the Society for Cinematographic Instruction in Medicine and Surgery took over the distribution of Eastern's dental films in 1925.[114] While Eastern continued to distribute medical films after then—and to retain hopes of breaking into the market of medical film production—it efforts do not seem to have met with much success. Sometime in the late 1920s, Eastern abandoned the medical film market altogether.

Tichenor entered the second market—that of health education films aimed at the general public—in 1919 or 1920, shortly after his first encounter with medical films. Here he found a very different market to that of the medical film. As with medical films, physicians and health educators had been interested in movies as tools of public education long before Tichenor or Eastern took an interest in the field, and this interest persisted into the postwar period.[115] But for Tichenor, the field was not hampered by the sorts of problems that dogged the medical field. While commentators worried about problems of distribution, and while sponsors were often cautious about the cost of films, these concerns did not seem, to Tichenor, to stifle the commercial market in health films as they did in the area of medical education. On the contrary, many film companies poured into the field, and Tichenor found himself struggling to differentiate his company from its many competitors. Tichenor did not worry so much about stimulating a market in health films as establishing a place for Eastern within it. Thus, where Tichenor's principle objective in the case of medical films had been to cultivate the market as a whole, in the case of health films it was to establish Eastern within a rapidly growing market.

Tichenor was not alone in seeing an expanding market in health education films. In 1926 Thomas C. Edwards (the acting executive officer of the National Health Council [NHC]) argued that at the end the First World War there had been less than 25 health films "of any value,"[116] whereas by 1926 there were at least 300 such films. At the same time, the ways of distributing such films had multiplied. In 1918 they had been quite limited, but by 1926 they could be obtained from a bewildering range of organizations (including semicommercial firms, YMCAs, state boards of health, universities, voluntary health organizations, life insurance agencies, and industrial groups) and were viewed by millions of people.[117] In an effort to identify films "of any value," the NHC published a list of health education films in 1921, which by 1928 had gone through five editions, expanding from a short typescript to 98 pages in 1926 and 178 pages in 1928.[118]

During the 1920s, Eastern produced health films on cancer, clean water, occupational health, and the work of the state nurse. Eastern also produced a variety of other films that touched on health themes such as automobile safety, the safe handling of explosives, and fire prevention. The boundary between health and other types of film such as accident prevention could be quite porous, as was the boundary between medical and health films. Edwards, for example, included many films within the health education category that Tichenor regarded as more properly part of the medical education market, such as *Gastric Motor Phenomena* (n.d.), on the motor phenomena of the stomach and duodenum.

At first Tichenor tended to rely on his clients to distribute his health films. Eastern's two cancer education films—*Reward of Courage* (1921) and *A Fortunate Accident* (1925)—were distributed through the American Society for the Control of Cancer (ASCC), which was rapidly building up a network of regional cancer organizations.[119] *The Danger That Never Sleeps* (1921) was distributed through the fire insurance industry as part of a broader educational program that sought to promote fire safety awareness. *Why Hurry?* (1926) was part of an accident prevention campaign. *How Jimmy Won the Game* (ca. 1926) was part of a campaign by the explosives industry to encourage children to beware the dangers of explosives.[120] Finally, *Your Glass of Water—Are You Sure It's Safe?* and *Sunshine Lady* were part of the Pennsylvania Sesqui-Centennial Commission's sponsorship of films on "the way to health for her [Pennsylvania's] citizens."[121]

Part of the appeal for Tichenor of working with health and other campaigns was that they already had (or were developing) their own public educational programs. Much of the organization of distribution was already in place. Films could be screened alongside a health lecture or a lantern slide show. They could be included in health exhibitions and could supplement newspaper, poster, and other media publicity. They could be shown in workplaces, classrooms, hospitals, public health events, town halls, women's organizations, theaters, libraries, and so on. All that was needed was a projector, a power supply, a white wall or screen, and a projectionist. Health organizations thus often came with their own ready-made distribution network. Tichenor welcomed such networks but did not rely entirely on sponsors for distribution: "the wide-spread distribution you secured for it [*The Danger That Never Sleeps*]," W. E. Mallalieu, general manager of the National Board of Fire Underwriters, wrote to Tichenor in 1922,[122] "impresses us as being unusual, as does your continued interest in the production."

Tichenor's reluctance to rely entirely on others to distribute his films became increasingly apparent during the 1920s. From about 1922–23, he began to describe Eastern as a distributor as well as producer of health films. In some cases, it seems to have acted as a distributor for other production companies. In addition, the library at 220 West Forty-Second Street came to serve as a source of revenue for the company. Its growing collection of health films was increasingly rented out to other organizations. The films themselves were constantly relabeled, one year having the Eastern label and another year that of another company. Thus, *An Unbeliever Convinced*, produced by the Essanay Film Company in about 1919, was listed as an Eastern Film Corporation film in 1928.[123] *What Price Recklessness?* was listed as an Eastern Film Corporation film in 1928 but as that of the Carter Cinema Producing Company in 1930.[124] Those for which there was no demand could be used as a source of stock footage, cut up, or copied, and patched together into new films. Scenes from health films might reappear in other films that had nothing to do with health.

Most of the health education movies that Eastern made and distributed have not survived, but descriptions of some of them have. Most were wrapped in a dramatic narrative, often a conversion account, in which those who followed the sponsor's advice were saved and those who did not suffered a terrible fate. For example, the cancer film *Reward of Courage* (1921) involved the conversion of a businessman to the sponsor's recommendations regarding cancer, after which he saves his wife from a quack and encourages her to undergo successful treatment for cancer from a recognized surgeon.[125] In the fire and accident prevention movie, *The Danger That Never Sleeps* (1921), some children are amazed to see the figure of Columbia come to life in a fire prevention poster and are persuaded by her to become Knights of Carefulness, pledged to safeguard others, to learn and to recognize dangerous conditions at home and in the city, and to teach others to make carefulness a habit.[126] In *A Fortunate Accident* (1925), a woman is saved from cancer when a young physician accidentally discovers a lump in her breast and persuades her to seek early treatment for the disease.[127] In a different way, the community chest propaganda film—*When It Strikes Home* (1920s)—uses a dream sequence to convert a workman who doesn't believe in contributing to funds for the general welfare. He falls asleep and has a dream that demonstrates the need for such a fund.[128] In *How Jimmy Won the Game* (ca. 1926), Jimmy learns about the dangers of blasting caps from his father, a quarry boss, and stops Jack, the star pitcher of the school baseball team, from exploding a blasting cap, thereby helping to win a baseball game by ensuring that Jack can pitch his team to victory.[129]

On the other side of coin, there were also stories that demonstrated the folly of not converting or converting too late. In the fire prevention movie *An Unbeliever Convinced* (ca. 1919) a building owner refuses to comply with city fire prevention regulations. His building burns and his daughter perishes.[130] *What Price Recklessness?* (1920s) told the story of a young man who is willfully reckless, only to have his comeuppance. While working at the grinding wheel without the protection of goggles, the wheel flies apart and he is blinded for life.[131] In *Why Hurry?* (1926), an accident prevention movie for children, a series of accidents befall the Heedless family, every one of which could have been avoided. Among the accidents are auto and trolley accidents, a home fire, asphyxiation, shock and resuscitation; also, the film includes a story of a man who while speeding in his car runs down his own mother.[132]

The End of Eastern

Tichenor's enthusiasm for medical and health films did not survive the 1920s. In the mid-to late 1920s, Eastern got into financial difficulties, and Tichenor began to look elsewhere for business opportunities and abandon his interest in sponsored films. The company's prospects briefly improved in 1926 when the state of Pennsylvania hired Eastern to make all the movies for its sesquicentennial celebrations, and Eastern opened new offices in Philadelphia.[133] The celebrations included vast exhibition spaces in which the sesquicentennial commission created a special motion picture room where visitors could watch a series of twenty-one specially produced movies on various aspects of the government, natural resources, and other features of life in Pennsylvania.[134] The motion picture exhibit was later shown in Pennsylvania schools.[135]

Tichenor tried to build on the success by coediting in November 1926 a special issue of the *Annals of the American Academy of Political and Social Science* on "the motion picture in its economic and social aspects" with contributions from Krows, Montague, Terry Ramsaye, Julius Klein, and others, including Tichenor himself.[136] Widely cited, the volume focused mainly on educational, advertising, and training films and the industry that produced and distributed them.

Despite these efforts, Eastern's problems continued. Krows suggests that one reason was the "ruinous competition of talking pictures"[137]—perhaps a reference to Tichenor's investment in the "failed" sound technology of Phonofilm—which he claims was beginning to tell on Eastern by 1930. It should be noted, however, that silent films remained popular among the sponsors of "special purpose" films well into the 1930s, partly because they were often cheaper to produce than sound films and partly because some educators felt that introducing a commentary into sound films usurped their teaching role.[138] There remained a market in silent movies, even if it was not the market it once had been.

A second reason for Eastern's problems may have been Tichenor's marketing model—for most sponsored films this involved rock-bottom prices, no payment until the client was satisfied, and a year in which to pay.[139] Such a business strategy might have worked well when the economy was good, but it created problems as things soured at the end of the 1920s. The market in educationals and industrials began to dry up, and this (combined with the fact that at some point in the 1920s Peck decided not to pour more money into Eastern and that Tichenor failed to find an investor to replace him) meant that it became increasingly difficult to keep the company going. Tichenor and Peck remained partners, and Tichenor persuaded him to support other business ventures in the 1920s and 1930s. But at some point Peck lost faith in Eastern.

Tichenor himself increasingly focused on other media interests. In 1922 he established the magazine *Aero Digest,* and he soon acquired (partly with support from Peck) a raft of other publications including *Sportsman Pilot* (1929?), *Fore An' Aft* (1930; a yachting publication), *Spur,* and *Plumbers' and Heating Contractors' Trade Journal.* According to *Time,* Peck and the New England banking house of Bodell & Co. were stockholders in Angus Co., the publishers in 1932 of *Spur,* which had earlier ceased to pay dividends. Together with Tichenor, already a small stockholder, they secured control of Angus and vested it in Tichenor. This acquisition gave Tichenor control of *Plumbers' & Heating Contractors' Trade Journal,* for Angus published this journal along with *Nation's Schools* and *Modern Hospital.* Tichenor promptly sold the last two back to their former owner. Then he scooped up *The Port* (a little-known monthly published by the Port of New York Authority, which he planned to build into a review of port news the world over) and the *Outlook and Independent* (1932), which he renamed *New Outlook.*[140]

This is not to say that Tichenor completely abandoned an interest in movies. *Aero Digest* was based at the same offices in 220 West Forty-Second Street that housed Tichenor's film companies, and at times Tichenor would mix his interests in Eastern and airplanes.[141] Even after the demise of Eastern, he remained involved in the industry. In 1936 he was Mayor Fiorello LaGuardia's mediator in a dispute with theater exhibitors.[142] But publishing and airplanes came to take up much of his energy, and without his attention, Eastern faded. It seems likely the company ended sometime in the early 1930s.[143]

Conclusion

The forgoing highlights the complex meanings of the category of the public health film for commercial producers and distributors of such films. Tichenor had little interest in these forms of film until the late 1910s and early 1920s, and when he did take an interest in them, it was only as part of a broader effort to get a return on his failing investment in features and comedy productions and to sustain his involvement in filmmaking until he could triumphantly return to the world of entertainment film. Public health education films were thus a means to financial and business ends for Tichenor, no more special than any other form of sponsored film, and less desirable in his view than his true love of entertainment movies. Indeed, in some ways his turn to sponsored films did not involve a break from entertainment films. Tichenor often told would-be clients of sponsored films that entertainment could enhance the educational value of their movies, and that a well-made sponsored motion picture could find theatrical distribution without any payment from the sponsor; this even as the lines between theatrical and nontheatrical film hardened in the 1910s and 1920s. Likely Tichenor believed his own claims, though others doubted the value of entertainment in education. It may also be that Tichenor thought that producing entertaining sponsored films would pave the way to a return to the theatrical film world—at least until those hopes disappeared in the late 1920s and sponsored films themselves became less financially viable. The skills and resources that were necessary to produce an entertaining public health film might also be used in features and comedy.

The public health film might have been a means of sustaining Tichenor's business interests in film, but this did not mean it was indistinguishable from other special interest films. As a businessman, Tichenor had to understand the market in public health films, and as we have seen, he saw it as an established and growing market, which meant, for Tichenor, figuring out how to carve out a place for Eastern within it. However, while the nature of the market served to distinguish public health films from medical education films—quite a different, less-established, less dynamic market in Tichenor's view—this nature did not distinguish it from other forms of film. To Tichenor the market in public health films was not that dissimilar to other markets, such as for accident prevention films, social service films, and movies for advertising and political campaigns, which meant that he promoted those products in similar ways to public health films. It is true that sometimes he cultivated clients in established markets by offering philanthropy. However, this philanthropy served a different purpose to its use in less developed markets such as medical education. If in medical education it served to promote the market as a whole, in health education it aimed more to establish Eastern within these developed and growing markets.

There were other ways in which Tichenor's corpus of public health films overlapped with other forms of film. One concerned the company's working arrangements. When Eastern contracted to make a film, Tichenor or his subordinates would assign some of its permanent staff to the movie. This meant that a camera operator, actor, scenarist, editor, or producer who made political films at one time might later make a public health film, a commercial advertisement, a medical education film, or an entertainment film. This tendency to assign staff to different types of film meant that techniques and approaches to filmmaking were routinely transferred from one type of film to another, as were the material resources belonging to Eastern—its props, stages, lighting equipment, processing laboratories, and extensive film library. Thus, props appeared and reappeared in different movies, footage from Eastern's film library was cut and spliced into different motion pictures, and filmmaking techniques and narrative forms—such as the conversion narrative—developed for one form of movie were later transferred to others.

Tichenor himself constantly blurred the different categories of film in his writings. Not only did he blur the categories of entertainment and sponsored film; not only did he see the market in public health films as comparable to others such as accident prevention films; he also saw the category as overlapping in different ways with other sponsored films. As I have noted, he argued that movies that sold commercial products and those that "sold" ideas or practices such as going to the doctor had similar objectives. They both aimed to change or reinforce people's behaviors. From such a perspective, public health films were part of a larger category of film for Tichenor: "special interest" or "purpose" films that included commercial advertising, political campaign movies, medical training, and educational or didactic movies—all distinct types of film, but types that overlapped around the central problem of changing or reinforcing behaviors and ideas. Even their subject matter was not always the defining feature of a public health film for Tichenor. There were areas such as accident prevention that sometimes seemed to fit into the category of the public health film and sometimes to be regarded as a separate category. Both accident prevention and welfare movies might contain a public health message while including much else that had little to do with public health.

Tichenor himself sometimes portrayed Eastern's public health films as a small if well-defined corpus, embedded in a series of progressively larger corpi, much as the smallest Russian doll is hidden within a series of progressively larger dolls. From this perspective, Eastern's public health films were part of a larger corpus of Eastern's sponsored films (that also comprised medical education, advertising, and political films), itself part of the larger corpus of Eastern's total film output (both sponsored and entertainment films), which was itself part of the still larger corpus of Tichenor films (the output of all Tichenor's companies), itself perhaps part of the still larger corpus of silent films produced by the network of Tichenor's various business associates and employees (including Jesse L. Lasky, Cecil B. De Mille, George Lessey, Lambert Hillyer, and Oliver Hardy, among others). From such a perspective, the corpus of public health films is a very small part of a much larger corpus of films that comprise perhaps many of the films of the 1910s and 1920s. Tichenor was after all central to the network of entertainment filmmakers of the 1910s and continued to maintain such contacts into the 1920s, even as he expanded his interest in sponsored films. But as the foregoing suggests, such a portrayal does not fully capture the protean nature of the public health film from a business perspective. Tichenor might sometimes have portrayed the public health film as a well-defined type, but in practice it was always shading into other categories of film.

Tichenor himself worked aggressively during the late 1910s and the 1920s to drum up clients for public health sponsored films, to turn their messages into something that worked as a film, and to make a return for Eastern and its investors. Yet it seems likely that his recruitment methods created risks for the company. As noted above, it was always possible that a sponsor would express dissatisfaction and refuse to pay for the film, or that Eastern's "philanthropy" would fail to develop a market or be unsuccessful in creating a space for the company within such a market. Such problems could be expected at any time and, as long as the company produced a profit overall, individual losses on a particular film or in a particular market could be absorbed. However, as economic times got harder at the end of the 1920s and Eastern's financial problems mounted, losses threatened to overwhelm profits even in the long term, and Tichenor came to view the company and the market in sponsored film as no longer viable. If in the early 1920s Tichenor had seen the market for health education films as an established market (and the key task was to find a place for Eastern within it), in the late 1920s it was in his view an overcrowded market (and the key questions were how to get out of it and where else to develop business opportunities).

Notes

My thanks to Judith Freidman, who scoured Rhode Island newspapers for mentions of Tichenor and Eastern; Shera Moxley who identified the records on Amber Star in the archives of the Rhode Island Supreme Court; and Ray Lewis, the owner the Capeville Flea Market, who gave me some Tichenor memorabilia in addition to some other materials that he sold me. My coeditors, Anja Laukötter and Christian Bonah, helped me improve and cut what remains a very long essay. Other help is acknowledged in the endnotes.

1. Some of the best discussions of commercial film interest in medicine and health are over sixty years old: Adolf Nichtenhauser, "A History of Motion Pictures in Medicine" (unpublished manuscript, ca. 1950), Adolf Nichtenhauser History of

Motion Pictures in Medicine Collection, MS C 380, Archives and Modern Manuscripts Program, History of Medicine Division, National Library of Medicine, Bethesda, MD. Arthur Edwin Krows, "Motion Pictures—Not for Theaters," *Educational Screen* (September 1938–June 1944). There is virtually no discussion of the commercial side of medical/health film production in the following: Lester D. Friedman, ed., *Cultural Sutures: Medicine and Media* (Durham, NC: Duke University Press, 2004); Graeme Harper and Andrew Moor, eds., *Signs of Life: Medicine and Cinema* (London: Wallflower Press, 2005); Leslie Reagan, Nancy Tomes, and Paula A Treichler, eds., *Medicine's Moving Pictures: Medicine, Health, and Bodies in American Film and Television* (Rochester NY: University of Rochester Press, 2007).

2. Forty-six commercial companies distributing educational films are listed in Metropolitan Life Insurance Company. Welfare Division, National Health Council, *Film List Including Information on Visual Aids and Their Producers and Distributors*, 5th ed. (New York: Prepared and printed by Welfare division, Metropolitan Life Insurance Company, 1928), 165–78.

3. According to the 1930 census, Tichenor was born in 1882, while other sources suggest 1880. I haven't had much luck in tracing any family member or business associates of Tichenor. However, a scrapbook belonging to a Frank A Tichenor was found during a house clearance in Exmore, Virginia, and was acquired in around 2008 by Ray Lewis, who owns the Capeville Flea Market, 26175 Lankford Hwy, Cape Charles, VA 23310. Lewis sold some items—mainly aviation memorabilia—from the scrapbook on EBay under the name Figscollectibles. I visited the flea market on December 20, 2010, and viewed the remains of the scrapbook. Most of the material from it had already been sold, and Lewis told me that much of it had been removed before he obtained it. What was left comprised mainly clippings of Tichenor's interests in aviation and some envelopes, drawings, and other memorabilia (including some movie memorabilia) from Tichenor and his son Frank A Tichenor Jr. It is unclear to which Tichenor the scrapbook belonged or whether it was his wife's or the family scrapbook. Citations to material obtained from it are labeled "Tichenor scrapbook."

There are several Tichenor family listservs, but as of September 4, 2016, appeals for information to these had met with no response: Tichenor Families in America at http://85213.forums.motigo.com/; the TICHENOR-L Archives at http://lists5.rootsweb.ancestry.com/index/surname/t/tichenor.html; Tichenor Family Genealogy Forum, http://genforum.genealogy.com/tichenor/. Tichenor does not appear in Harold A Tichenor, *Tichenor Families in America* (Napton, MO: privately printed, 1988).

4. Visugraphic produced a number of educational movies, including medical movies such as *This Great Peril* (1929). See Arthur Edwin Krows, "Motion Pictures—Not for Theaters," *Educational Screen* 18, no. 10 (December 1939): 362–63.

5. Coronet (based in Providence, RI), produced *Unhooking the Hookworm.* Kirsten Ostherr, "Cinema as Universal Language of Health Education: Translating Science in Unhooking the Hookworm (1920)," in *The Educated Eye: Visual Culture and Pedagogy in the Life Sciences*, ed. Nancy Anderson and Michael Dietrich (Hanover, NH: Dartmouth College Press, 2012).

6. On Bray see Donald Crafton, *Before Mickey: The Animated Film, 1898–1928* (Chicago: University of Chicago Press, 1993), 137–68, esp. 158–60 for his turn to

nontheatricals. For brief histories of other educational film companies, some of which made medical movies, see Paul Saettler, *The Evolution of American Educational Technology* (Greenwich, CT: Information Age Publicizing, 2004), 99–106.

7. See, for example, (1) The Legend Film Corporation incorporated c. 1920: Arthur Edwin Krows, "Motion Pictures—Not for Theaters," *Educational Screen* 18, no. 10 (December 1939): 364–65; and (2) Vitagraph: Richard Koszarski, *Hollywood on the Hudson: Film and Television in New York from Griffith to Sarnoff* (New Brunswick, NJ: Rutgers University Press, 2008), 108–12.

8. Another entrepreneur who tried to mix theatricals and nontheatricals was Ernest Shipman of the Legend Film Corporation. See Peter Morris, *Embattled Shadows: A History of Canadian Cinema 1895–1939* (Montreal: McGill-Queen's University Press, 1992), chap. 4.

9. Arthur Edwin Krows, "Motion Pictures—Not for Theaters," *Educational Screen* 20, no. 9 (November 1941): 384.

10. "One Hundred Thousand Photoplay Fans and Five Thousand Exhibitors," *Ogden Standard* (Ogden City, UT), July 12, 1913, 2. I'm grateful to Dennis Gallagher, the archivist at Villanova University for the following information: "Frank A. Tickenor (*sic*) (listed Francis Aloysius Tichenor, New Jersey). First time name appears is in the catalog for 1895–1896. The last time the name appears is in the catalog for 1900–1901. His name does not appear in the graduation list. Furthermore, his name is not listed in the catalog for 1902–1903." Dennis J. Gallagher email to David Cantor, sent June 22, 2009. Note that Tichenor is then based in New Jersey.

11. The 1909 date comes from "Frank A Tichenor," *Moving Picture News*, June 21, 1913, 13, which claims he had been in the film industry for four years. His interest in films seems to predate this however. Terry Ramsaye notes that he watched Sigmund Lubin's *Passion Play* (1898), though the date of this viewing is not specified. Terry Ramsaye, *One Million and One Nights: A History of the Motional Picture through 1925* (New York: Simon and Schuster, 1986), 377.

12. "Jesse L. Lasky Enters M.P. Field," *New York Clipper*, December 20, 1913, 15. For similar comments, see "About Photoplays and Photo Players," *Anaconda Standard* (MT), April 26, 1914, 11. "Tichenor & Lincoln Working Wonders," *Cedar Rapids Republican* (Cedar Rapids, IA) April 22, 1914, 11.

13. "About Photoplays and Photo Players," *Anaconda Standard*, 11.

14. This company was established on March 29, 1910, to purchase, lease, and manage moving picture theaters and manufacture moving picture machines and films, with a capital, $5,000. Tichenor was a director along with Maurice Daniels and Mary E. Losee. "New Corporations," *New York Clipper*, April 16, 1910, 232. Three years later, the company claimed to be the largest manufacturer of slides in the world and, as its name change suggests, it had also begun to make and distribute film for motion pictures. For Tichenor's involvement with the company, see "Frank A Tichenor," *Moving Picture News*, June 21, 1913, 13, and "Photo Play Productions Co. Enters Feature Film Field," *New York Clipper*, April 4, 1914, 14. For an advertisement listing Tichenor as president, see *Printer's Ink* 84 (1913): 267.

15. "One Hundred Thousand Photoplay Fans and Five Thousand Exhibitors," *Ogden Standard* (Ogden City, UT), July 12, 1913, 2. "The First International Exposition," *Moving Picture World*, July 19, 1913, 324–27. "One Hundred Thousand Photoplay Fans and Five Thousand Exhibitors Attend New York Convention and

Exposition and Honor Frank A. Tichenor, Whose Foresight and Energy Carried the Project to Success," *Columbus Daily Enquirer*, published as *The Columbus Enquirer-Sun*, March 1, 1914, 6. A copy of a pamphlet and an uncorrected proof of the same from this exhibition is "First International Exhibition of the Motion Picture Art in Conjunction with the Third Annual Convention of the Motion Picture Exhibitors League of America. New Grand Central Palace, New York, July 7 to 12, 1913" (Source: Tichenor scrapbook). Board of directors: chairman, Frank Tichenor; secretary, F. E. Samuels; treasurer, L. F. Blumenthal; president ex-officio, S. H. Trigger; others, M. Needle, L. Rosenthal, and J. King.

16. "Jesse L. Lasky Enters M.P. Field," *New York Clipper*, December 20, 1913, 15.

17. One report suggests he might have starred in one Photo-Play Productions' movie, *A Prince of Good Fellows* (1914). "'Frank A. Tichenor,' Starring in 'A Prince of Good Fellows'" *Newark Advocate* (Newark, OH), July 14, 1914, 6.

18. On Photo-Play's five-reel production, see "Tichenor Explains in Detail Why 'Littlest Rebel' Should Set New Mark in Production of Features," *New York Clipper*, May 2, 1914, 15. "The Littlest Rebel," *New York Clipper*, August 29, 1914, 14. For further reports of the film, see an advertisement for it in *New York Clipper*, April 18, 1914, 10. "'The Littlest Rebel,' The Stage Success . . . ," *Ogden Standard* (Ogden City, UT), April 15, 1914, 8. "Tichenor & Lincoln Working Wonders," *Cedar Rapids Republican* (Cedar Rapids, IA), April 22, 1914, 11. "Gossip of the Latest Movies," *Hamilton Evening Journal* (Hamilton, OH), April 11, 1914, 2. "Film Flashes," *San Antonio Light* (San Antonio, TX), May 3, 1914, 21. "Press Finds Child Actress in Movie," *Duluth News-Tribune* (Duluth, MN), September 17, 1914, 12. "About Photoplays and Photo Players," *Anaconda Standard* (Anaconda, MT), April 26, 1914, 11. For the list of stars, see "M.B., St. Paul," *Photoplay Magazine* 10, no. 1 (June 1916): 156. For an advertisement, see *New York Dramatic Mirror*, May 6, 1914, 43.

19. It should be noted that the Farnums had no place in *The Littlest Rebel*; Edward K. Lincoln, one of cofounders of the company, took the lead role of Captain Herbert Carey. For a biography of Lincoln, see "E. K. Lincoln" in *The First One Hundred Noted Men and Women of the Screen*, ed. Carolyn Lowrey (New York: Moffat, Yard and Co, 1920), 100–101. For Lincoln's criticisms of stage actors who try to make films, see "Jolting the 'Legits,'" *New York Tribune*, April 12, 1914, 9. The film appears to be lost, but photographic scenes from it illustrate the novelization of the play published as a Photo Drama edition: Edward Peple, *The Littlest Rebel* (New York: Grosset and Dunlap, 1914).

20. Arthur Edwin Krows, "Motion Pictures—Not for Theaters," *Educational Screen* 18, no. 7 (September 1939): 242. On the founding of Photo-play, see "Photo Play Productions Co. Enters Feature Film Field," *New York Clipper*, April 4, 1914, 14. See also the notice on "Photo Productions Company, Inc., Manhattan, N.Y.; $25,000; Arthur G. Hamilton, Edward K. Lincoln and Frank A. Tichenor, New York," *Bulletin of Photography* 14 (1914): 214. A 1915 entry for Photo-Play goes as follows: "Photo-Play Productions Company, 220 West 42nd Street, New York: Purchases motion picture rights of well-known stage successes. Frank A. Tichenor is general manager and Edgar Lewis is producer," in *1001 Places to Sell Manuscripts: The American Writer's Year Book and Directory to Markets for Manuscripts*, comp. William R. Kane (Ridgewood, NJ: The Editor Company, 1915), 237. The notice of bankruptcy is in "Bankruptcy Notices," *New York Times*, May 5, 1915, 18, and the sale of its assets in

"Bankruptcy Sales," *New York Times,* June 23, 1916, 20. For more information on Photo-Play's problems, see "Holds for Mrs. Van Heusen," *New York Times,* January 6, 1915, 9; "Movie Promoters in Row," *New York Times,* December 9, 1914, 14; "Justice Greenbaum Denies Injunction in Photoplay Productions Case," *New York Clipper,* March 20, 1915, 13.

21. General was incorporated in 1910 to distribute films produced by licensees of the Motion Picture Patents Company (founded 1907), which licensed and enforced key patents in the film industry. A story goes that as General got into trouble after antitrust rulings in 1914, Tichenor fought to save $30,000 he had invested in General and in the process began a long business relationship with Peck, who had also invested in the company. Scott Curtis, "A House Divided: The MPPC in Transition," in *American Cinema's Transitional Era: Audiences, Institutions, Practices,* ed. Charlie Keil and Shelley Stamp (Berkeley: University of California Press, 2004), 239–64. See also Eileen Bower, *The Tranformation of Cinema, 1907–1915* (Berkeley: University of California Press, 1994). "Frank A. Tichenor, Publisher, was 69," *New York Times,* May 5, 1950, 21. See also "Funeral Service for Frank Tichenor," *Box Office,* May 13, 1950, 49, and "Tichenor, Aero Digest Editor, Is Dead in East," *Chicago Daily Tribune,* May 5, 1950, B12.

22. Arthur Edwin Krows, "Motion Pictures—Not for Theaters," *Educational Screen,* 18, no. 7 (September 1939): 242–45, 243.

23. "Eastern Film Corporation to Announce Releasing Affiliation Shortly," *New York Clipper,* September 4, 1915, 16. There is another story in which the Broadway impresario Lee Shubert, a famous Broadway impresario, organized the Eastern Film Corporation, where Arthur E. Seger became famous as the original movie character Buster Brown. Tec 5 Firman B. Loree, "Sergeant Romped on Screen as Original Buster Brown," *Paris News* (Paris, TX), January 29, 1945, 7. However, I have been unable to find any other link between Segar, Buster Brown, or Shubert and Eastern.

24. A 1915 advertisement in *Moving Picture World* went "WANTED good scenarios for clean, high grade, one and two reel comedy and drama productions. Slapstick *not* wanted. Novelty sought. Highest prices for best work." Advertisement from Eastern's scenario department, *Moving Picture World,* 25, no. 4 (July 24, 1915): 737. "Rhode Island. Eastern Film Corporation," *The Editor: Journal of Information for Literary Workers,* July 31, 1915, 137.

25. "Eastern Film Corporation," *The Editor: Journal of Information for Literary Workers,* September 11, 1915, 262.

26. "Rhode Island. Eastern Film Corporation," *The Editor: Journal of Information for Literary Workers,* July 17, 1915, 89. "Rhode Island. Eastern Film Corporation," *The Editor: Journal of Information for Literary Workers,* July 31, 1915, 137. On Murillo, see "Mary Murillo, Script Writer Extraordinary," *Moving Picture World,* March 16, 1918, 1525. "A Successful Irish Scenario Writer: Mary Murillo Talks about Herself," *Irish Limelight* 1, no. 10 (October 1917): 9. Luke McKernan, "Searching for Mary Murillo," *The Bioscope,* November 5, 2009, http://bioscopic.wordpress.com/2009/11/05/searching-for-mary-murillo. Luke McKernan, "Mary Murillo Career Overview," Women and Silent British Cinema, 2007, http://womenandsilentbritishcinema.wordpress.com/the-women/mary-murillo/mary-murillo-career-overview/. See also Antonio Ríos-Bustamante, "Mary Murillo: Early Anglo Latina Scenarist," *Romance Languages Annual* 7 (1995): 604–9.

27. "Eastern Film Corporation to Announce Releasing Affiliation Shortly," *New York Clipper*, September 4, 1915, 16.

28. Ibid.

29. Ibid. Other actors seem to have come from New York or local Rhode Island theaters. See, for example, "'The Parish Priest' Played at St. Michael's," *Evening Tribune* (Providence RI), November 24, 1915, 7.

30. "Important Changes in Eastern Film of Providence," *New York Clipper*, October 23, 1915, 40. Sally A. Dumaux, *King Baggot: A Biography and Filmography of the First King of the Movies* (Jefferson, NC: McFarland, 2002), 89. Tichenor may have met Baggot a few years before. "Action and Interest of New Photoplays and the newest radiations of Film Stars," *Ogden Standard* (Ogden City, UT), September 27, 1913, 2.

31. "Hillyer, Lambert," in *Motion Picture Studio Directory: Trade Annual 1921*, ed. William Allen Johnston (Chicago: Motion Picture News, Inc, 1921), 266.

32. Arthur Gelb and Barbara Gelb, *O'Neill: Life with Monte Cristo* (New York: Applause Theater Books, 2000), 479.

33. The original intention was to film *Mr. Pratt, The Old Home House*, and *Partners of the Tide*. See "Eastern to Film Joe Lincoln Stories," *Moving Picture World*, August 21, 1915, 1305. In 1915 the company acquired an old whaling bark called *Morning Star* that it planned to use in these films, and later a fishing schooner called *Moselle*. Eastern acquired *Morning Star* in 1915 and sold it in 1916. "Old Whaling Bark will be Used for Movie Scenes," *The Day*, August 11, 1915, 9. "Jibboomer's Observations," *The Day*, May 29, 1916, 2. The *Morning Star* was a three-mast old whaling bark (238 gross tonnage), built in Dartmouth, MA, in 1853. Department of Commerce, Bureau of Navigation, *Seagoing Vessels of the United States with Official Numbers and Signal Letters, 1916: Part VI of the Forty-Eighth Annual List of Merchant Vessels of the United States for the Year Ended June 30, 1916* (Washington, DC: Government Printing Office, 1916), 26. In 1916, the captain of the schooner reported that thieves had broken into the boat and commited a robbery. See "'Movie' Boat Robbed," *Providence Journal* (RI), February 3, 1916, 9. On the *Moselle*, see "Fishing schooner for 'Movies,'" *Evening Tribune* (Providence, RI), September 27, 1915, 14. "Eastern Film Company Buys Schooner Moselle," *Providence Journal*, September 27, 1915, 12. The company also turned out many comedies. One comedy actress—Vivian Ogden—later recalled making eighteen comedy pictures for Eastern in twenty weeks in 1915. "Screen Stars Busy Completing Promising List of New Plays," *Lincoln Sunday Star* (Lincoln, NE), October 11, 1925, 8.

34. "Eastern Burns House for 'Cap'n Eri,'" *Moving Picture World*, September 25, 1915, 2203. "Eastern Film Corporation Making Spectacular Production," *New York Clipper*, September 18, 1915, 15.

35. "Written on the Screen," *New York Times*, November 7, 1915, X11. It is possible that the *Conquest* was in fact the *Moselle* that Eastern had purchased a few months earlier, also captained by Charlie Chaplin. "Eastern Film Company Buys Schooner Moselle," *Providence Journal*, September 27, 1915, 12.

36. "Eastern Film Corporation Making Spectacular Production," *New York Clipper*, September 18, 1915, 15.

37. Kathleen Karr, "Hooray for Providence, Wilkes-Barre, Saranac Lake and Hollywood," in *American Film Heritage: Impressions from the American Film Institute Archives*, ed. Tom Shales and Kevin Brownlow (Washington, DC: Acropolis Books,

1972), 108. The actress Helen Lowell sued Eastern for $20,000 for breach of contract. "Court Brevities," *Evening Tribune* (Providence, RI), November 13, 1915, 3.

38. Bostwick's position was split between W. P. Barrett (business manager) and George Lessey (director of production). "Important Changes in Eastern Film of Providence," *New York Clipper*, October 23, 1915, 40.

39. Ibid.; Dumaux, *King Baggot*, 89.

40. Ríos-Bustamante, "Mary Murillo: Early Anglo Latina Scenarist." Bert Ennis, who had been in charge of publicity and sales, seems to have added the scenario department to his responsibilities. "Important Changes in Eastern Film of Providence," *New York Clipper*, October 23, 1915, 40. "Bert Ennis Is in Town . . . ," *New York Clipper*, December 18, 1915, 5.

41. Anthony Slide and Alan Gevinson, *The Big V: A History of the Vitagraph Company* (Metuchen, NJ: Scarecrow Press, 1987), 136.

42. "L.W.P. Writes," *The Editor: Journal of Information for Literary Workers*, January 1, 1916, 30.

43. "Up and Down the Street and in the Lobbies," *Evening News* (Providence, RI), April 19, 1916, 8.

44. *Acts and Resolves Passed by the General Assembly of the State of Rhode Island and Providence Plantations at the January Session, A.D. 1917* (Providence, RI: E. L. Freeman Company Printers, 1917), 562–63. Information on Peck and Young comes from Dintenfass's petition in the Rhode Island Supreme Court archives, Supreme Court Judicial Records Center, Pawtucket, RI.

45. According to Simon Louvish, Amber Star was the parent company of Vim. Simon Louvish, *Stan and Ollie, The Roots of Comedy: The Double Life of Laurel and Hardy* (New York: St. Martin's Press, 2002), 106. John McCabe, *Babe: The Life of Oliver Hardy* (London: Robson, 2004), 31.

46. Mark Dintenfass to Louis Burstein, October 24, 1916, Supreme Court, Providence County, 1917, Dintenfass v. Amber Star Films Corp., Supreme Court Judicial Records Center, Pawtucket, RI.

47. Ibid.

48. "Dintenfass v. Amber Star Film's Corp. et al. (no. 271)," Supreme Court of Rhode Island, January 17, 1917, *Atlantic Reporter* 99 (December 7, 1916–March 22, 1917) (St. Paul, MN: West Publishing, 1917), 516–18.

49. In court documents, Dintenfass claimed that the others had tricked him by telling him he did not need to attend a key meeting at which he was removed from the presidency. He also claimed that the plaintiffs had caused Vim to enter into contract with the Eastern Film Corporation, in which Peck and Tichenor were interested as stockholders and which was largely beneficial to Eastern and against the interests of Vim. See the Dintenfass's petition in Supreme Court, Providence County, 1917, *Dintenfass v. Amber Star Films Corp.*, Supreme Court Judicial Records Center, Pawtucket, RI.

50. In 1917 Tichenor appointed F. E. Samuels, who had previously been the secretary and manager of the Annual Ball of the New Jersey State Exhibitor's Ball to act as his assistant detail and manager. Samuels was to remain in Florida for the winter, returning in May 1917 to the "summer studio" in Providence, RI. "Exhibitor's Ball Assured Success," *Moving Picture World*, January 27, 1917, 507.

51. “New Incorporations,” *New York Times,* January 14, 1917, E5. According to the *Times,* the company was incorporated with $5,000 by R. Wright, C. Kingsley, and H. Schwab at 74 Broadway.

52. Vim had employed nearly fifty people plus extras in 1916, with a regular weekly payroll of approximately $3,800. Richard Alan Nelson, “Before Laurel: Oliver Hardy and the Vim Comedy Company, a Studio Biography,” in *Current Research in Film: Audiences, Economic, and Law,* vol. 2, ed. Bruce A. Austin (Norwood, NJ: Ablex Publishing Corporation, 1986), 136–55, esp. 142. It is unclear what happened to the New Jersey studios.

53. “Jaxon Film Corporation Enters Field,” *Moving Picture World* 31 (1917): 1934. See also newspaper clipping, “Jaxon Film Corporation,” Folder “Jaxon Film Corp.,” Richard Alan Nelson Collection, 1898–1980, Florida State University Strozier Library Special Collections, Tallahassee, FL.

54. “General Film Announces ‘Sparkles,’” *Moving Picture World,* July 7, 1917, 111. “Jaxon Film Corp,” *Moving Picture World,* July 14, 1917, 283. “Jaxon Comedies,” *Moving Picture World,* July 21, 1917, 532. “Jaxon Comedy” (a report on “Play Ball”), n.d., newspaper clipping Folder “Jaxon Film Corp.,” Richard Alan Nelson Collection, 1898–1980, Florida State University Strozier Library Special Collections. Jaxon also announced that its films would be distributed not through General, but on the open market through the medium of independent exchanges. It was a surprising move, given Tichenor’s association with General and the fact that General was desperate for product in 1916–17. The two companies came to terms a couple of months later, and General became Jaxon’s distributor: “‘Pokes and Jabs’ Comedies on the Open Market,” *Moving Picture World,* April 14, 1917, 298. “Many Inquiries on ‘Pokes and Jabs,’” *Moving Picture World,* April 28, 1917, 646. “‘Pokes and Jabs’ Popular,” *Motography* 17, no. 17 (1917): 896. Newspaper clipping, “A Radical Departure,” April 20, 1917, Folder “Jaxon Film Corp.,” Richard Alan Nelson Collection, 1898–1980, Florida State University Strozier Library Special Collections. “More Comedies for General,” *Motography* 17, no. 26 (1917): 1388. “Group Bookings for ‘Pokes and Jabs,’ *Motography* 17, no. 26 (1917): 1390. “More Comedies for General,” *Moving Picture World,* June 23, 1917, 1955. “General Film Announces ‘Sparkles,’” *Moving Picture World,* July 7, 1917, 111. “Sparkle Comedies,” *Moving Picture World,* July 7, 1917, 130. “Debut of ‘Sparkle Comedies,’” *Motography* 18, no. 1 (1917): 23. On General’s distribution of comedies, see Kalton C. Lahue, *World of Laughter: The Motion Picture Comedy Short, 1910–1930* (Norman: University of Oklahoma Press, 1972), 11–42.

55. *The Film Daily Year Book of Motion Pictures* 41 (New York: Film Daily, 1933), 619. Before 1921 Tichenor had allowed the lease on the Florida studio to lapse so he could concentrate on studio work in Rhode Island. Nevertheless, he kept close connections to the company: General continued to distribute its films (including the twelve-chapter action spy serial, “A Daughter of Uncle Sam” (1918), and its New York offices were Tichenor’s 220 West Forty-Second Street address. Nelson, “Before Laurel,” 144. “Walter A. Morton Becomes Over-Sea K. of C. Secretary,” *Moving Picture World,* October 19, 1918, 360.

56. “Amber Star Film Corporation,” *The Editor* 45, no. 1 (January 13, 1917): 22. *The Julius Cahn-Gus Hill Theatrical Guide and Moving Picture Directory* 20 (1921): Moving Picture Section, 333a.

57. On the problems of the film industry in Jacksonville, see Stuart B. McIver, *Dreamers, Schemers and Scalawags*, vol. 1 (Sarasota, FL: Pineapple Press, 1988), 36. Richard Alan Nelson, *Florida and the American Motion Picture Industry, 1898–1980*, vols. 1 and 2, *Dissertations on Film* (New York: Garland Publishing, 1983).

58. Karr, "Hooray for Providence," 108. "Eastern Film Company's Building on Elmwood Avenue Destroyed by Fire Yesterday," *Providence Journal*, August 24, 1917, 3. "Fire Destroys Big Film Company," *Lowell Sun* (MA), August 23, 1917, 7. "Movie Plant Destroyed," *Fitchburg Daily Sentinel* (MA), August 23, 1917, 5. The *Insurance Press* recorded the loss as $100,000. *Insurance Press*, January 30, 1918, 48g. But for a different estimate, see "$35,000 Insurance Loss on Film Plant," *The Standard*, September 1, 1917, 227: "Following is a list of companies and amounts involved in the loss on plant of the Eastern Film Company, practically destroyed by fire at Providence, RI, August 23, property loss $60,000: on brick studio, $25,000; on engine and boiler, $4,500; on car shop, $1,000; on contents, $4,500; in the following companies: Northern, Eng., $10,000; Springfield F. & M., $7,000; Phila. Und., $7,000; Home Und., $7,000; Niagara, $3,500; Guaranty Und., $500; total, $35,000."

59. Koszarski, *Hollywood on the Hudson*, 102.

60. Ibid.

61. James Irving, *How to Sell Manuscripts* (Auburn, NY: The Authors' Press, 1920), 47.

62. "Charles Beahan Produces Movie to Show Here," *Clearfield Progress*, December 17, 1921, 6. According to IMDB, the cast included Frank Brownlee, M. A. Kelly, Lark Bronlee, William Crowell, Joseph S. Chailee, and Richard Martin. IMDB misdates the movie as 1920.

63. "Tichenor Leaves General," *New York Dramatic Mirror*, March 25, 1919, 25.

64. The first advertisement for this company appeared in 1919. *Motion Picture News*, November 15, 1919, 3567. On its business policy, see "Noticed and Noted," *New York Times*, July 4, 1920. The movies distributed by the Photo Products Export Company included *Beyond the Great Wall* (1920), an Eastern Film Corporation movie, directed by A. B. Heath (Arch Heath). *The Rich Slave* (1920), a Jaxon Film Corporation movie. *The Final Curtain* (1916), originally produced by George Kleine and distributed by Kleine-Edison Features and reissued by Photo Products Export Company in 1920. *The Destroying Angel* (1915), originally produced by Thomas A. Edison, Inc., and distributed by Kleine-Edison Feature Service. (The Photo Products Export Company bought the rights to the film in November 1920 and announced plans to reissue it, but it is not known whether the film was actually rereleased.) *The Devil's Prayer-Book* (1916) (also known as *The Law of Blood*) originally produced by George Kleine and distributed by Kleine-Edison Feature Service and reissued on a state rights basis in 1920 by Photo Products Export Company. *The Spendthrift* (1915), originally produced by George Kleine and distributed by George Kleine and reissued on the state rights market by Photo Products Export Company in November 1920. *When Love Is King* (1916), originally produced by Thomas A. Edison Inc. and distributed by Kleine-Edison Feature Services and rereleased by Photo Products Export Company in 1920. The Photo Products Export Company also released at least two educationals, *The Good Sport* (n.d.) and *The Matinee Girl* (n.d.). See Gladys Bollman and Henry Bollman, *Motion Pictures for Community Needs: A Practical Manual of Information and Suggestion for Educational, Religious and Social Work* (New York: Henry Holt, 1922),

177, 182. Perhaps *The Good Sport*, Thomas A. Edison, Inc. Released by George Kleine, 1918. For further information on Photo Products Export Company, see *Federal Trade Commission Decisions* 5 (1922–23), 225. See also "State Righter Nearly Ready," *New York Clipper*, June 30, 1920, 33.

65. "Completing Rubaiyat. Prospect of Trade Preview Has Aroused Interest," *Los Angeles Times*, April 2, 1922, III 30. "The Silent Drama," *Morning Oregonian* (Portland), April 9, 1922, 1.

66. Allan R. Ellenberger, *Ramon Novarro: A Biography of the Silent Film Idol, 1899–1968: With a Filmography* (Jefferson, NC: McFarland, 1999), 21, 60, 203. André Soares, *Beyond Paradise: The Life of Ramon Novarro* (New York: St Martin's Press, 2002), 23–25, 94–95, 369–70. David S. Shields, *Still: American Silent Motion Picture Photography* (Chicago: University of Chicago Press, 2013), chap. 6.

67. Gerben Bakker, "Selling French Films on Foreign Markets: The International Strategy of a Medium-sized Film Company," *Enterprise and Society* 5 (2004): 72.

68. The Simplex Projection Studios at 22 West Forty-Second Street—possibly the Simplex Projection Rooms that Tichenor had rented out for showing films—are listed under "Film Libraries" for nontheatrical films in *The Film Daily Year Book of Motion Pictures* (New York: Wid's Films and Film Folk, Inc. 1925), 608.

69. "Forty Million Feet of Motion Pictures in Our Film Library," *Printers' Ink*, April 7, 1927, 238.

70. Leo Enticknap, "De Forest Phonofilms: A Reappraisal," *Early Popular Visual Culture* 4 (2006): 273–84. Donald Crafton, *The Talkies: American Cinema's Transition to Sound, 1926–1931* (Berkeley: University of California Press, 1997), 63–93.

71. Tichenor may have had connections with De Forest earlier than 1928. His close colleague, the banker Frederick W. Peck, was a partner/founder of De Forest Phonofilms Inc. (est. 1924) (Crafton, *The Talkies*, 564n7), which went bust in 1926 after releasing a number of films, mainly short recordings of vaudeville acts, musical numbers, political speeches, and operatic arias. Some of these films, including movies of Eddie Cantor and President Coolidge, are available on the Internet and can be found through a Google Video search for "Phonofilm."

72. "Ticherer—Frank A," *Billboard*, May 20, 1950, 53. (Note the misspelling of Tichenor's name.) Arthur Edwin Krows, "Motion Pictures—Not for Theaters," 23, no. 1 (January, 1944): 19.

73. Frank A Tichenor, "Motion Pictures as Trade Getters," *Annals of the American Academy of Political and Social Science* 128 (November 1926): 84–85.

74. On Tichenor's involvement in making political campaign films, see Arthur Edwin Krows, "Motion Pictures—Not for Theaters," *Educational Screen* 18, no. 7 (September 1939): 243. Tichenor had filmed political campaigns before the creation of Eastern. See, for example, the story of how Theodore Roosevelt loaned him a coat while he was filming Roosevelt's presidential campaign in a freezing 1912. "'Outlook' Saved by Man Once Aided by 'TR.' Frank A. Tichenor Buys Magazine in Which 'Teddy' Once Was Interested," *Binghamton Press*, July 2, 1932, 1. It may be that Tichenor covered the 1912 election for the Manhattan Slide and Film Company. The Library of Congress has a lantern slide showing a campaign poster for Woodrow Wilson and Thomas R. Marshall, "For President Woodrow Wilson, for Vice-President Thomas R. Marshall," New York City: Manhattan Slide Company, Inc. [1912], LC Control No.: 2007680381. According to his obituary, Tichenor was also closely

connected to three Republican presidents—Theodore Roosevelt, Warren Harding, and Calvin Coolidge. According to Krows, Tichenor directed Coolidge's campaign film in the 1924 election. Arthur Edwin Krows, "Motion Pictures—Not for Theaters," *Educational Screen* 18, no. 1 (January 1939): 16.

75. "One Hundred Thousand Photoplay Fans and Five Thousand Exhibitors," *Ogden Standard* (UT), July 12, 1913, 2.

76. "Moving Picture Show to Be Given Prison Inmates," *Providence Journal*, August 20, 1915, 11. "Moving Pictures for State Institutions," *Evening Tribune* (Providence, RI), August 20, 1915, 13. "'Movies' at the Prison," *Evening Tribune* (Providence, RI), September 27, 1915, 9. By 1916 the *Delinquent* noted that inmates of the Rhode Island State Prison were writing moving picture stories for Eastern, which had awarded prizes totaling thirty dollars. About one hundred stories were submitted for examination. "Notes," *The Delinquent* 6, no. 1 (January 1916): 16. "Prison Inmates Awarded Prizes for Movie Stories," *Providence Journal* (RI), February 12, 1916, 4. "Plans for Baby Week," *Sunday Tribune* (Providence, RI), February 13, 1916, 13. "Fall River Fire Scenes Shown in Motion Pictures," *Providence Journal* (RI), February 17, 1916, 8.

77. Tichenor's interest in industrials and educationals is indicated by three purchases in 1920 from the National Board of Review: "A Garden of American Motion Pictures 1918–1919"; "The Best Motion Pictures for Church and Semi-seligious entertainments"; and "Motion Picture Films Valuable for Education." See Frank A. Tichenor to National Board of Review, March 3, 1920, National Board of Review of Motion Pictures records, 1907–71, box 4, Jaxon Film Corp., Manuscripts and Archives Division, The New York Public Library.

78. Arthur Edwin Krows, "Motion Pictures—Not for Theaters," *Educational Screen* 18, no. 7 (September 1939): 242–45.

79. On rentals see Karr, "Hooray for Providence," 108. Firms that rented space included the Atlantic Film Corporation, the Coronet Film Company and the Truart Motion Picture Corporation. See "Atlantic Film Co. to Produce," *New York Clipper*, March 14, 1917, 32. "Making Pictures in R.I.," *Variety*, September 5, 1919, 64. Karl Klark, "Providence," *Variety*, October 31, 1919, 52. On the fire, Krows claims the fire destroyed about two-thirds of the equipment, perhaps because, according to a 1915 report, the wardrobes and property departments were in the old brewery building, where the fire was concentrated. "Movies with the Providence Label," *Providence Sunday Journal*, May 30, 1915, 5. The scenario editor was also located in the old brewery. Eastern's main building was a new construction, well apart from the brewery, and back up against Roger Williams Park, which served as background in one of the first pictures.

80. Tichenor, "Motion Pictures as Trade Getters." "Advertising Agencies and Commercial Motion Pictures," *Printers' Ink*, April 14, 1927, 218.

81. Tichenor, "Motion Pictures as Trade Getters," 84.

82. Ibid.

83. "Changing Habits and Commercial Motion Pictures," *Printers' Ink*, May 5, 1927, 190.

84. See the advertisements in *Educational Film Magazine* 6, no. 3 (September 1921): 23; *Educational Film Magazine* 6, no. 4 (October 1921): inside back cover; and *Educational Film Magazine* 6, no. 5 (November 1921): 20. For a related series of advertisements, see the ones that Eastern sent to *Advertising and Selling Fortnightly*

in 1924–25. "Have You a Commercial *Motion Picture Film* for which You Would Like *Distribution?*," *Advertising and Selling Fortnightly*, December 3, 1924, 42; "No Motion Picture Theatre *Accepts a 24 Sheet Poster* as Suitable for Showing *On its Screen!*," *Advertising and Selling Fortnightly*, December 17, 1924, 51; "Motion Pictures *for Special Purposes* Motion Picture *Editing, Titling, Printing, etc.*," *Advertising and Selling Fortnightly*, December 31, 1924, 49; "What Can *Motion Picture Advertising* do for *Your Business?*," *Advertising and Selling Fortnightly*, January 14, 1925, 16; and "Motion Pictures *Make a Powerful Weapon* for the Salesman—*We Make Them!*," *Advertising and Selling Fortnightly*, January 28, 1925, 61. See also "Motion Pictures and the Salesman," *Printers' Ink*, April 21, 1927, 230.

85. "Motion Pictures *for Special Purposes* Motion Picture *Editing, Titling, Printing, etc.*," *Advertising and Selling Fortnightly*." For another advertisement describing how Eastern's cameramen traveled, see "In Four Corners of the Earth—Eastern's Cameramen," *Printers' Ink*, April 28, 1927, 206.

86. W. M Gregory, "Problems Concerning the Educational Motion Picture," *Moving Picture Age* 5, no. 1 (January 1922): 20–21, 25–27. Before the war, the General Film Company had established an educational department selling scraps of feature films for other companies to turn into educational movies, part of a broader "reclamation" initiative that helped set the stage for the problems about film quality in the postwar years. Arthur Edwin Krows, "Motion Pictures—Not for Theaters," *Educational Screen* 18, no. 5 (May 1939): 154–56. For a contemporary discussion of companies offering reedited films, see Don Carlos Ellis and Laura Thornborough, *Motion Pictures in Education: A Practical Handbook for Users of Visual Aids* (London: George E. Harrap, 1923), 25–26.

87. Evart G. Routzahn and Mary Swain Routzahn, *The ABC of Exhibit Planning* (New York: Russell Sage Foundation, 1918), 85–86.

88. Thus, in 1918 the Routzahns worried about the small number of good films generally accessible through commercial agencies or other centers that circulated films for educational or social welfare. Routzahn and Routzahn, *The ABC of Exhibit Planning*, 85–86. On the Routzahns as publicity specialists, see Scott M. Cutlip, *Fund Raising in the United States: Its Role in America's Philanthropy* (New Brunswick, NJ: Transaction Publishers, 1990), 233–35. See also Thomas C. Edwards, "Health Pictures and Their Value," *Annals of the American Academy of Political and Social Science* 128 (November 1926): 135. "Have You a Commercial *Motion Picture Film* for which You Would Like *Distribution?*," *Advertising and Selling Fortnightly*, December 3, 1924, 42.

89. Tichenor, "Motion Pictures as Trade Getters," 85–87.

90. "'Movies' at the Prison," *Evening Tribune* (Providence, RI), September 27, 1915, 9.

91. Arthur Edwin Krows, "Literature and the Motion Picture," *Annals of the American Academy of Political and Social Science* 128 (November 1926): 72. His example was motion picture adaptations of literary works.

92. David Cantor, "Uncertain Enthusiasm: The American Cancer Society, Public Education, and the Problems of the Movie, 1921–1960," *Bulletin of the History of Medicine* 81 (2007): 39–69; David Cantor, "Choosing to Live: Cancer Education, Movies, and the Conversion Narrative in America, 1921–1960," *Literature and Medicine* 28 (2009): 278–332. See also Laukötter, this volume.

93. Arthur Edwin Krows, "Motion Pictures—Not for Theaters," *Educational Screen* 18, no. 7 (September 1939): 243.

94. Quotation in Eastern advertisements in *New York Times,* December 12, 1926, E14. See also advertisement in *New York Times,* December 1, 1926, 47.

95. Arthur Edwin Krows, "Motion Pictures—Not for Theaters," *Educational Screen* 18, no. 7 (September 1939): 243.

96. For references to this company, see Nichtenhauser, "A History of Motion Pictures in Medicine," 1:135–41. Adolf Nichtenhauser Medical Film Materials 1933–55, box 5, folder "Clinical Film Company," New York, NY. For its 1917 catalog, see Clinical Film Libraries (Clinico-Clinico Motion Pictures Catalogue-Surgical Medical Dental, ca. 1917 in General Medical Products Information Collection (GMPI), OHA 168, Otis Historical Archives, National Museum of Health and Medicine, Armed Forces Institute of Pathology, Silver Spring, MD. OCLC includes a reference to an eleven-page pamphlet, Clinical Film Company, *Clinico Films: The Modern Method of Clinical Study,* ca. 1915, OCLC: 122523595. However, I have been unable to find a copy of this last pamphlet. Don Carlos Ellis and Laura Thornborough, *Motion Pictures in Education: A Practical Handbook for Users of Visual Aids* (New York: Crowell, 1923), 112–13.

97. Arthur Edwin Krows, "Motion Pictures—Not for Theaters," *Educational Screen* 20, no. 9 (November 1941): 383.

98. James S. Edlin, "Cinematography: Its Uses in Teaching Medicine and Surgery—A Prophecy in Fulfilment," *International Journal of Surgery* 35 (1922): 191–94. "Society for Cinematographic Instruction in Medicine and Surgery," *Medical Woman's Journal,* 28 (1921): 240. "Cinematographic Instruction," *Boston Medical and Surgical Journal* 186 (May 25, 1922): 714. See also James L. Edlin to Simon Flexner, September 5, 1921, Simon Flexner Papers (BF 365), Society for Cinematographic Instruction in Medicine and Surgery, American Philosophical Society Library, Philadelphia PA.

99. Edlin, "Cinematography: Its Uses in Teaching Medicine and Surgery,"193.

100. Joseph Franklin Montague, "What Motion Pictures Can Do for Medical Education," *Annals of the American Academy of Political and Social Science* 128 (November 1926): 141.

101. Nichtenhauser, "A History of Motion Pictures in Medicine," 2:146–50. Colleen Bradley-Sanders, Archivist, Frederick L. Ehrman Medical Library, New York University Medical Center, New York City), email to David Cantor, February 8, 2010.

102. Arthur Edwin Krows, "Motion Pictures—Not for Theaters," *Educational Screen* 20, no. 9 (November 1941): 384. Montague, "What Motion Pictures Can Do for Medical Education." J. F. Montague, "A One Year's Report on the Successful Employment of Motion Pictures in Medical Education," *New York State Journal of Medicine* 27 (1927): 176–77. Nichtenhauser, "A History of Motion Pictures in Medicine," 2:146–50.

103. Arthur Edwin Krows, "Motion Pictures—Not for Theaters," *Educational Screen* 20, no. 9 (November 1941): 384.

104. Anonymous review of "Taking the Doctor's Pulse," *Educational Screen* 8 (1929): 110. "Medical Movies May Make Vivisection Unnecessary," *Educational Screen* 7 (1928): 19. J. F. Montague, "Inside Information on Your Health," *Amateur Movie Makers* 2 (December 1927): 36ff. J. F. Montague, "The Possibilities of Medical

Movies," *Camera: A Practical Magazine for Photographers* 36 (1928): 185–87. He also illustrated his lectures with clips from his films. Reprts of his Lectures are in "American Proctological Society," *Western Medical Review* 29 (1924): 502 and "British Association of Dermatology and Syphilology," *British Journal of Dermatology and Syphilology* 36 (1924): 377.

105. Christopher Lawrence and George Weisz, eds., *Greater Than the Parts: Holism in Biomedicine, 1920–1950* (New York: Oxford University Press, 1998). David Cantor, ed., *Reinventing Hippocrates* (Aldershot, UK: Ashgate, 2002).

106. J. F. Montague, *The Origin of Rectal Specialists and the Future of Proctology* (New York: J. F. Montague 1920), 36.

107. J. F. Montague, *Taking the Doctor's Pulse and Another Essay* (Philadelphia: J. B. Lippincott, 1928), 37.

108. Montague, "What Motion Pictures Can Do for Medical Education,"141.

109. Nichtenhauser, "A History of Motion Pictures in Medicine," 3: 93–96.

110. For a general account of developments in the United States in the late 1920s and early 1930s, including the Eastman-American College of Surgeons collaboration, see Nichtenhauser, "A History of Motion Pictures in Medicine," 3:91–185.

111. For details of Eastman's involvement in film, see Kirsten Ostherr, *Medical Visions: Producing the Patient through Film, Television, and Imaging Technologies* (New York: Oxford University Press, 2013).

112. Quotation in J. F. Montague, "An Open Letter to the Medical Profession. A Plan for Unfolding the Project of Applying Motion Pictures to Medical Education," Typescript, Yale University Library (date stamped March 25, 1927), New Haven, CT. Call Number: Hist R835 M54 1927+ Oversize Notes, p. [1]. My thanks to Toby Appel for sending me a copy. For reports of this lecture, see "The Application of Moving Pictures to Medical Education," *Medical Herald and Physiotherapist* 46, no. 4 (April 1927): 114. "Motion Pictures in Medical Education," *New York Medical Week* 6, no. 16 (April 16, 1927): 16. "Medical Film Foundation Is Suggested," *Photo-era Magazine* 59, no. 10 (July 1927): 51.

113. Montague, "An Open Letter to the Medical Profession," 3. J. F. Montague, "A Plan for Unfolding the Project of Applying Motion Pictures to Medical Education," *Journal of the Iowa Medical Society* 17 (1927): 204. J. F. Montague, "A Plan for Unfolding the Project of Applying Motion Pictures to Medical Education," *Eye, Ear, Nose and Throat Monthly* 6 (1927): 328.

114. "Additions to List of Technical Films," *Journal of the American Dental Association* 12 (1925): 101.

115. Martin S. Pernick, "Thomas Edison's Tuberculosis Films: Mass Media and Health Propaganda," *The Hastings Center Report* 8, no. 3 (June 1978): 21–27; Martin S. Pernick, *The Black Stork: Eugenics and the Death of "Defective" Babies in American Medicine and Motion Pictures since 1915* (New York: Oxford University Press, 1996). See also Susan E. Lederer and Naomi Rogers, "Media," in *Medicine in the Twentieth Century*, ed. Roger Cooter and John Pickstone (Amsterdam: Harwood Academic Publishers, 2000), 487–502; Lisa Cartwright, *Screening the Body: Tracing Medicine's Visual Culture* (Minneapolis: University of Minnesota Press, 1995); Nichtenhauser, "A History of Motion Pictures in Medicine." Leslie Willis Sprague (director, Industrial Service Section, Community Motion Picture Bureau, New York City), "Motion Pictures in Public Health," *Nation's Health* 1, no. 4 (August 1919): 330–32. Leslie Willis Sprague,

"Uses of Motion Pictures in Industrial Medicine," *Nation's Health* 1, no. 5 (September 1919): 396–98. Leslie Willis Sprague, "Uses of Motion Pictures in Industrial Diseases," *Nation's Health* 1, no. 6 (October, 1919): 496–98.

116. Thomas C. Edwards, "Health Pictures and Their Value," *Annals of the American Academy of Political and Social Science* 128 (November 1926): 135. It should be noted that Edwards's notion of a health film probably included some movies that Tichenor would have classed as medical. Edwards, "Health Films and Their Value," 134.

117. Ibid., 135.

118. Ibid., 137. Metropolitan Life Insurance Company, Welfare Division, Motion Picture Bureau, *National Health Council: Film List, Advance Copy Subject to Suggestions and Revisions* (New York: Metropolitan Life Insurance Company, 1926.). Metropolitan Life Insurance Company, Welfare Division, *National Health Council Film List Including Information on Visual Aids and their Producers and Distributors*, 5th ed., prepared and printed by Welfare Division, Metropolitan Life Insurance Company (New York: Metropolitan Life Insurance Company Press, 1928). For a report on this publication, see "Films on Health," *Educational Screen* 4, no. 9 (November 1925): 540. In 1926 the American College of Surgeons had also begun to list health films of which it approved alongside the medical films already mentioned.

119. Cantor, "Uncertain Enthusiasm"; Cantor, "Choosing to Live"; David Cantor, *The Reward of Courage (1921): A Rediscovered Cancer Film of the Silent Era* (Bethesda, MD: National Library of Medicine, 2013).

120. "The Danger That Never Sleeps," *Educational Film Magazine* 6, no. 4 (October 1921): 14. "Safety Motion Picture," *Safety Engineering* 52, no. 2 (August 1926): 61. "Eastern Safety Conference to Meet in Newark," *National Safety News* 13, no. 4 (April 1926): 49. "How Jimmy Won the Game," *Engineering and Mining Journal* 124 (1927): 868. "Safety Film of Institute of Makers of Explosives," *Chemical Digest* 5, no. 12 (1928): 1681.

121. *Report of the Sesqui-Centennial Commission of the Commonwealth of Pennsylvania*, January 14, 1927, 55. Note that the chair of the Commission, Clyde L. King is a collaborator with Tichenor in Clyde L. King and Frank A. Tichenor, eds., *The Motion Picture in Its Economic and Social Aspects, Annals of the American Academy of Political and Social Science* 128 (November 1926). For descriptions of these movies, see "Proving Popular," *Listening Post* 5, no. 1 (January–February, 1927), 18. For a showing of Sunshine Lady, see "The Northumberland County Public Health Association," *Listening Post* 5, no. 1 (January–February, 1927), 22. They were added to the State Health Department Library. "The Moving Picture Service," *Pennsylvania's Health* 5, no. 5 (September–October, 1927), 17.

122. W. E. Mallalieu to Frank A. Tichenor, January 7, 1922, National Board of Review of Motion Pictures Records, 1907–71, box 4, Jaxon Film Corp., Manuscripts and Archives Division, The New York Public Library.

123. Clinton Rogers Woodruff, "Wanted: Civic Dramatists: The Place of Movies in Education for Democracy," *National Civic Review* 11 (1922): 381. Metropolitan Life Insurance Company, Welfare Division, *National Health Council: Film List Including Information on Visual Aids and Their Producers and Distributors*, 5th ed. (New York: Prepared and Printed by Welfare Division, Metropolitan Life Insurance Company, 1928), 62.

124. Note that a 16mm film with this title was produced by the Carter Cinema Producing Corporation of New York in Victor Animatograph Corporation, *Victor Directory of Film Sources*, 2nd ed. (Davenport, IA: Victor Animatograph Corporation, December 1930), 26. And a 35mm film also called *What Price Recklessness?*, from the Motion Picture Institute of New York, is listed in James A. Fitzgerald, Carl A. Hoffman, John R. Bayston, *Drive and Live* (Chicago: Johnson Publishing Company, 1937), 257. Metropolitan Life Insurance Company, Welfare Division, *National Health Council: Film List Including Information on Visual Aids and Their Producers and Distributors*, 5th ed. (New York: Prepared and Printed by Welfare Division, Metropolitan Life Insurance Company, 1928), 60.

125. Cantor, *The Reward of Courage* (1921).

126. "The Danger That Never Sleeps," *Educational Film Magazine*.

127. "'A Fortunate Accident': The New Cancer Film," *Campaign Notes of the American Society for the Control of Cancer* 7, no. 2 (1925): [4].

128. Metropolitan Life Insurance Company, Welfare Division, *National Health Council: Film List Including Information on Visual Aids and Their Producers and Distributors*, 5th ed. (New York: Prepared and Printed by Welfare Division, Metropolitan Life Insurance Company, 1928), 85.

129. A 1928 version of the movie is available at through the Internet Archive at https://archive.org/details/HowJimmyWonTheGame (accessed May 30, 2013).

130. John Joseph Phelan, *Motion Pictures as a Phase of Commercial Amusement in Toledo, Ohio* (Toledo, OH: Little Book Press, 1919), 90. Metropolitan Life Insurance Company, Welfare Division, *National Health Council: Film List Including Information on Visual Aids and Their Producers and Distributors*, 5th ed. (New York: Prepared and Printed by Welfare Division, Metropolitan Life Insurance Company, 1928), 62. For showings of this movie, see "National Fire Prevention Association," *Municipal Journal and Public Works* 46, no. 18 (May 3, 1919): 331. "Fire Prevention Meeting," *Safety Engineering* 37 (1919): 267. Montana State Fire Marshall, *Annual Report* 7 (1920): 32. Eastern seems to have kept connections with organizations concerned with fire prevention. In 1927 it was listed as an associate member of the National Fire Protection Association. See the Association's *Yearbook* (1927): 58.

131. Metropolitan Life Insurance Company, Welfare Division, *National Health Council: Film List Including Information on Visual Aids and Their Producers and Distributors*, 5th ed. (New York: Prepared and Printed by Welfare Division, Metropolitan Life Insurance Company, 1928), 60.

132. Metropolitan Life Insurance Company, Welfare Division, *National Health Council: Film List Including Information on Visual Aids and Their Producers and Distributors*, 5th ed., 65. G. G. Weaver and E. S. Ejricsson, comps., *Bibliography of Technical and Industrial Motion Picture Films and Slides* (New York: New York State Department of Industrial Teacher-training, 1934), 128. For screenings of this movie, see "Safety Film to be Screened," *Rochester Democrat and Chronicle and Rochester Herald* (New York), November 22, 1926, 25. "To Use Movies in Teaching of Safety Methods," *Rochester Democrat and Chronicle and Rochester Herald*, January 14, 1927, 34. "Safety Motion Picture," *Safety Engineering*, "Eastern Safety Conference to Meet in Newark," *National Safety News*.

133. The earliest mention of this office is April 1926. See J. K. Holbrook (Eastern Film Corporation) to Mr. H. H. Shenk, April 23, 1926, Record Group

25, Records of Special Commissions: Series 95, Sesquicentennial Commission for the Commonwealth of Pennsylvania, Pennsylvania State Archives, Harrisburg, PA. According to this and a later letter in 1927, the address of its offices in Philadelphia was 1013 Commercial Trust Building, SE corner, Fifteenth and Market Streets.

134. *Report of the Sesqui-Centennial Commission of the Commonwealth of Pennsylvania*, January 14, 1927, 55.

135. H. H. Shenk (Sec. Executive Committee and State Librarian of Pennsylvania) to Mr. Jordan (Curator, Independence Hall, Philadelphia), May 6, 1926, Pennsylvania State Archives, Record Group 25, Records of Special Commissions: Series 95, Sesquicentennial Commission for the Commonwealth of Pennsylvania. "Visual Education," *Pennsylvania School Journal* 75, no. 8 (February 1927): 431.

136. King and Tichenor, *The Motion Picture in its Economic and Social Aspects*.

137. Arthur Edwin Krows, "Motion Pictures—Not for Theaters," *Educational Screen* 23, no. 4 (April 1944): 162.

138. On criticism of sound film from teachers, see John E. Devine, *Films as an Aid in Training Public Employees, A Report to the Committee on Public Administration of the Social Science Research Council* (n.p., 1937), 46.

139. Arthur Edwin Krows, "Motion Pictures—Not for Theaters," *Educational Screen* 18, no. 7 (September 1939): 243.

140. "Out Steps Tichenor," *Time*, July 11, 1932, 25. On Tichenor's acquisition of Fore An' Aft see *Printers' Ink* 153, no. 1 (1930): 85.

141. "U. OF M. Notes," *Daily Kennebec Journal* (ME), February 4, 1925, 12.

142. "Exhibitor Unit Guns Roar Warning to Union Pickets," *Box Office*, May 9, 1936. "Mayor's Threat to Close Theatre Spurs Mediation," *Box Office*, November 14, 1936, 11. For Tichenor's connections with La Guardia, see also Lowell M. Limpus and Burr W. Leyson, *This Man La Guardia* (New York: E. P. Dutton, 1938), 377. Tichenor seems to have been involved in film arbitration into the 1940s as his membership of the American Arbitration Association suggests. See *International Motion Picture Almanac, 1942–1943* (New York: Quigley Publishing, 1942), 854.

143. Eastern and Tichenor are listed in *The Film Daily Year Book of Motion Pictures* (New York: J. W. Alicoate, 1929), 561. Its last appearance in *The Film Daily Year Book of Motion Pictures* is the 1930 edition (New York: J. W. Alicoate, 1930), 635, where the Eastern Film Studio in Providence is listed with Frank A. Tichenor (chief studio executive), J. H. Gerhardt (general studio manager), Arthur Edwin Krows (general production manager), and Frank R. Follette (head, Camera Department).

Chapter Two

In the Service of Industry and Human Health

The Bayer Corporation, Industrial Film, and Promotional Propaganda, 1934–42

Christian Bonah

Public relations (PR) was central to a transformation in the relationship between business and the public during the early twentieth century. Where once businesses had focused their appeal to the public on the products they manufactured and sold, from 1918 onward, guided by the new field of public relations, they also began to sell what they stood for: their image as a corporation.[1] Image-building campaigns were intended to enhance the social and moral legitimacy of giant companies, faced with attacks on monopolistic and commercial practices and allegations of social irresponsibility.[2] They deployed a panoply of tools to analyze and manage public opinion, promote corporate cohesion, and establish a corporate soul that would serve to counter the attacks upon them and promote their business interests as a whole.[3]

Motion pictures were a key tool used by corporations in such image-building campaigns. "Scenes of art and industry" had appeared as early as 1907 in Pathé film catalogues. However, industrial pictures really emerged after World War I, adapting wartime propaganda techniques to commercial interests. By the 1920s and 1930s, they were firmly established as one of "new techniques" of public relations and one of the most prolific formats in film history. Indeed, film was more than just a technique. It also allowed public relations experts to create a new rhetoric of persuasion in public relations that aligned new visual aesthetics with industrial modernization and modern lifestyle.[4] Corporations were not alone in doing this, and indeed they and their public relation experts used film to create image-building campaigns that portrayed businesses as somehow much more than commercial organizations; they were presented as socially responsible organizations that were engaged in promoting education, health, cultural enrichment, and even religion. In the dark days of the Great Depression, such image-building campaigns served to counter threats to commercial independence, prosperity, and even survival by creating an image of the corporation as committed to a service ideal.

In the case of the pharmaceutical industry—the focus of this chapter—image-building campaigns were developed to meet the challenges faced by that sector in particular. The turn-of-the-century birth of modern pharmaceutical companies that manufactured ready-made, prepackaged standardized drugs had ushered in profound changes in the therapeutic market previously dominated by small corporations that provided pharmacists with the raw materials with which to make up a prescription.[5] Increasingly, pharmacists no longer made up a prescription but dispensed preprepared drugs such as the German synthetic pharmaceuticals Phenacetin (1888), Aspirine (1899), Veronal (1904), and Plasmochin (1927), all Bayer products. This development, combined with the growing acceptability of pharmaceutical patenting and the spreading use of trademarks, ushered in a period of fierce pharmaceutical market competition.[6] It was here where the "unseen engineers" of PR and the rising "friendly pharmaceutical giants"[7] met to mould public attitudes and thinking and to fight what certain observers have characterized as "pharmaceutical wars."[8]

One of these rising pharmaceutical companies, often described as the world's pharmacy in the interwar period,[9] was the Germany-based Bayer Corporation. Created in 1863 as a chemical dyestuff manufacturer, it became a joint stock company in 1881 and entered the therapeutic market with its first pharmaceutical product, the fever-lowering Phenacetin, in 1888. Between 1881 and 1913 Bayer, in cooperation with university-based research, multiplied its synthetic drug production and developed into a pharmaceutical company with an international sales organization, sometimes criticized for its "unfair monopolization of commonly made chemical substances" through patenting and trademarking before the First World War.[10] As of 1913, the company had earned 80 percent of revenues from exports, and central to its success was its sophisticated engagement with scientific marketing.[11] Industrial-medical films became part of the Bayer public relations efforts in the 1920s, and the following contribution explores how Bayer engaged with film advertisement in the interwar period.

In particular, the essay uses Bayer to provide an insight into the relationship between propaganda and advertising in this period. Since World War II, the term *propaganda* has become associated with the misuse of techniques of mass persuasion. But this was less the case between the world wars. Thus, in his 1928 essay *Propaganda*, Sigmund Freud's nephew Edward Bernays (1891–1995) helped pioneer the technique of shaping and manipulating public opinion.[12]

He saw conscious and intelligent manipulation as an important element in democratic society. In a chapter on business and the public, he suggests that "the development of public opinion for a cause or line of socially constructive action may very often be the result of a desire on the party of the propagandist to meet successfully his own problem [in Bayer's case, of selling drugs] which the socially constructive cause would further."[13] Bayer provides a little-studied but exemplary illustration of Bernays's assertion that shows how social issues of human health were addressed, framed, and staged by Bayer PR counselors. My focus is a corpus of films produced by Bayer, analyzed here not merely as material objects (films) but in their "complex constellation of media, techniques, forms of knowledge, discourse and social organization."[14]

Pharmaceutical advertising was tricky, since drug consumption usually passed through the hands and pens of an intermediary, the physician. Since the beginning of the century, professional associations of physicians and pharmacists had tried to limit direct-to-consumer advertising, often portrayed as irrational or compromising, the province of the "quack." A consequence was that so-called ethical drug companies had directed pharmaceutical advertising only to physicians through professional channels, except for goods of ambiguous status as drugs (toothpaste, vitamins, talcum powder, or cod liver oil, etc., production of which was expanded), or to promote in general the expansion of laboratory-based pharmaceutical research and development, and production. It was with these tasks in mind that pharmaceutical corporations increasingly created internal public relations departments or hired outside PR experts.

One of the problems facing these PR firms was how to balance corporate commercialism and the public service ideal, "to serve mankind," as a slogan coined by E. R. Squibb & Company in 1921 put it.[15] Squibb might have invented the slogan in the pharmaceutical sector, but it was by no means alone among corporations in promoting this image of itself. Among those that jumped on the bandwagon was Bayer, which had been involved in the American and worldwide markets since the 1890s. The story goes that the company's propaganda department used film, among other visual media, to foster an image of honesty, integrity, high quality control, and a dedication across the world to the ideal of serving the public: as one film announced, "in the service of humanity." Initially, films produced by Bayer were addressed to medical and professional audiences. In the 1930s Bayer extended the scope of its motion pictures to target the general public, commissioning a series of image-building films to enhance the corporation's reputation. The set of five image-building (*Wert-Werbungsfilme*) films produced between 1934 and 1942 forms the corpus and the core of my analysis.

Bayer's in-house advertising journal *Zepro-Nachrichten* (Zepro-news) captures something of the company's vision of corporate propaganda. In May 1934, shortly, after the journal was established, an editorial noted that

> inconsistency of demand in the pharmaceutical sector creates the necessity for inexhaustible and intensive propaganda for the pharmaceutical industry. . . . At the same time pharmaceutical propaganda is the point where advertisement

> departs from purely economic premises to become a factor of culture in a very common sense. The propagandist of Bayer products can be aware that he is acting in the service of human health. He is fulfilling the task of informing/ educating about possibilities of prophylaxis and participates in improving health of populations. His work has thus a character of social-hygiene and of social ethics.[16]

Underlying the quotation was a new concept of promotional strategy: *Wert-Werbung*, literally "value advertisement."[17] The concept initiated by Bayer in the late 1920s proposed promotional strategies that were quite distinct from classic product advertisement.[18] The basic idea was to produce marketing strategies that promoted corporate name, brand, and image building. It was intended to market not so much individual products as the general quality and trustworthiness of the company. Enhancing consumer trust[19] in a company and its name was essential at a time when patenting drugs was no longer enough to assure financial returns on R&D investments, when trademarks became widely accepted on an ever more competitive interwar drug market[20] and when Bayer had lost many of its drug patents after World War I.[21]

A significant aspect of the promotional strategy pursued by Bayer was the use of film. The pharmaceutical company started film production around 1924, and from 1926 shared a specially equipped in-house film unit with Hoechst (IG-Farben) that recruited Oskar Wagner as its film director from the German film company Universum Film AG (UFA), the major film studio in Germany, often regarded as the home of the German film industry from the Weimar Republic and through to World War II. In 1934 Bayer established its own independent *Filmstelle*, a unit for film planning and production, which produced around seventy films between 1934 and 1944 (see appendix 2.1). In addition, in the 1930s Bayer developed and operated *Tonfilmwagen*, sound-film trucks that toured remote areas across the world for public film shows (fig. 2.1).

Until recently, sponsored films were largely neglected by film and medical historians alike. Yet vast numbers of such films were produced, almost from the beginnings of the motion picture industry. Film archivists estimate that the industrial and advertising "genre" alone accounts for more than four hundred thousand films produced between 1910 and the 1960s and, as such, is the largest genre of films known.[22] They can be defined as films made by a particular sponsor for a specific purpose other than as a work of art or entertainment. Films were generally designed to serve a specific pragmatic purpose often for a limited period of time.[23] It is well-known that in general most sponsored films have not survived. But the Bayer films are an exception. Bayer has corporate archives that are freely available to the historian and the public, and most significantly it has a qualified and ambitious archivist who has collected, safeguarded, stored correctly, and digitized the overwhelming part of the company's audio-visual heritage and memory amounting to over 1,500 films today.[24]

Recent scholarship in the field of industrial, sponsored, nonfiction, and most recently "utility" film has suggested that rather than focus on individual

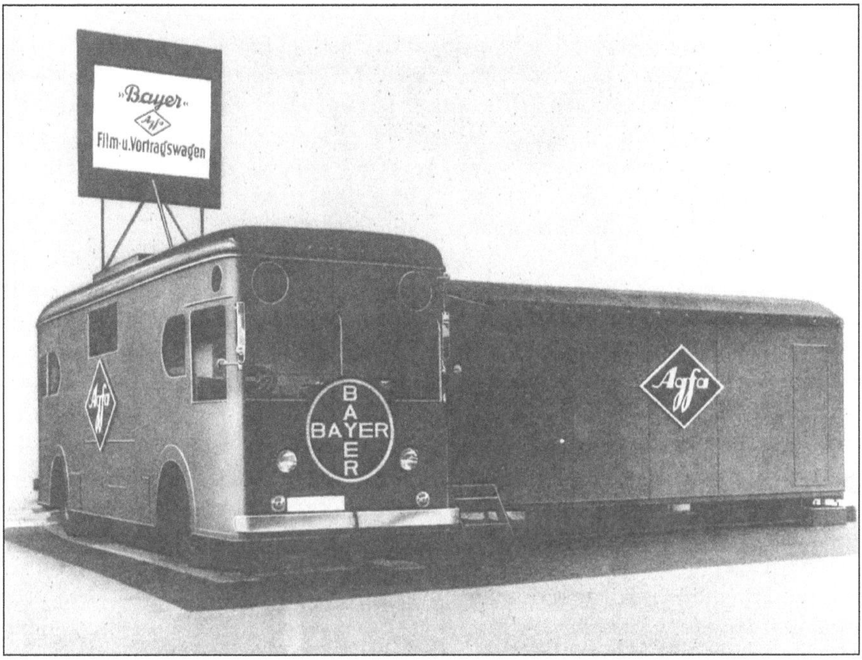

Figure 2.1. The Bayer film truck (*Tonfilmwagen*) in the journal *Zepro-Nachrichten*. "The Giant of the Backroad [*Der Riese der Landstrasse*]," *Zepro-Nachrichten* 2 (1936): 7–8. Bayer AG, Corporate History and Archives.

films, sponsored films should be explored as a series of comparable films, generally a series of films produced or disseminated by a particular sponsor.[25] A so-defined corpus allows us to gain film contextual knowledge by referral between films composing the series. Furthermore, while traditional film studies have tended to focus on the work of a particular director, scholars of sponsored films increasingly supplement such an approach with a focus on the corporate context of production and screening.[26] Such an approach aims to explore the place of film within a wider landscape of corporate communication that often involves different media forms and techniques, the so-called multimedial alliance (Medienverbund), defined as a "network of competing, but also mutually interdependent and complementary media or media practices."[27] Historically, this reflects the fact that many of these films were made and used in concert with campaigns that orchestrated a range of media productions ranging from posters, pamphlets, and magazine articles to lectures, radio, and the films. If films are analyzed in their filmic context in a first part of this contribution, their embedding in campaigns is addressed in a second part.

Studies of the sponsored film have also raised questions about the use of retrospective classifications such as industrial, educational, or documentary film. This chapter echoes such concerns by focusing on Bayer film production as presented in the company's archives. From production to distribution and screening, films are analyzed here as an archaeology of how they were conceived, produced, and used in practice. The group of films retained may be defined as a corpus for analytical purposes (in contrast to genre and subgenre distinctions), since they correspond to a specific corporate practice within a given period of time and place. The role of the corpus approach consists, therefore, in a choice that taking the serial analysis approach seriously at the same time reflects upon significant units for series to be analyzed as corpus.[28]

Drawing widely on the Bayer pharmaceutical film production until 1945, this chapter will first describe how Bayer established its internal film production unit and then will outline film production for the pharmaceutical company until 1945. Bayer's total output might be regarded as a corpus in itself, but it is beyond the scope of this essay to do more than sketch out the story of Bayer's involvement in film. Instead, it will focus on a subset of the Bayer corpus, what the company referred to as image-building (*Wert-Werbungsfilme*) films.[29] Specifically, it focuses on five image-building films, analyzing how Bayer mobilized serious or avant-garde film techniques and prominent film directors including Walter Ruttmann and Ulrich Kayser, whose work for the pharmaceutical industry has generally received little attention.[30] Such an account will show how these directors, and the film and production techniques they employed, served Bayer's promotional strategies. Finally, I will analyze the screening of one of these films to gauge how such occasions were used to create media events that served as a promotional strategy.

One further point requires clarification. By using the term *propaganda*, the quoted editorial, aligned political propaganda, advertising, and health education as ways of communicating good health.[31] But in Germany in 1934 such comments struck a sensitive chord, raising the question of the impact of National Socialism (NS) on the corpus of pharmaceutical propaganda films produced in Germany. Indeed, a legacy of such concern is that until the 1960s, historians of documentary film under NS (influenced by critical theories of totalitarianism and fascism and their National Socialist propaganda analysis) tended to catalogue all films produced during the NS regime as "Nazi-films," understood as an essential instrument of mass manipulation. In essence, film critique served as a critique of fascism.[32] The problem with such views is that they tend to reproduce and accept the rhetoric of NS propagandists about their power.[33] In the 1980s, social historians introduced new concepts such as Germany's "ambiguous modernity" and "reactionary modernism" that paved the road for consideration of the complex association of traditional, regressive, and nationalist values with the extensive techno-scientific modernization of German society under NS. Informed by such approaches, studies of "documentary film under NS"[34] show how filmmakers employed modern media techniques and call for a more differentiated analysis.[35] Regarding propaganda as a concept, the following study thus engages in a double disentanglement. First, rather than regard Bayer's films as NS films, this chapter problematizes the relationship between the corpus of Bayer industrial films produced under NS and NS political propaganda. It does this by focusing on the sponsors' and film directors' political commitments, opportunism, retreat into "inner emigration," or resistance as will be suggested in the cases of Ruttmann and Kayser. Second, rather than considering information, education, and propaganda as distinct and opposing outcomes, it returns to an archaeology of practices and films that were considered as propaganda. These practices have a problematic relationship to propaganda, sometimes part of it, sometimes not, and need to be situated in particular contexts.

Origins of the Bayer Film Unit and Film Production

Starting in the interwar years, a growing number of Western industrial corporations began to produce commercial films that mixed education and science with advertising and promotional propaganda.[36] In the case of Bayer, the story begins in 1924 when the company asked Krupp (the steel company based in Essen)[37] to produce two films: one, an industrial film on the Bayer production sites in Leverkusen and Elberfeld, internally known as the "Caspari-Film";[38] the second, Bayer's first scientific advertisement/teaching film on the biology of moth (see appendix 2.1). Other early Bayer films included animated cartoons for aspirin promotion in Latin America produced by Bayer subsidiaries in New York.

Bayer's early efforts in film production were transformed in the mid-1920s, when it began collaboration with the pharmaceutical company Hoechst. The roots of this collaboration go back to a visit in 1925 by Alexander von Rothe, director of the medical film institute of the Berlin Charité and member of the UFA *Kulturfilmabteilung*, to various pharmaceutical corporations, including Bayer and Hoechst, in order to create a society for medical teaching films.[39] Following the visit, the director of the pharmaceutical department of Hoechst, Dr. L. Lautenschläger, agreed to develop the pharmaceutical part of the Charité film collection and started to produce scientific advertisement/teaching films on the physiological action of drugs, which included techniques of micro-cinematography and animation to depict microbes, parasites, and insects such as amebia, taenia, anopheles, or ascaris.[40] The following year, 1926, Hoechst created its own *Filmstelle* under the direction of Hoechst pharmaceutical department collaborator Wilhelm Rahn.[41] The same year, Rothe's first assistant, the veterinarian, parasitologist, and film director Oskar Wagner left UFA to organize film production for the chemical and pharmaceutical company in its newly created Hoechst Film Unit.

Except for two films produced in 1927,[42] Bayer was not until 1931 involved in choosing which scientific films were to be produced, leaving the lead to the Hoechst film department. But the collaboration with Hoechst became increasing difficult after the restructuring of Bayer's organization in 1929. Until then scientific advertisement films were the responsibility of Hoechst's and Bayer's scientific pharmaceutical departments, since they were conceived as instruction for physicians. However, when the different sales departments of Bayer were reorganized and merged in 1929, film advertisement became their responsibility, and disagreements between Hoechst and Bayer arose over the production of popular advertisement films that departed from the editorial line of professional training films and seemed to break with Hoechst's understanding of the ethical limits to direct-to-consumer drug promotion.

A catalyst for the breakup was the commission by Bayer director Rudolf Mann of five popular advertisement films for aspirin products. They were to be produced by the leading German advertisement filmmaker Julius Pinschewer in Berlin,[43] along the lines of films produced by New York subsidiaries of Bayer and that had attracted the attention of directors at Bayer's Leverkusen operation. The result was that Hoechst distanced itself from these direct-to-consumer promotional films, and Hoechst executives instructed their film unit to keep Hoechst products clear from such "unethical" undertakings. A second breaking point in the joint Hoechst-Bayer film venture occurred when festivities for the seventieth anniversaries of Bayer's general director of the administrative board, Carl Duisberg, and its director of the sales organization, Rudolf Mann, led to the production of two corporate anniversary films: a cartoon version of the curriculum vitae of Duisberg and the Julius Pinschewer synthesis of the Bayer sales organization worldwide, a tribute to Mann (see appendix 2.1). These were corporate cohesion films, and once again they went beyond scientific advertisement for physicians' instruction.

After these two events, Hoechst and Bayer film production began to drift apart. Hoechst may have taken a lead in the "propagandistic application"[44] of teaching/scientific advertisement films and their production, but Bayer Leverkusen became increasingly interested in producing its own films intending to produce them differently. From 1931 onward, the creation of an advertisement unit directed specifically at physicians within the scientific department paved the road for the production of a film on sleeping sickness,[45] a remarkable promotional black and white sound cartoon for aspirin by Pinschewer loosely reminiscent of the Dumas novel *The Three Musketeers*[46] and eventually to the creation of an independent film department, the *Filmzentrale* Bayer Leverkusen, which appeared for the first time in the organizational chart of the corporation in January 1934. Responsible for popular and scientific film production under the direction of Bayer employee Dr. Spielmann, the department occupied the fifth floor of the Bayer building on the prestigious Kurfürstendamm in Berlin in order to be close to Germany's major film production facilities and to attract qualified personnel such as the professional film technician (cutting and mounting) Eva Mord. Bayer's involvement in films went far beyond the initial Hoechst university-industry collaboration to produce corporate sponsored teaching/scientific advertisement films (see appendix 2.1).[47] Bayer harnessed film production to its far-reaching global concept of image-building (*Wert-Werbung*) transgressing and amalgamating the genres of artistic and spectacular film with advertisement film addressed to general audiences. Finally, Bayer film production included so-called supporting program films characterized in the 1935–36 Bayer film catalogue as "special films" (*Sonderfilm*) conceived as pure entertainment.

The year 1938 brought a significant change to the so far rather unhampered development of Bayer film production. Declining economic conditions in National Socialist (NS) Germany led to restrictions that stalled film production and led to layoffs.[48] The same year, the Berlin film unit stopped foreign language sound synchronization (for films to be shown to non-German audiences) and was reduced to a pure distribution office. With the outbreak of war in the summer of 1939, the Bayer directorate opened a film production facility in Denmark under an independent company VEPRO A.S. (Verdens Propaganda Aktie-Selskab). In collaboration with a group of Copenhagen cartoon animators, VEPRO produced several animated films between 1939 and 1944 for Bayer.[49] Film production also continued at Bayer throughout World War II.[50] It included shots of the Bayer plant in Elberfeld by the cameraman Hans Gottschalk[51] and a new malaria film, initiated in Leverkusen in 1940, eventually named *Feind Malaria* (1942)—and discussed later in this essay. The arrival of American troops in Leverkusen (where film production had been relocated with the outbreak of war) on April 14, 1945, brought the Bayer film production under National Socialism to an end and opened a new era of reconstruction under the guidance of an allied control commission. A list of films produced between 1924 and 1944 by the film units of Hoechst and Bayer, during and after their collaboration, figures in appendix 2.1.

The story of Bayer film production is thus one of collaboration with Hoechst followed by separation. Its involvement in film screening was different. It began to reorganize film screening at about the time it was involved in joint film production with Hoechst. Pictures were initially produced on 35mm film stock (Normalfilm, NF) and screened on mobile Kino-Box projectors. In 1925 Leverkusen equipped its administrative building auditorium with a film cabinet, entrusting screenings to a foreman of the electrical workshop. From the late 1920s, the company organized screenings of a selection of pharmaceutical films for clinicians in major cities coupled with explanatory lectures that were reported in the professional and general press. The growing use of film and Bayer's turn to an autonomous film unit eventfully justified the hiring of a projectionist in the early 1930s and the equipping of a major meeting room in the Leverkusen pharmaceutical plant as a film theater in 1935.[52] In January 1930, the Bayer Leverkusen directorate decided that only 16mm films and projectors such as the AGFA Movector 16A should be used from then on for popular and mobile film projections and that they should be screened with a sound attachment, meaning a synchronous record player.[53] Popular film projection developed significantly, especially with the acquisition of sound trucks, of which thirty were in use in 1939 in Latin America. A German version of a "Tonfilmwagen—a film theatre on wheels," including an adaptable one-hundred-seat big top tent—was developed in 1935 (fig. 2.1). Film production and use increased to the point that guidelines for film use were issued, and film inventories led to a first Bayer film catalogue compiled and published in 1935–36.[54]

Pharmaceutical Propaganda in the Interwar Period

Underlying Bayer film production was its creation of a central department for propaganda conceived as an organizational response to the "necessity for inexhaustible and intensive propaganda for the pharmaceutical industry" due to the inconsistency of demand in the pharmaceutical sector. As noted in the introduction to this chapter, the term *propaganda* did not imply anything pejorative. Bayer was using the term in a way that was consistent with how many European and North American industries used it, namely as referring to activities that sought to enhance sales by the use of "modern" techniques of persuasion.[55] Bayer propagandists defined their activities at the time as "the alert, conscious and intended effect on the unconscious, it is the systematic persuasion of the masses with a specific goal."[56]

Confidential corporate memos from the mid-1930s indicate how the Bayer film unit imagined its role within the corporation's propaganda department. At the same time, they allow us to gauge why Bayer was so attracted to film as a medium of promotion and why the company turned to image-building—*Wert-Werbungs*—film. One explanation by Bayer representatives for their turn to film were claims of film's novelty and modern character that legitimized film production and projection. Another was pragmatic—the huge size of the film audience. A Bayer film catalogue editorial from 1935–36 illustrates the point.[57] Based on 1933–34 film statistics, the director of the film unit argued in this editorial that almost 247 million spectators were attracted to movie theaters in Germany that year. This meant an average of 6.8 visits per year for every German. In a global perspective, he concluded, figures indicated that 185 million spectators entered a movie theater every week throughout the world in 1934.

But the turn to film was more than just about existing film audiences; films opened access to hitherto inaccessible populations or geographic localities. Issue 4 of *Zepro-Nachrichten* acknowledged that audio-visuals—in 1934, soon after the adoption of film—had been able to reach audiences that other forms of communication generally failed to reach. Sound film, the editorial argued, "added living images to auditory impressions that can be understood by everyone, even illiterates."[58] Where the print media was limited to those who could or wanted to read, films—in the view of the *Zepro-Nachrichten* writers—attained "new continents" of rural populations, be they in peripheral regions of Germany, foreign audiences elsewhere, or the illiterate. As a consequence, Bayer invested heavily in mobile film projection units and automobiles. They traveled throughout many countries carrying the Bayer gospel of "it's good, it's Bayer" and "trust the Bayer-Cross" to remote places.[59]

It was here that Bayer's use of propaganda in relation to film departs from later pejorative uses of the term.[60] Film was one of several tools that aimed to create receptive audiences for ideas, practices, or products. As the introduction to the 1935–36 Bayer film catalogue put it, "The intimate expectations for entertainment conveyed by the spectators, the cosy atmosphere of the dark movie theater surrounding him/her, and music and images will amend any critical

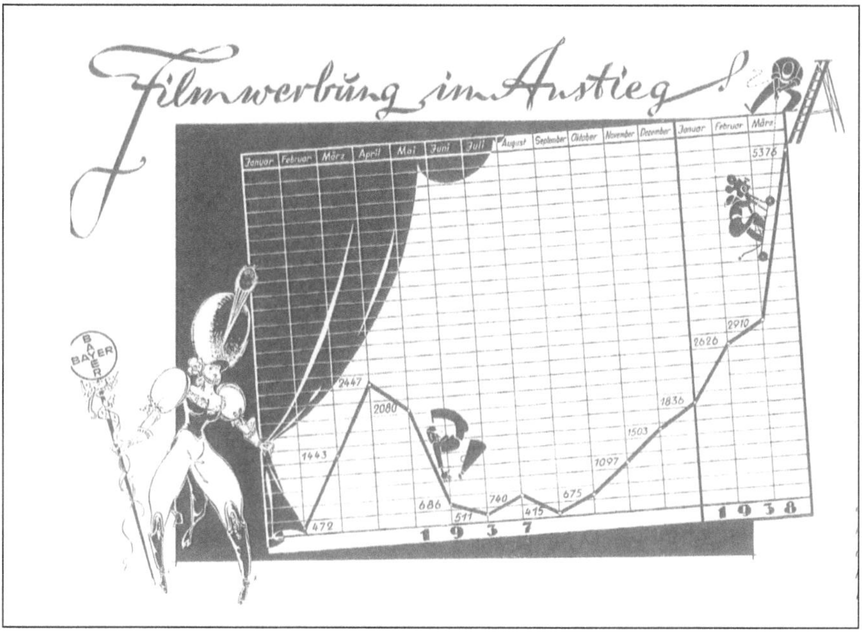

Figure 2.2. "What represents film? Figures indicate it." Audience development of German cinema spectators in 1937–38 and its use as argument by the Bayer film unit. *Zepro-Nachrichten* 2 (1938): 10. Bayer AG, Corporate History and Archives.

awareness thus enhancing the suggestive power of advertisement."[61] Attaining mass audiences, capturing new parts of society, and enhancing receptiveness and thus the management of public opinion were the three key elements of Bayer pharmaceutical propaganda as it pursued "systematic persuasion of the masses with a specific goal." In this strategy, the 1935–36 film catalogue introduction concluded, "Film is one of the most significant means of promotion of our time. . . . It is absolutely necessary."[62]

Defining a Corpus beyond Industrial Utility Film: Bayer Image-Promotion Films, 1934–42

A focus on practices not only destabilizes the concept of propaganda but also allows us to question preexisting categorizations such as they have evolved in film history around "documentary," "industrial," or "advertising" film, just as much as it also destabilizes the categories of "(fascist) propaganda film," "experimental film," or "politically progressive" filmmaking. More positively it allows us to develop film history as media archaeology. This means confronting the supposedly natural objects (a corpus of propaganda films) with the situated practices that correspond to them and make them exist (objectify them), and finally to explain these practices not by a unique motive but through all the contingent and concomitant practices they are rooted in.

Bayer's own way of categorizing film is captured in its 1935–36 guidelines for film screenings, which also shows how they related to other film categories and to Bayer's promotional strategies.[63] Bayer's guidelines insist that in order to meet its ambition to "interest the public and enhance the reputation of our corporation," the film screening needed to carefully adapt film programs to specific audiences. It needed to create a tailored event. Bayer identified five categories of spectators as target audiences: (1) universities, (2) medical societies and similar associations, (3) schools, (4) a select audience referring to individuals identified by the company as a special target for marketing, and finally (5) general screenings for everyone. Each of these categories of audiences and occasions of events had corresponding categories of films produced by the corporation. The Bayer Film Unit distinguished between (1) popular advertisement films, (2) scientific demonstration films, (3) Kulturfilm, (4) image-building films (*Wert-Werbungsfilme*), and finally (5) special films.

1. *Popular advertisement films* were either very short, one-minute films (30m) (conceived as "a speaking one image ad," that aimed to catch the spectator's eyes and ears through visuals, music, and slogans) or somewhat longer advertisement films that lasted for from three to five minutes (80–120m) and which could promote a product through a plot. These popular versions of films were deemed important since they could achieve wide distribution. They were screened in movie theaters not in the main program but as part of the supporting program, for which Bayer had to pay, and by mobile projection units that traveled throughout the countryside organizing projections in remote areas little exposed to movies at the time.

2. *Scientific demonstration films* provided a means to "present in easily accessible and convincing ways instructive knowledge to specific audiences."[64] These films represented a particularly significant part of Bayer film production in that they were not only instructional films but doubled as science-based advertisements for Bayer or its products. In contrast to the popular films, Bayer felt that they were best targeted at specific audiences, often physicians, and screening took place at special events not as part of the regular cinema schedule.

3. Kulturfilm was defined by the propaganda department as an intermediary form situated between "strictly scientific films only useful for experts" and feature/theatrical entertainment films. Their task was to instruct in a popular and comprehensive way. Ideally suited for image-building purposes, such films could highlight both the production process and products of the corporation and, because advertising was not explicit, they were distributed for free in preprograms. Not only did this mean that distribution was wide and inexpensive, but Kulturfilm (like *Wert-Werbungsfilme* below) deliberately mixed popular education and corporate promotion selling a label as Kultur. The distribution of these films was aligned with the established Kulturfilm genre,[65] and the films

were included in regular movie theater programs, thereby profiting from movie theater tax reductions.

4. *Image-building films* sprang from the concept that general advertising was just as important as product-specific advertising. This so-called representational advertising was supposed to convey to the public an idea of the importance of the pharmaceutical sales community/corporation and how it tackled the immense task of serving the public's health. The Bayer propaganda department planned to produce a high-budget *Wert-Werbungfilm* general film every one or two years. If Kulturfilms were defined by their distribution practices and limited length, image-building films were defined more by their corporate sponsor's intention and production investment. A regular practice consisted of transforming the long image-building films into reedited shortened versions distributed as supporting program Kulturfilm.

5. *Special films* were described as films the sole intention of which was to increase the entertainment aspect of film events or to obtain access to audiences that otherwise would have been difficult to reach. These film productions were conceived as pure entertainment for popular Bayer film events that comprised a mix of advertisement films, popular music during breaks, and special (entertainment) films. These films did not mention Bayer or its products and were usually tuned to major cultural or sporting events (see appendix 2.1).

From the company's internal classification above, it becomes clear that what historians label industrial or corporate film comprises a variety of very different types of films.[66] Thomas Elsaesser has argued that to read and interpret nonfiction film, the historian needs to ask three questions: who commissioned the film? what was the occasion for its production and screening? and who was the audience and to what use was it put?[67] In the case of Bayer, the answers to these questions reinforce the five categories of film that Bayer itself differentiated. It is difficult to lump popular advertisement shorts of a minute or two intended to present one product to a general audience on the occasion of product specific sales promotion on the one hand with twenty-minute instructional films addressed to physicians for their information about disease definition and new treatment schemes, or with high budget one-hour prestigious image-building films screened in regular movie theater programs.

Recent scholarship on utility films[68] further develops the idea that "the different exhibition frames played a decisive role in determining the meaning and reception of a film."[69] Yvonne Zimmermann has argued in this context that industrial films are multi-intentional and multifunctional and may serve advertising, information, instruction, and education all together, but in specific settings according to different target groups. In the case of utility films, it follows that it is more their use that defines them than their aesthetics or the author behind them. Corpuses of films should then be selected accordingly.

The re(de)fined unit of analysis chosen as our corpus is a series of image-building films (*Wert-Werbungsfilme*) produced by Bayer over a period of eight years—between 1934 and 1942—in cooperation with the UFA Kulturfilmabteilung.[70]

Their purpose, as the Bayer promotional department commented, was to "fulfill in an ideal manner the task to present the Bayer organization and its achievements. They move our corporation center stage and represent a strong support for all our other means of propaganda."[71] The films were intended to create particular events in the public sphere every one or two years. Like Kulturfilm, Bayer conceived these motion pictures as an intermediary form situated between strictly scientific films only useful for experts and pure feature/theatrical entertainment films. They were distributed either to prestigious movie theaters as part of the regular schedule or to special events created by the Bayer Corporation independently. From an aesthetic and technical point of view, *Wert-Werbungsfilme* combine elements of industrial production film (Werksfilme) and instructional film (Lehrfilm) and promotional pictures. What distinguished them most was that Bayer wanted them to be of high quality and to be extended treatments of the subject; therefore, the corporation devoted large budgets to their production.

Beyond Genres: The Bayer Image-Building Film Corpus, 1934–42; Creating and Exploiting Ambiguities

Between 1934 and 1942, five prestigious *Wertwerbungsfilme* were produced by Bayer in collaboration with the UFA. All films are black-and-white sound productions. The series began with the huge budget, UFA-coproduced film *Stored Sun Energy* (1934). This 35mm sound production was directed by Ulrich Kayser, a UFA film director who had been producing nature and animal films since the 1920s (including microcinematography in collaboration with Herta Jülich), and nationalistic Kulturfilms that after 1933 blurred seamlessly into NS Kulturfilm propaganda glorifying modern agriculture, blood and soil, and traditional values.[72] The script for *Stored Sun Energy* came from Karl Spielmann, the director of the Bayer film department that was created the same year. This was how the Bayer-UFA cooperation was conceived: Bayer provided the script, UFA the film expertise.

According to the Bayer film catalogue, the film represented "a new type of film" giving an internal view of the organization of the giant pharmaceutical company.[73] Live-action and cartoon animation sequences illustrate how coal, formerly only a product used to power factories, was now conceived as a storehouse of enormous quantities of energy from the sun and of healing forces. Contrasting traditional medieval mystical healing arts with modern scientific pharmaceuticals, the film visualizes different diseases, their hidden causes, and the pharmaceuticals used to fight against them. Echoing a form of commissioned industrial film that Yvonne Zimmermann describes as consensus-building media that promote public acceptance of modernization,[74] the film stages mighty industrial cranes, bulldozers, and mixing containers preparing substances that become tablets inscribed with the Bayer cross, each the material result of the entire production chain. According to the Bayer's public relations film strategy, *Stored Sun Energy* was shortened and transformed into a Kulturfilm

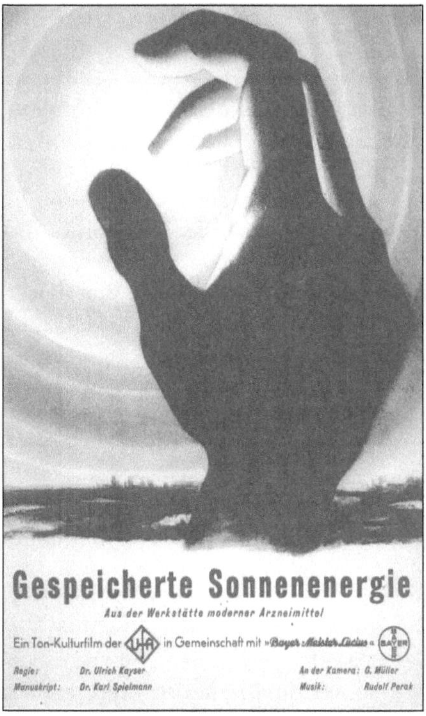

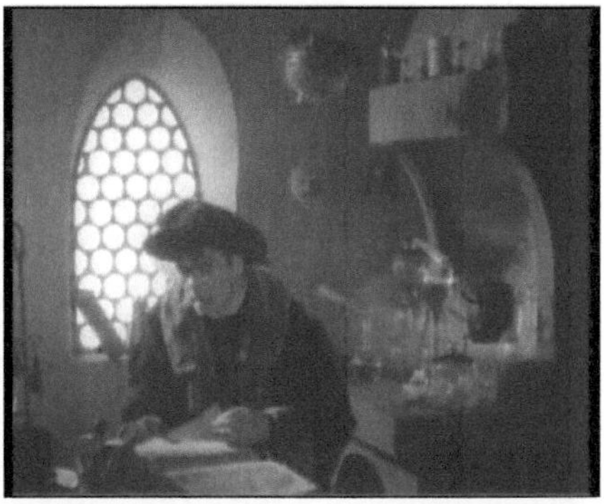

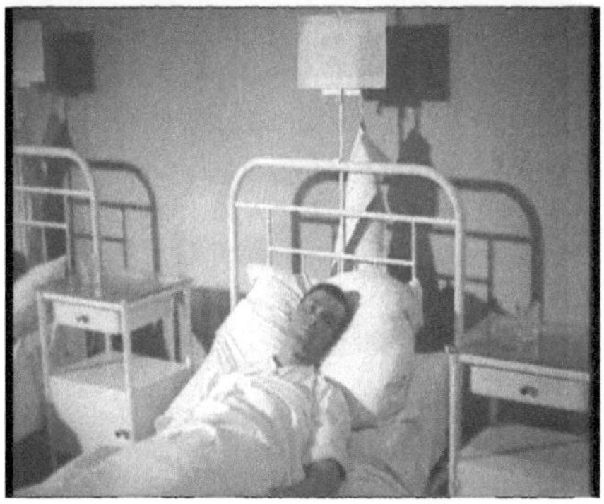

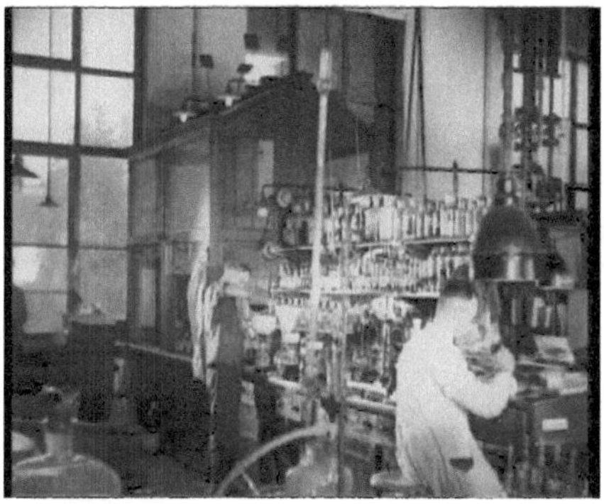

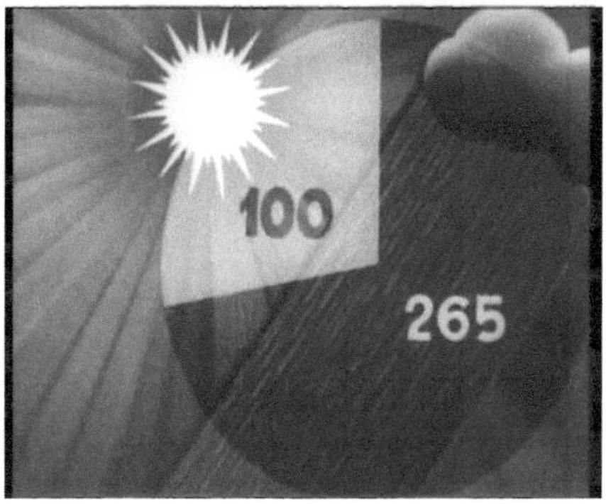

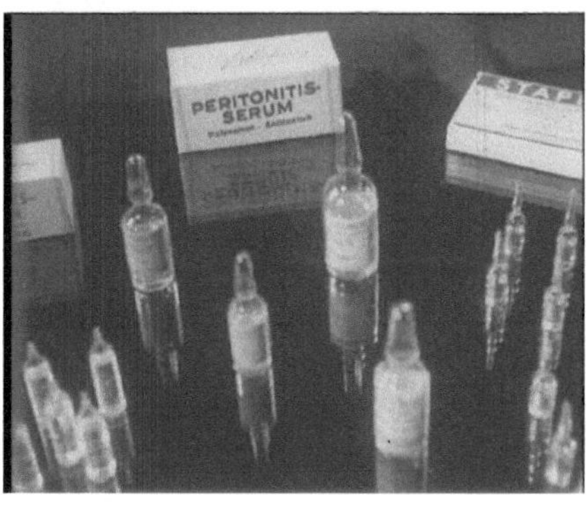

Figure 2.3a–f. Film announcement, and film stills from *Gespeicherte Sonnenernergie* (*Stored Sun Energy*, 1934), Bayers's first image building film. Stills illustrate the integration of elements from health education, industrial, teaching, and *Kulturfilm* genres. Bayer AG, Corporate History and Archives, A Werksfilme Allgemeines 92-1 vol. 1.

that appeared under the title *From the Workshop of Modern Medicaments* (1935). In this form, the film was screened during its first year in more than six hundred movie theaters in over nine thousand shows as a supporting program (and tax-reducing) Kulturfilm without any payment from the company. (As noted above, in the Bayer film classification, Kulturfilm not only meant a film genre but a form of distribution.) A much shortened, popular advertisement version of the film was produced and widely circulated as *Under the Bayer Cross* (1935).

Malaria (1934) was the second of the big-budget productions that Bayer coproduced with UFA reprising their earlier collaboration in which Bayer/Karl Spielmann provided the script and UFA/Ulrich Kayser made and directed the film. Bayer produced different versions of *Malaria*, including two expanded teaching/scientific advertisement films (scientific demonstration films in Bayer categories, see appendixes 2.1 and 2.2). *Plasmochin* (1934) was described as the physician-oriented chemical-compound-centered version presenting one of Bayer's leading synthetic anti-malarial drugs of the same name. *Malaria Experimental Research and Clinical Results* (1934) was the disease- and public-health oriented re-montage of the Bayer-UFA image-building film produced by its scientific-pharmaceutical (not the advertisement) department in Leverkusen.

Several industrial films dedicated to malaria and its public health treatment had been produced in the early 1930s amongst others by the Shell Corporation.[75] The Bayer film had some aesthetic similarities to these earlier films, and the ways it structured the presentation of the disease, its containment, and its treatment were also similar. The Bayer film takes the spectator first to malaria-infested regions, where it staged the way the disease devastated landscapes and cities as the population flees from the scourge. Combining animation, micro-cinematography, and depiction of clinical settings and practice, the film instructs the viewer about forms of the disease, its clinical symptoms, the life cycle of the pathogen, and disease transmission—much as educational pictures had done before. The second part of the film presents methods of environmental containment (such as swamp drainage and the chemical spraying of water surface). These methods served to set up the story Bayer really wanted to get across, that of new anti-malarial treatments developed by Bayer. Thus, the film shows the scientific development of Plasmochin, Chinoplasmin, and Atebrin[76] in Bayer laboratories in Leverkusen (borrowing this time from the manufacturing film genre), where spectators witness in detail the troublesome and demanding efforts that preceded the development of Bayer preparations. The film ends with the presentation of the three Bayer products and their precise treatment schemes leading to the illustration of abandoned land being repopulated, restoring the health and wealth of large regions of the globe impressively underscored by triumphant musical arrangements. In certain aspects, *Malaria* echoes Kayser's aggressive agitation film *Land unterm Kreuz* (1927) that argued for the German annexation of what Germans called Upper Silesia from Poland. Where the latter promotes "justifications" for the reinvestment of "politically" abandoned land east of the German Reich, *Malaria* portrays the scientific battle for the restoration of a "sanitarily" abandoned land in southern colonies.

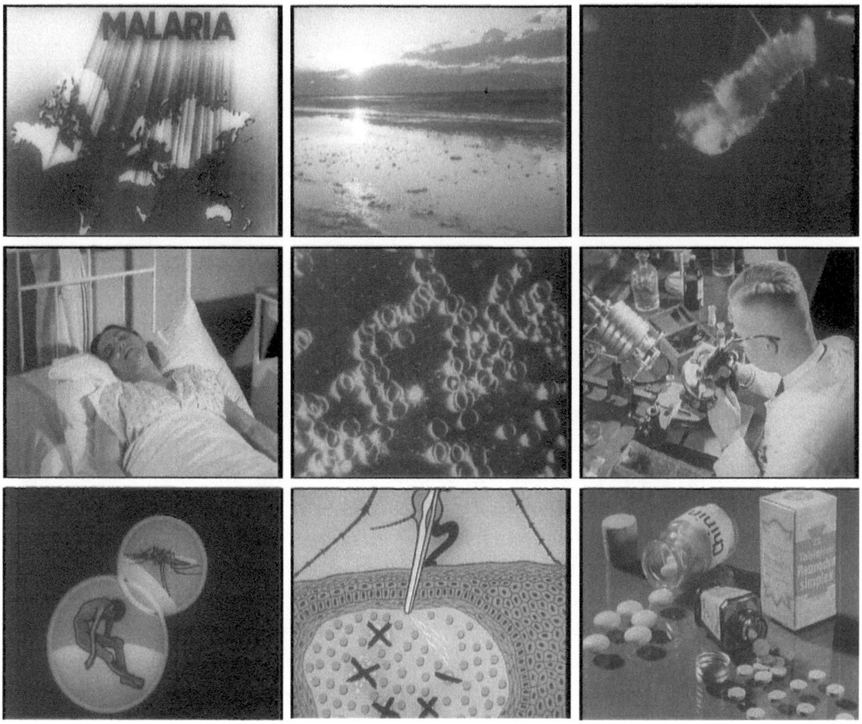

Figure 2.4a–i. Film stills from Bayer's second image building film *Malaria* (1934) illustrating the by then typical integration of health education, industrial, teaching, and *Kulturfilm*. Bayer AG, Corporate History and Archives.

The third film, *Creeping Poison—Burden of Humanity* (1936), aims to illustrate the long fight of humanity against syphilis that finally, after afflicting populations for centuries, "has been vanquished."[77] The film moves from describing traditional therapeutic approaches to a long historical sequence illustrating the genesis and development of the revolutionary chemotherapy Salvarsan produced by Bayer. The second part of the film mimics health education films in that it portrays both clinical symptoms and the development of the disease through three stages. The film is the third in a row of the by-then-established production team associating Bayer/Karl Spielmann providing the script and UFA/Ulrich Kayser directing the film. The film concludes with the presentation of Salvarsan products and their industrial preparation and clinical use that aims to show its audience of physicians and patients the unlimited faith Bayer had in these preparations.

A fourth film production, *Under the Banner of Trust* (1937), breaks with the script-production division of labor established in the three earlier films. This time, Bayer instead brought in acclaimed avant-garde film director Walter Ruttmann,[78] known especially for his 1927 experimental film, *Berlin: Symphony of a City. Under the Banner of Trust* starts with sick patients in a ward and their worried family members at home. Ruttmann takes the spectator through the world of workers in the factory who are addressed by their director—evoking Fritz Lang's *Metropolis*—in order to then turn to the presentation of sophisticated, powerful, modern, and technical mass-production assembly lines for standard drugs, once again illustrating and negotiating modern drug development. What drugs achieve is quickly hinted at when the disease name "malaria" appears on the screen followed by a microscope, lab, and mass preparation facilities and workers. Ruttmann guides the spectator through a world of impressive machines and workers who display extreme concentration, thoroughness, and precision. Products are portrayed as sophisticated and relentlessly monitored: the name of the game is quality. From the world of the factory, the film and its drugs return to the bedsides of ailing patients and their physicians. The film ends with a staged airplane view of the world as a globe in which Leverkusen is connected with humanity throughout the world by the slogan "quality made in Germany—drugs made by Bayer." In 1938, still crediting Ruttmann as director, Bayer remounted a twenty-minute Kulturfilm version of the film with the evocative title *In the Service of Humanity* (*Im Dienste der Menschheit*, 1938).

Ruttmann had experimented with very early sound film (*Deutscher Rundfunk*, 1928),[79] and after a gap of several years in which he was unable to make films, from 1933 on directed industrial and commissioned films like *Steel* (*Acciaio/Stahl—Arbeit macht glücklich*, 1933) for the Italian steel industry. He returned to Germany where he collaborated on *Blood and Soil: Foundations for A New Reich* (*Blut und Boden: Grundlagen zum Neuen Reich*, 1933), directed *Old Germanic Agriculture* (*Altgermanische Bauernkultur*, 1934) and participated in Leni Riefenstahl's *Triumph of Will* (*Triumph des Willens*, 1935). In 1935 UFA appointed Ruttmann as a film director in its advertisement department (UFA Werbeabteilung), where he produced several city and advertising films and more and more overtly propagandistic films for German armament and military sponsors. His output in 1938 was predominantly industrial documentary films produced under NS: he directed *Mannesmann* (1938); *Henkel, a German Industry at Work* (*Henkel, ein deutsches Werk in seiner Arbeit*, 1938), and *Under the Banner of Trust/In the Service of Humanity* (1938) for Bayer. The two Bayer films were thus part of the larger conversion of Ruttmann from a pacifist left-wing experimental film director to an aligned National Socialist propaganda documentary filmmaker whose films can be described as evoking "reactionary modernism."[80] His 1938 industrial Bayer films conceived as industrial work symphonies were highly reminiscent of his avant-garde city films, and they were the last films in which he kept a certain distance from official and more explicit NS political and war propaganda. (Compare his 1938 Bayer films with his 1940 films *German Armory/Deutsche Waffenschmieden, 1940* and *German Tanks/Deutsche Panzer*, 1940). The year 1938 was not only the final year in which Ruttman's film production was marked more by its Weimar avant-garde origins than its NS accommodation; it was also the final year of the Bayer-UFA collaboration. In the last image-building film of our corpus, UFA disappeared from the film credits and was replaced by NS military institutions.[81]

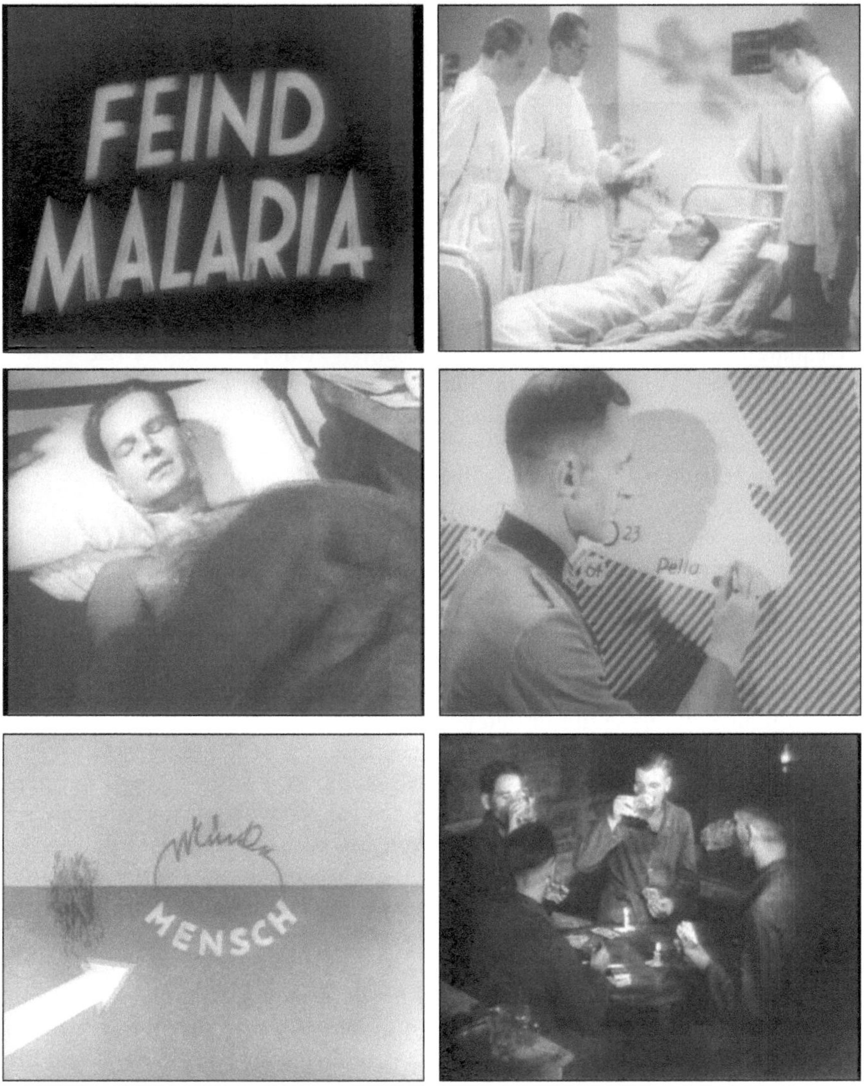

Figure 2.5a–f. Film stills from *Feind Malaria* (*Enemy Malaria*, 1942) illustrating the transition to emotional storytelling as the film production shifted after 1939 from collaboration with UFA to the Academy for Military Physicians. Flash-back elements and biographical storylines transform the former *Kulturfilm* mimicking film form. Bayer AG, Corporate History and Archives.

The fifth film in our corpus *Enemy Malaria* (*Feind Malaria*, 1942) was produced in 1942–43 by Bayer—by then integrated into the IG Farben trust—in association with the Academy for Military Physicians (Militärärtzliche Akademie) and the German Wehrmacht.[82] Film credits of the version located in the Bayer archives do not indicate the director, scriptwriter, or cameraman (see appendix 2.2). Not surprisingly, the thirty-four-minute film is produced exclusively in German.

Despite the similarity in title to the 1934 production, the film is almost a completely new creation, clearly under the direction of the Military Academy. In less than two minutes, the film moves quickly through epidemiological, historical, and geographic information in order to then take root in a fictive plot played by actors from the Military Academy (the same actors had earlier figured in the syphilis prevention film, *A Word from Man to Man* (*Ein Wort von Mann zu Mann*, 1941).[83] Situated in a hospital ward, the fiction tells the stories of two patients admitted for suspected malaria. Ward investigations and activities are interrupted by flashbacks illustrating patient statements and looping with educational sequences, both animated and documentary, explaining the cause, diagnosis, and treatment of different malaria types. Produced in 1942, the film is constructed as a demonstration of the rational and efficient organization "that has taken its weapons from the enemy malaria."[84] The second part of the film is increasingly oriented to the prevention of malaria among troops and the management of occupied/conquered territories for malaria eradication. Losing some of the fictional structure and story, it integrates a long documentary sequence on larvae life in water, reminiscent of microscopic scientific film sequences produced since the late 1920s in malaria films.[85]

The five *Wert-Werbungsfilme* had much in common, thus justifying their constitution as a corpus.[86] They all integrated typical elements of three established documentary subgenres: (1) *health education films* that had appeared during the first decade of the twentieth century in many European and North American countries[87] to promote strategies of disease control through campaigns addressing war on tuberculosis, venereal diseases, alcoholism, malaria, etc., were defined and screened as "the art to propagate, to disseminate, to vulgarize and to spread, in one word to popularize, an idea utilizing factual knowledge";[88] (2) *manufacturing films* that concerned work and factory processes and were established as short film category prior to 1914 by producers such as Pathé, Gaumont, Raleigh & Robert, and Charles Urban;[89] and (3) *scientific research and teaching films* that used motion pictures as an educational medium in classrooms and lecture halls.[90] Generally, the five films resembled Weimar Kulturfilm in their production form, and all except the last were shortened and transformed into Kulturfilm versions for distribution purposes.

These five films thus did not generally fit one genre but, rather, often comprised an amalgam of styles. Film historians have often used the concept of genre as a device by which to structure film analysis. In practice, the corpus of *Wert-Werbungsfilme* was on a continuum in which film directors produced pictures that deliberately entangled different forms of film (health education, manufacturing research/teaching, on the one hand; entertainment, instruction, and advertisement on the other), sometimes veering more toward one form than another, at different times in each film, and in different films. The films had factual content along the lines of what Timothy Boon has described in reference to Paul Rotha as "films of facts."[91] They point to the moment where the cult of techno-science and the popularization of scientific facts cemented trust in science and technology as value-free, objective elements in "the service of humanity" but also promoted corporate identities and reputation in the form of filmed factory tours.[92] Walter Ruttmann's 1938 Bayer film exemplifies and illustrates this tendency. Recent German documentary film studies of "reactionary modernist" film under NS have characterized as the "new objectivity" the cult of technology of the sort that Ruttmann promoted in this film.

Such themes were also evident in other Bayer image-building films. These films often reduced subjectivity and multiplicity of points of view to a universal faith in science and technology expressed through an iconography that equated the progress of humanity with the investing in and deployment of science and technology. These films appear not to speak from somewhere in the name of someone (such às Bayer). It was precisely through the disappearance of situatedness and subjective authorship that these films sought to lead the spectator to the conviction that nature and industrial culture spoke through facts themselves (a propaganda of facts). Production, mise-en-scène, and projection of these corporate films combined to use techno-scientific suggestions to mobilize spectator-citizens to support seemingly unquestionable "crusades for health," where in the end Bayer products were naturalized as facts themselves (corporate propaganda with facts).

Thus, the Bayer image-building film corpus functioned both as corporate propaganda of facts and as a propaganda with facts, where the corporation precisely situated itself at the intersection of the two. This chapter argues that mimicking established film genres (health education, manufacturing, and research/teaching film), Bayer image-building films appealed to contexts of use where apparent use, at first glance information or education, was mixed with the hidden agenda of corporate promotion. These industrial films were in accordance with Yvonne Zimmermann's affirmation multi-intentional and multifunctional serving advertising, information, instruction, or education all together where "the different exhibition frames played a decisive role in determining the meaning and reception of a film."[93]

Yet by deliberately creating and exploiting genre ambiguities, Bayer image-building films were, as the director of the advertising agency Werbekunst Epoche Reklame, Max Friedländer, suggested in 1929 for advertisement film, "indeed perhaps a bit of a traitor; they approached their public under the cover of disinterested expressions, they spoke of general human [or scientific] subjects, waited until the spectators became interested or amused, and then fired at the unprepared audience, like a bomb, their well-known projectile, the poignant conclusion, that amounts to an incredible remedy or a radical insect powder."[94]

This was not only the point, as *Zepro-Nachrichten* put it, "where advertisement departed from purely economic premises to become a cultural factor in a very common sense," but also where utility film analysis needs to carefully distinguish between the film sponsor's intentions in making the film and their intentions in screening it. In particular, it needs to focus on how the screening of film adapted (and sometimes subverted) Bayer's intentions in producing films and created a second promotional goal, "the alert, conscious and intended effect on the unconscious" that Bayer film propagandists were looking for. The following section will explore how Kultur, promotion, and propaganda were intertwined visually in the Bayer films in order to achieve—or not—what the 1935–36 in-house guidelines for film events requested: "The highest principle for every projection has to be that it is attractive to the audience present in order to match the prestige of our company."[95] Furthermore, it seems appropriate to pursue how film's utility aesthetics were entangled with screening practices.

Spectator Bonding: Of Visual Chains, Transitions, and Emotional Storytelling

It has been shown so far that Bayer's commercial propaganda films mixed and mimicked a variety of utility film subgenres, including the genres of health education, manufacturing, and research/teaching film. But mixing and mimicking other genres and styles created problems for Bayer in that the jumble of styles could undermine the message it wanted to get across as much as it could reinforce it. Film often worked by associating different images to create a visual argument of sorts, but the use of many different styles and genres within a commercial film risked creating associations that Bayer did not endorse. In what follows, I will examine some of the techniques that Bayer deployed in its films to try to control the audience response. My focus will be on one theme that recurs in many of the image making films—malaria.

Malaria as a disease was first understood in contemporary scientific terms in 1898, when Walter Ross established the life cycle of the malaria parasite Plasmodium and its transmission through an intermediary host, the anopheles mosquito. At the center of the 1934 *Malaria* film lies the visual presentation first of the plasmodium life cycle, then of the plasmodium-anopheles-human transmission cycle. Alternating and superposing live-action and animation sequences, the film carefully translates scientific evidence into images and their commentary. The film's central innovation is created when drawings produced in the Bayer film unit especially equipped for animation[96] link transmission cycles to an image that associates them with the formation of an endless chain of human contamination (see fig. 2.6). There are thus two intersecting chains here—the visual chain within the film and the biological chain of contamination— that the motion picture uses to depict and explain the burden and the endless chain of contamination that needs to be broken if the scourge is to be beaten.

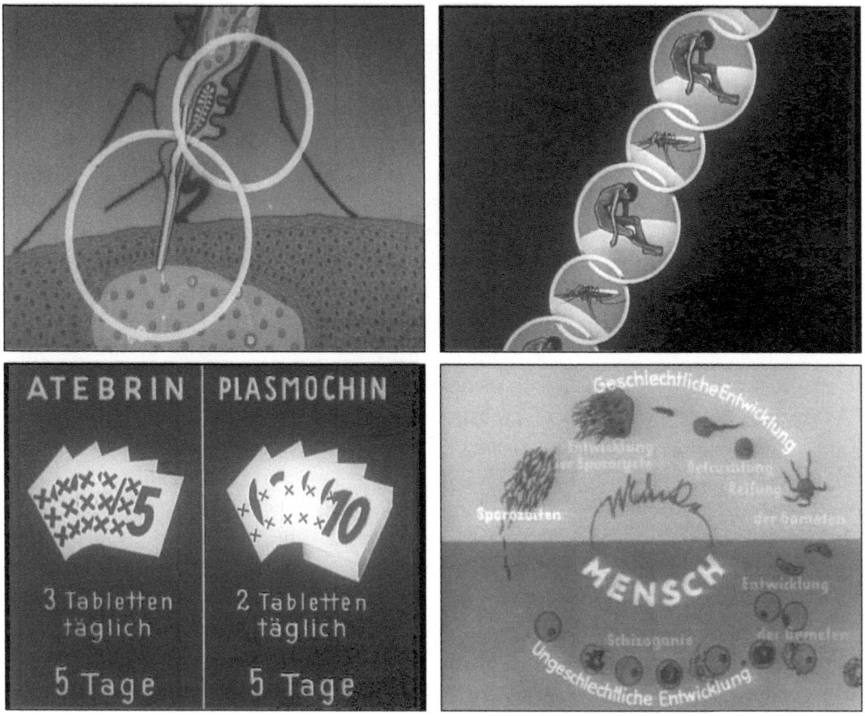

Figure 2.6a–d. Film stills 2.6a–c from *Malaria* (1934), illustrating the visual chain aesthetics moving from scientific microcinematography to animation mosquito lifecycles, the chain of human contamination, and breaking the chain by Bayer pharmaceuticals. In contrast film still 2.6d from *Feind Malaria* (1942) does not reproduce the chain reaction but rather insists on an immanent contamination cycle. Bayer AG, Corporate History and Archives.

As mentioned above, films work by associating images. And indeed, in the last part of the film, breaking the chain is visually associated with Bayer pharmaceuticals. Their presentation borrows aesthetic and formal film elements from advertisement film when individual products are presented and from physician teaching films when treatment schemes with details like "three tablets a day for five days" are provided (see figs. 2.3 and 2.4). If mechanical approaches like mosquito nets and environmental solutions like swamp drainage, typical of malaria health education films of the 1920s and early 1930s,[97] are presented, the breaking of the constructed endless visual chain is only associated and visualized in connection with the explanation of how the Bayer anti-malarial drugs work. The drugs, as suggested in the 1929 citation by Max Friedländer, were fired "at the unprepared audience, like a bomb" after the film's initial mimicking of a classical health education film.[98]

The visual chain was one method of trying to create an association between Bayer and the defeat of malaria. But it was not used in all anti-malaria films.

Thus, despite the fact that *Stored Sun Energy* (1934) visualizes anti-malaria drugs as a group of the prominent Bayer products and lends the initial opening image to *Malaria*, the visual chain of endless human contamination is not used in the film. Its central message lies somewhere else, since the film is conceived as a manufacturing film displaying the harmony of research and production as well as of workers and machines in accomplishing the task of producing drugs as industrial goods to save humanity. Also, *Feind Malaria* (1942) does not import the 1934 animation sequences either but rather proceeds to a complete and new set of animation in order to explain the life cycle and the disease. In this renewed version, the life cycle revolves around an individual but does not lead to the visual chain or to the actions/products that might break it (fig. 2.6). Furthermore, where the 1934 *Malaria* film uses a purely visual image without legends, *Feind Malaria* uses a mix of image and text.

Bayer thus used a variety of techniques to shape its audience response from a series of visual associations to a mix of commentary and visuals. But it did not rely entirely on the production techniques to shape audience responses. It also tried to shape responses by controlling the context in which they were screened and by monitoring audience responses. Thus, in the case of the 1934 *Malaria* film, Bayer used a variety of means of screening the films, including the use of film trucks as film theaters on wheels to reach out to remote areas and populations, thereby connecting them to the Bayer visual chain. Translated into at least five other languages, the film was projected on promotional tours in city, town, and countryside as part of Bayer prestige communication strategies. In other settings, Bayer screened the films and the visual chains within them through specific high-profile events. In 1937 *Zepro-Nachrichten* reported how the 1934 *Malaria* film had been shown to the entire army corps in Milan and Naples.[99] The program showed an Italian film company Luce-distributed short war movie, *Hours of War in the African Sky*,[100] before the screening of *Malaria*. The show ran for eighteen evenings, attracting over eighteen thousand spectators to movie theaters rented for the occasion in fascist Italian cities, and the *Zepro-Nachrichten* report praised the use of targeted invitation letters to bring audiences to the event. Military music accompanied the shows and military corps arriving at the theater created traffic jams "that attracted the attention of even the most indifferent citizens that something was happening there. Arising questions allowed to repeat time and again the words Bayer, film and Malaria and led to vivid exchanges."[101] The dispositive[102] achieved its ultimate goal of linking public attention and Bayer products when, on April 2, 1937, the Italian crown prince and his wife attended the event.

To assess the effectiveness of propaganda, Bayer's guidelines for film projections included a section "after the show" indicating that the number of audience members should be counted, conversations among the masses leaving the show should be reported, and employees should seek direct conversation with spectators to obtain their "untainted judgement" on their impression of the show and whether they had been persuaded as to the message of the film.[103] Based on such techniques, the *Zepro-Nachrichten* report on the Italian film events

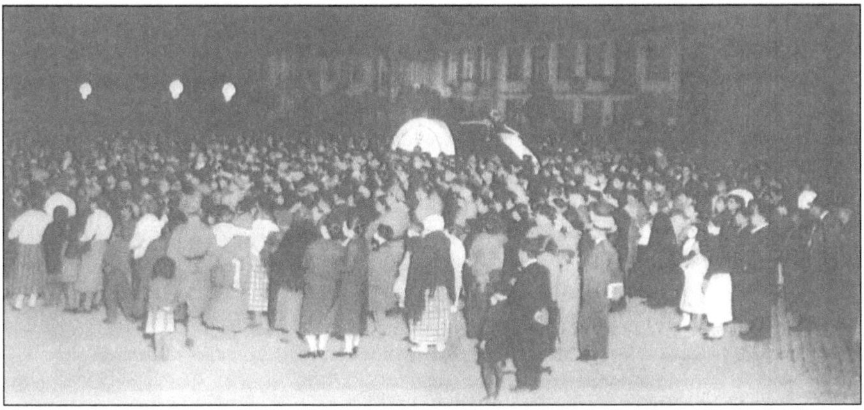

Figure 2.7. Crowd at the entrance of public film show of *Malaria* creating a public event. *Zepro-Nachrichten* 3 (1937): 27. Bayer AG, Corporate History and Archives.

concluded that the film succeeded in making the public aware of Bayer, an awareness that suggested "a bright and influential line" orienting future film propaganda. Put another way, the 1934 *Malaria* film suggests that Bayer image-building films from visual aesthetics to screening events sought to create a third type of chain (in addition to the visual chain and the biological chain of contamination) in which media events sought to link audiences to scientific facts, themselves present as a visual chain within the film. Through its control of both production and screening, Bayer was to be the glue that held both these chains together: the visual chain within the film and the link between the audience and scientific fact.

A second area where Bayer's films sought to shape audience responses concerns filmic transitions. Corporate-sponsored research/teaching, scientific advertisement, and image-building films often assembled very heterogeneous sequences mixing live-action, fiction, animation, and scientific elements. In such circumstances, the mastering of transitions between these sequences was essential to assure narrative continuity for spectators. At the same time, these transitions established associations and created translations. The association of images in films works through the mastery of transitions between them, and sometimes they don't work. Thus, reproducing an often-articulated criticism of teaching and Kulturfilm, *Stored Sun Energy* is punctuated by cumbersome transitions moving from one sequence to the next, which often interrupt the filmic harmony of illusions. It remains largely a didactic explanation illustrated with images rather than a cinematographic oeuvre as such. Often the images only illustrate what the off-screen commentator asserts. In one sequence near the beginning, for instance, the film presents a traditional mystical past in which strange healing figures produce obscure remedies. In a poorly constructed fictional scene where a commentator reads the text "Roots and burls are collected in the ghostly woods in the moonlight" actors poorly play out the spoken words.[104] Similarly, the music in this sequence simply accompanies the live-action visuals filling the silence rather than structuring the film. While we have little information on audience responses to the film, the transitions in *Stored Sun Energy* (from documentary factory views, animated scientific drawings, and fictional vignettes to products like Aspirin, Pyramidon, Adalin, Vigantol, and Salvarsan among other preparations as well as sera production by Behring in Marburg) interrupt the continuity of the film, presenting the spectator with a series of images that function like a series of self-contained expositions rather than a coherent visual argument.

By contrast, for the spectator, the 1938 Ruttmann film makes more sophisticated use of the visual medium. Ruttmann's mastery of visual transitions leads the spectator rather than leaving guidance to the commentary. Reassembling several of the shots used in *Stored Sun Energy*, Ruttmann gives great care to transitions between sequences, and he almost completely omits off-screen commentary *In the Service of Humanity*, except for technical scientific explanations. As in *Berlin Symphony of a City* and subsequent industrial films, music is the dominant nonvisual tool for associating images and becomes a way of structuring the film. When spoken texts are necessary, they are associated with the image of the person depicted. In the case of the opening scene of the factory director's speech, Ruttmann rarely illustrates the speaker. Instead, he films the sequence from the director's perspective, with the camera depicting the crowd of workers and uses close-ups of their facial expressions to visualize their reception of the words. Declarations and comments in *Stored Sun Energy* become a never-ending visual tide in Ruttmann's film of rotating machines and ballets of tablet dances with Bayer products blinding in and fading out at the same rhythm. Drugs make appearances just like the machines illustrating a body of resolute and united workers succeeding in the great pharmaceutical symphony. Transitions extend their visual representation when the machines' back-and-forth movement is extrapolated to represent oscillation between ailing patients, treating physicians, and the production of the drugs that will heal them: Bayer pharmaceuticals. Similarly, the machine sequences swing back and forth between the industrial plant and the physician's office. The final visualized transition is that of a sleeping sickness epidemic in Africa, first announced by bushmen's drums, then by western telegraphs leading finally to Leverkusen drug production and distribution including the latest Bayer investment: the Bayer airplane for universal and urgent drug delivery. Telecommunications, drug production, and transport systems melt into a cult celebrating modern science and technology typical of German documentary during National Socialism. Colonial subjects in faithful recognition await drugs for a relief from ailment. At the center and conclusion, the Bayer airplane flies around the cartoon world parachuting drugs "in the service of humanity." While we know little about which sequences were most appealing to audiences—those in *Stored Sun Energy* or in *In the Service of Humanity*—they provide an indication of the range of approaches that Bayer used to sway audiences, from a mix of visuals linked by commentary to a more sophisticated visual approach that sought to tell a story primarily through the transitions from one image in a sequence to another.

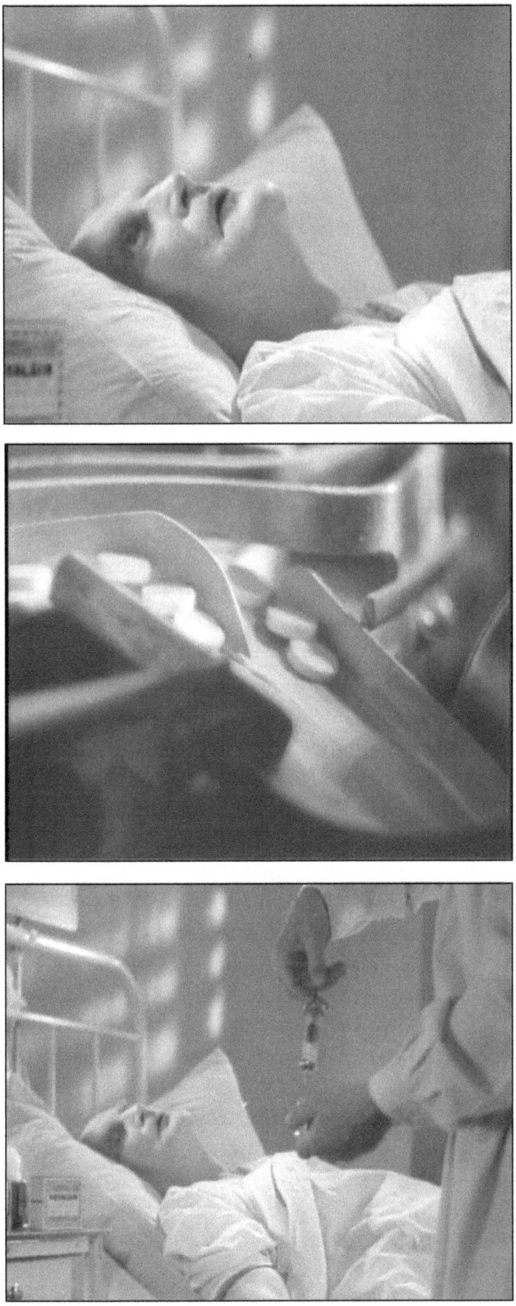

Figure 2.8a–c. Mastery of filmic transitions in Walter Ruttmann's *In the Service of Humanity* (1938). Bayer AG, Corporate History and Archives.

A third area where Bayer sought to shape audience responses brings us back to the post-1938 fracture. It will be recalled that the first four Bayer films were reminiscent of Kulturfilms using animation and verbal commentary. After 1938 there emerged a different pattern of filmmaking exemplified by the 1942 *Enemy Malaria* production: emotional storytelling. In this film, visual chains of the sort employed in the 1934 *Malaria* film are absent and transitions are less carefully managed and more abrupt than in the 1938 Ruttman film. As in other NS health propaganda films like *A Word from Man to Man* (1941), the film *Feind Malaria* is organized around a fictional story of individual characters that is neither documentary nor animation but rather fictional entertainment. It begins with a short classical Kulturfilm opening about history, land, victims (a military cemetery), and marching troops during the 1941 Balkan offensive that employs pre-1938 visual associations but then moves to a story that seeks to evoke an emotional response from the audience through its identification with the characters in the film. The movie starts in a military hospital in occupied territory where the fictional physician asks an individual patient, "So Lohmann, how did this all begin?"[105] Structuring the plot, the patient then plays and narrates (illustrated through flashbacks comprising fiction and long animated and microcinematographic scientific explanation sequences) his illness in parallel to the story of his hospital treatment. The emotional underpinnings of the patient's perspective and his suffering, counterbalanced by the caring physician's knowledgable explanations, significantly changes how the film appeals to the spectator. Imagined as military personnel, the spectators are given the central message that the military campaign against the enemy malaria can be and has been won.

Enemy Malaria does not import from the earlier films the powerful and impressive images of machines and factories that seek to overwhelm the spectator with their size and strength. Rather, the military sanitary campaign is center stage, with maps depicting malaria-infested areas and a military organization fighting the biological enemy with weapons ranging from preventive Bayer Atebrin and Plasmochin administration to mechanical protection by mosquito nets, chemical treatment of landscapes, and swamp drainage. In contrast to the 1934 film, Bayer chemicals are individually presented but represent only one aspect of the overall malaria campaign. Audiences are asked to identify with German soldiers, the only figures given any individuality in the film, while local "native" populations are considered only as reservoirs of infection: malaria infestation in these populations serves as a way of indicating the risk to the German troops. Bayer's chemicals function rather as icons of domination and elements of systematic organization, a way of rationalizing society and space, much as the military, which produced the film, sought to dominate and organize local populations. Visually, even the animation sequences (which illustrated the science of malaria and its eradication) indicate how NS health education propaganda under war conditions after 1939 reoriented its principle structure around the emotional stories of individuals and the organizational system ruling the social body. The life cycle animation sequence in *Enemy Malaria* is not a visual chain of the sort found in the 1934 film but a circle revolving around one individual. The film tries to evoke individual emotions and promote transformation in "socially irresponsible attitudes of individuals" that represent reservoirs for transmission. Despite its inclusion in the list of Bayer-produced image-building films, *Feind Malaria* illustrates the rupture that entry into war produced in our corpus, where after 1939 corporate film clearly was subordinated to military imperatives, becoming thus officially part of mainstream NS political propaganda mobilizing soldiers and nourishing the imagery of the advent of a new NS order symbolized by the musically orchestrated micro-cinematographically filmed dramatized hatching of a mosquito egg into a full-fledged entity.

Conclusion

The foregoing has highlighted the limitations of using the label "industrial" or "corporate" film to capture the Bayer films of the 1930s and 1940s.[106] While they were produced by an industrial corporation, the company itself did not use the label. Instead, it divided its films into five different categories, defined in part by the audiences they were intended to reach and the type of message the company wanted to project: popular advertisement films, scientific demonstration films, Kulturfilm, image-building films (*Wert-Werbungsfilm*) and special films. Some of these films had a public health component. However, Bayer's fivefold classification of its films also problematizes the term *public health education film* in relation to Bayer's output. Such a label does not fully capture what the company hoped to achieve in producing and releasing them. While audiences might learn something about the causes of disease and illness and interventions against them, the company wanted much more of its films. As recent analyses of utility film have argued, industrial film is highly situational.[107] Bayer's films illustrate the point: they were shaped both by the intentions of its producers and sponsors (Bayer and UFA) and also by the ways in which they were distributed and screened.

Bayer's image-building films provide a window onto these issues. These films do not fit easily into any one film category: they comprised a mix of influences from different film genres—research films, (health) educational films, industrial films, and Kulturfilm. Such film genres were, of course, not Bayer's invention. They had been used by a variety of different organizations—government public health agencies, the military, and private health organizations, among others—to promote their various agendas long before Bayer became interested in them. Bayer's innovation was twofold: it brought them together to form a new type of film (the image-building film) and turned them into corporate tools for wide-ranging global promotional strategies. In this endeavor, it relied on experienced and renowned filmmakers from the UFA culture and education unit. As such this story is not only about how Bayer's industrial *Wert-Werbungsfilme* imported, mimicked, and transformed established medical-subject-related documentary-film genres of the 1920s and 1930, but also about how this process of imitation and transformation was aided by one of the leading film companies in Germany.

The 1938 Bayer production *In the Service of Humanity* illustrates a further point of this essay: that industrial image-building films communicating good health deliberately created audio-visual ambiguities that could be harnessed to corporate interests and matched to drugs' inherently ambiguous status as both medical and public health tools and as economic goods.[108] The silver-screen propagandist of Bayer products suggested that he was primarily "acting in the service of human health," fulfilling the task of informing/educating the public about possibilities of prophylaxis and so positioning Bayer as a participant in efforts to improve the health of populations, or in other terms as an ethical drug manufacturer and civil servant. Yet at the same time, I argue, he was persuading the spectator of Bayer films of the value of the company and its products. Bayer's products might have been largely absent from the films, but individual Bayer products (and Bayer itself) were invisibly promoted by suggestion and association. Mimicking health education and Kulturfilm, Bayer image-building films were media containers for corporate messages.

A focus on Bayer's corpus of image-building films also shows that production under National Socialism should be separated into two distinct periods with a watershed in 1939, when entry into war significantly changed conditions of production and films themselves. Prior to 1938, Bayer produced films in collaboration with UFA using film scripts provided by the company. Their directors might have had NS sympathies, but there were other reasons for hiring them: Kayser provided classical Kulturfilm expertise with National Socialist undertones; Ruttmann provided a combination of an alignment with official NS modernist aesthetics understood as an ensemble of aesthetic-societal practices with his technical mastery in creating visual chains and fluent transitions where film aesthetics became a tool of influencing audiences and spectator bonding. After 1939 film production was under the control of the Military Academy, and the character of this category of film changed dramatically. The style, purpose, occasion, and addressees of these films were now no longer shaped just by corporate agendas but also by demands and aesthetics of political and military health propaganda.

With German defeat in 1945, Bayer's image-building films were the target of Allied censors. The five films discussed here were shelved, and when Bayer film production resumed in the early 1950s, new productions replaced them. A 1952 production carrying the title *Malaria Bridges of Help* marked a change in corporate propaganda,[109] situating the company and its products in a larger discussion about developmental aid for less developed counties in the Southern hemisphere. Here the company sought to portray health issues as an apolitical concern that transcended the opposing ideologies of the Cold War. Health, a genuine humanitarian cause, became perfectly appropriated not only by the UN[110] and the WHO to reconstruct a democratic and peaceful Europe,[111] but also by Bayer to promote its commercial interests. Pharmaceuticals promotion for global markets no longer followed colonial orders or military mobilization but became part and parcel of humanitarian enterprises. From *In the Service of Humanity* to *Bridges of Help*, ambiguities remained in these postwar realignments. After all, as this analysis shows, image-building film when communicating good health not only depicted the sponsor as trustworthy but also, and this is what our utility film corpus analysis shows, deliberately created ambiguities that were adapted to and adaptable to the values of a time, whatever they were or are.

Appendix 2.1: List of Films Produced by Bayer between 1924 and 1945

Title	Year	Genre	Director	Product/subject	Sponsor	Length/ coproduction
Caspari-Film	1924	Industrial picture (Werkfilm)	Caspari	Industrial plant Leverkusen	Bayer/Krupp	4 reels
The moth / Die Kleidermotte	1924	SA/T	ND	Eulan	Bayer/Krupp	ND
Animated cartoons	1920s	PA	ND	Aspirin	Bayer subsidiaries US	ND
Desencin	1926	SA/T	O. Wagner	Desencin (blood pressure)	Hoechst/Bayer	ND
Rivanol	1926	SA/T	O. Wagner	Rivanol (disinfection)	Hoechst/Bayer	NF/SF 977m
Hypophysin	1926	SA/T	O. Wagner	Hypophysin (child birth)	Hoechst/Bayer	NF/SF 730m
Novocain	1926	SA/T	O. Wagner	Novocain (anesthetic)	Hoechst/Bayer	NF/SF 692m
Suprarenin	1926	SA/T	O. Wagner	Suprarenin (blood pressure)	Hoechst/Bayer	NF/SF 690m
Camphor Solution / Campherlösung Hoechst	1927	SA/T	O. Wagner	Campher-Sol.	Hoechst/Bayer	NF/SF 1042m
The new sleep medication Novonal / Das neue Schlafmittel Novonal	1927	SA/T	O. Wagner	Novonal (hypnotic)	Hoechst/Bayer	ND

(continued)

Title	Year	Genre	Director	Product/subject	Sponsor	Length/ coproduction
Examination of horses for Serum production Einstellung und Untersuchung der zur Serumgewinnung dienenden Pferde	1927	SA/T	ND	Diphtheria Serum	Hoechst/Bayer	ND
Tuberculin/Alt-Tuberkulin Koch	1927	SA/T	ND	Tuberculin	Hoechst/Bayer	NF 483m
Presentation of tetanus toxins for immunization of horses / Darstellung des Tetanus-Toxins zur Immunisierung der Pferde	1927	SA/T	O. Wagner / Pr. Bieling	Tetanus	Hoechst/Bayer	ND
Serum Film. Production of the Diphtheria antitoxin / Herstellung des Diphterie-Antitoxins (Behrings Diphterie Heilmittel Hoechst)	1927	SA/T	ND	Diphtheria Serum	Hoechst/Bayer	NF/SF 690m
Rats and fighting them Ratten und ihre Bekämpfung	1927	SA/T	ND	ND	Bayer: Plant protection Dept	ND
Images from German wine growing / Bilder aus dem deutschen Weinbau	1927	SA/T	ND	Nosprasit, Gralit, Aresin	Bayer: Plant protection Dept	SF 466m

Falstaff	1928	PA	Pinschewer	Cafiaspirina	Bayer	ND
Sinbad the Sailor / Sinbad der Seefahrer	1928	PA	Pinschewer	Cafiaspirina	Bayer	ND
The conquered Magician / Der besiegte Zauberer	1928	PA	Pinschewer	Cafiaspirina	Bayer	ND
Don Pancho	1928	PA	Pinschewer	Cafiaspirina	Bayer	ND
Bullfight / Stierkampf	1928	PA	Pinschewer	Cafiaspirina	Bayer	ND
Scorpion	1928	SA/T	ND	ND	Hoechst/Bayer	ND
Salvarsan, production and state evaluation and clinical use / Salvarsan, seine Herstellung, staatliche Prüfung und klinische Anwendung	1928	SA/T	ND	Salvarsan	Hoechst/Bayer/ Behring	NF/SF 1980m
Chemotherapeutic investigations on ameba dysentery / Chemotherapeutische Untersuchungen zur Amoebenruhr	1929	SA/T	ND	Rivanol	Hoechst/Bayer	NF/SF 770m
Bilharzia of poultry / Die Bilharzia des Wassergeflügels	1929	SA/T	ND		Hoechst/Bayer	NF/SF 345m
The garget / Der gelbe Galt	1929	SA/T	ND	Entozon Mastitis Streptococcus	Hoechst/Bayer	NF/SF 680m

(continued)

Title	Year	Genre	Director	Product/subject	Sponsor	Length/ coproduction
Production of the German immune serum against hog pest / Herstellung vom deutschen Immunserum gegen Schweinepest	1930	SA/T	ND	Serum	Hoechst/Bayer	
Excerpts from micro-cinematography / Aussschnitte aus unseren Mikro-Aufnahmen	1930	SA/T	ND	Infectious disease	Hoechst/Bayer	NF/SF 421m
Paradentosis / Paradentose	1930?	SA/T	ND		Hoechst/Bayer	NF/SF 325m
Results from hormone research / Ergebnisse der Hormonforschung	1930	SA/T	ND	Hormones	Hoechst/Bayer	NF/SF 1300m
Color and medicament substances / Farbstoff und Arzneistoff	1930	SA/T	ND	Antipyretics, Anesthetics	Hoechst/Bayer	
Novocain-Suprarenin-Carpule	1930	SA/T	ND	Novocain injection	Hoechst/Bayer	NF/SF 860m
Carl Duisberg The tale of your life Das Märchen eines Lebens	1931	A	ND	70th anniversary C. Duisberg	Bayer	

In one hour around the world In 1 Stunde um die Erde	1931	A	Pinschewer	70th anniversary R. Mann	Bayer	
Sleeping sickness / Schlafkrankheit der Menschen	1931	SA/T	Zschuke	Germanin Bayer 205	Bayer	130m
Biological evaluation of Digitalis Biologische Auswertung von Digitaliskörpern	1931	SA/T		Digitalis -Evaluation	Hoechst/Bayer	NF/SF 300m
Taenia taeniaformis, ein Bandwurm der Katze	1931	SA/T			Hoechst/Bayer	NF 155m
Experimental methods of circulation research / Experimentelle Methoden der Kreislaufforschung	1931	SA/T			Hoechst/Bayer	NF/SF 735m
Diphyllobothrium latum, the tapeworm of man, causal agent of bothriocephalosis anemia / Diphyllobothrium latum, der breite Bandwurm des Menschen, Erreger der Bothryociphalus-Anaemie	1931	SA/T			Hoechst/Bayer	NF/SF 352m
Three noblemen / Die drei Kavaliere	1932	PA	Pinschewer	Aspirin	Bayer	NF/SF 296m

(continued)

Title	Year	Genre	Director	Product/subject	Sponsor	Length/ coproduction
Beri-Beri	1932	SA/T			Bayer	SF
Opisthorchis felineus. Der Katzen-Leberegel	1932	SA/T			Hoechst/Bayer	
The physician (is right) / Der Arzt (hat Recht)	1933	PA		Eldoform	Bayer	NF/SF 40m
Big people, small people / Grosse Leute, kleine Leute	1933	PA		Eldoform / Helmitol	Bayer	NF/SF 40m
Syphilis and Salvarsan / Syphilis und Salvarsan	1933	SA/T		Salvarsan (updated)	Hoechst/Bayer	
Noise / Lärm	1933?	PA		Adalin	Bayer	NF/SF 30m
Sleep / Schlaf	1933?	PA		Adalin	Bayer	NF/SF 30m
Kidney / Niere (Animation / Trick)	1933?	PA		Helmitol	Bayer	NF/SF 40m
Sports / Sport	1933?	PA		Helmitol	Bayer	NF/SF 40m
Children / Kinder	1933?	PA		Kresival	Bayer	NF/SF 40m
Rain / Regen	1933?	PA		Kresival	Bayer	NF/SF 40m
White wonder / Das weisse Wunder	1933?	PA		Aspirin	Bayer	NF/SF 167m
Cortase	1933?	PA		Aspirin	Bayer	NF/SF 135m
The chain / Die Kette	1933?	PA		Aspirin	Bayer	NF/SF 113m
A horrible day / Un dia horoso	1933?	PA		Mitigal	Bayer	NF/SF 100m

Victory / Sieg	1933?	PA		Panflavin	Bayer	NF/SF 80m
Avertin	1933?	SA/T		Avertin	Bayer	NF/SF 1250m
Dyestuff and drugs / Farb und Arzneistoffe	1933?	SA/T			Bayer	NF/SF 788m
The German egg / Das deutsche Frischei	1933?	SA/T			Bayer	NF 1570m
Germanin	1933?	SA/T		Germanin	Bayer	NF/SF 165m
Hexeton	1933?	SA/T		Hexeton	Bayer	NF/SF 280m
Vigantol	1933?	SA/T		Vigantol	Bayer	NF/SF 933m
Dental products / Zahntechnische Produkte	1933?	SA/T		Xanthano, Moldano,Duroterm	Bayer	NF/SF 862m
Wheat diseases and fighting them / Getreidekrankheiten und ihre Bekämpfung	1933?	SA/T		Ceresan / agriculture	Bayer	NF/SF 910m
The man without memory / Der Mann ohne Gedächtnis	1933?	S			Bayer	NF/SF 1140m
A chapter in the productive battle / Ein Ausschnitt aus der Erzeugungsschlacht	1933?	SA/T		Ceresan / agriculture	Bayer	SF 112m
The Sacred Skirt / Der heilige Rock	1933	S			Bayer	NF/SF 285m

(continued)

Title	Year	Genre	Director	Product/subject	Sponsor	Length/ coproduction
Stored sun energy / Gespeicherte Sonnenenergie	**1934**	**WW**	**Ulrich Kayser**	**Pyramidon, Adalin, Vigantol**	**Bayer/UFA**	**NF 1036m**
Bayer I.G Farbenindustrie AG (adapted from Stored sun energy)	1934	Industrial picture	Ulrich Kayser		Bayer	NF/SF 1027
Diphtherie-Serum	1934	SA/T		Serum	Hoechst/Bayer	NF/SF 1063m
Pain and fighting it / Der Schmerz und seine Bekämpfung	1934	SA/T		Corbasil (Anaesthetics)	Hoechst/Bayer	NF/SF 684m
Malaria (and fighting it) /(und ihre Bekämpfung)	**1934**	**WW (SA/T)**	**Ulrich Kayser**	**Anti-malarials**	**Bayer/UFA/ (Hoechst)**	**NF 772m**
Malaria. Experimental research and clinical results (Plasmochin) / Experimentelle Forschung und klinische Ergebnisse (Plasmochin)	1934	SA/T	Ulrich Kayser	Plasmochin / Anti-malarials	Bayer	NF/SF 980m
Typhoral	1934	SA/T			Bayer/ Kinomat, Limberg & Peters	NF/SF 279m
Almighty sleep / Allmacht Schlaf	1934	SA/T			Bayer/UFA	

African adventure / Afrikanisches Abenteur	1934	PA		Plasmochin, Atebrin, Anti-malarials	Bayer	NF/SF 180m
African adventure / Afrikanisches Abenteur	1934	PA		Chinoplasmin, Anti-malarials	Bayer	NF/SF 175m
From the workshop of modern medicaments / Aus der Werkstatt moderner Arzneimittel	1935	SA/T K	Ulrich Kayser		Bayer/UFA	NF 382m
Under the Bayer Cross / Unter dem Bayerkreuz	1935	PA	Ulrich Kayser		Bayer	NF/SF 100m
Across Germany / Deutschland kreuz und quer	1935	S			Bayer	
Danger is everywhere / Gefahren überall	1936	PA			Bayer	
Creeping Poison – Burden of Humanity (Schleichendes Gift – Geissel der Menschheit	**1936**	**WW**		**Anti-syphilis**	**Bayer/UFA**	**NF/SF 827m**
Ascaris / Die Spulwurmkrankheit	1936	SA/T		Askaridol	Hoechst/Bayer	NF/SF 292m
Wonders revealed by the microscope / Wunder die das Mikroskop erschliesst	1936	SA/T		Microscopy	Hoechst/Bayer	
Blood / Das Blut	1936	SA/T			Hoechst/Bayer	

(continued)

Title	Year	Genre	Director	Product/subject	Sponsor	Length/ coproduction
Olympics / Olympiade	1936	S			Bayer	
Children games / Kinderspiele	1937	PA			Bayer	
Under the banner of trust / Im Zeichen des Vertrauen	**1937**	**WW**	**Walter Ruttmann**		**Bayer/UFA**	
In the Service of Humanity / Im Dienste der Menschheit	1938		Walter Ruttmann		Bayer/UFA	
Plant protection is required / Pflanzenschutz tut Not	1936/37	T		Nosprasit, Solbar, Ustin Venetan	Bayer Plant protection Dept	SF 365m
Results from vitamin research /Ergebnisse aus der Vitamin-Forschung	1937	SA/T			Hoechst/Bayer	
Inquiries on dental materials / Werkstoff-Untersuchung	1937	SA/T		Dental raw material evaluation	Hoechst/Bayer	
Entstehung und Bekämpfung der Leberegel-Seuche	1936/37	SA/T		Igitol	Hoechst/Bayer	NF 873m
The rapid Peter / Der schnelle Peter	1938	PA			Bayer	

War on flies: Mückenkrieg	1938	PA		Anti-malarials	Bayer
On physiology and pathology of digestion / Aus der Physizologie und Pathologie der Verdauung	1938	SA/T		Digestion	Hoechst/Bayer
The electron microscope in the service of medical research / Das Elektronenmikroskop im Dienste der medizinischen Forschung	1938	SA/T		Description of Electron microscope	Hoechst/Bayer
Cerebellum and psyche / Stammhirn und Psyche	1938	SA/T			Bayer / Studio Epkens (Köln)
Dental jaw surgery Kieferchirurgie	1938	SA/T			Bayer
Local anesthesia / Lokalanaesthesie	1938	SA/T			Bayer
Fruits in danger / Frucht in Gefahr	1938	SA/T			Bayer: Plant protection Dept
Chemotherapy of bacterial infections / Chemotherapie bakterieller Infektionen	1940 (?)	SA/T	Sergius Koncek		Bayer

(continued)

Title	Year	Genre	Director	Product/subject	Sponsor	Length/ coproduction
Teeth in danger / Zähne in Not	1940	SA/T			Bayer	
Emergency care in dental jaw surgery / Unfallbehandlung in der Kieferchirurgie	1942 (?)	SA/T			Bayer	
Adventure at the bottom of the sea / Abenteur auf dem Meeresgrund	1942 (?)	PA			Bayer / VEPRO A.S	
An old seawolf tells a story / Ein alter Seebär erzählt	1942 (?)	PA			Bayer / VEPRO A.S	
The wish ring / Der Wunschring	1942 (?)	PA			Bayer / VEPRO A.S	
The pub / Taverne	1942 (?)	PA			Bayer / VEPRO A.S	
Enemy Malaria / Feind Malaria	**1942**	**WW**			**Bayer/ Military Academy**	
Trachoma	1942	SA/T			Bayer	
Syphilis	1942	SA/T			Bayer	
Handicapped veteran's sport activities			Dr. Remberg		Bayer	

Legend: White = Bayer films; gray = Hoechst-Bayer films; bold = Wertwerbungsfilme forming the corpus analyzed in the present article.
R = Representational film (Repräsentationsfilm); SR = Sales representative film (Vertreterfilm); T = Training film (Lehrfilm); E = Fair exhibition film; M = Manufacturing film; A = Anniversary film; PA = Popular advertisement film (Populärer Werbefilm [1]); SA = Scientific advertisement

film (Wissenschaftlicher Werbefilm/Wissenschaftlicher Demonstrationsfilm [2]); K= Kulturfilm [3]; WW = Image-building representational film (Wertwerbungsfilm [4]); S=Special films (*Sonderfilm*); ND = No data.

Sources: The list of films produced by Bayer (and Hoechst) between 1925 and 1942 has been compiled from the following manuscripts in the Bayer Archives: Dr. Weintraud, *Chronologische Darstellung der Entwicklung der Bayer-Filmstelle,* unpublished typescript, forty-six pages, here pages 42–46. The list includes twenty-three "scientific films" produced between 1932 and 1942. Dr. Lautenschläger, *A Historical Note on the Development of the Filmabteilung des Werkes Hoechst* accounts for thirty-eight films produced by Hoechst between 1925 and 1941. Bayer Archives, A. Werksfilme Allgemeines, 92/1, vol. 1. *Bayer-Filme Aufstellung Jahreswende 1935–36,* Bayer Archives, A.3.Filmverzeichnisse, 92/1.1 Film Bayer Filmverzeichnis 1935/36–74.

The Bayer Archives hold an electronic database on their film collection. A chronological selection of films produced before 1945 yields 106 entries. The undated film list by Weintraud reflects films produced, but it is not exhaustive in view of short and minor advertisement films. The number of films from the present electronic database reflects films rescued and stored and thus accessible.

Classical studies of industrial film suggest five types of subcategories for industrial or corporate film, defined here as commissioned films used as industrial communication tools: representation film (presenting general aspects of the business), sales representative film (used with potential customers), training film (instructing employees), fair exhibition film (produced for trade exhibitions), and manufacturing film (showing manufacturing processes). Representation films or image films (*Repräsentationsfilm*) give an overview of a corporation, representative's film (*Vertreterfilm*) demonstrates the functioning of products, educational and training films (*Lehrfilm*) instruct employees, trade fair and exhibition films (*Ausstellungsfilm*) are made for these occasions, and manufacturing or process film (*Fabrikationsfilm*) shows the step-by-step manufacturing of goods. Yvonne Zimmermann, "'What Hollywood Is to America, the Corporate Film Is to Switzerland': Remarks on Industrial Film as Utility Film," in *Films That Work: Industrial Film and the Productivity of Media*, ed. Vinzenz Hediger and Patrick Vonderau (Amsterdam: Amsterdam University Press, 2009), 104–6. See also Manfred Rasch, *Industriefilm 1948–1959: Filme aus Wirtschaftsarchiven im Ruhrgebiet* (Essen: Klartext-Verlag, 2003); and Rasch, *Industriefilm 1960–1969: Filme aus Wirtschaftsarchiven im Ruhrgebiet; mit einem Nachtrag zu "Industriefilm 1948–1959"* (Essen: Klartext-Verlag, 2011).

An interwar classification of industrial film by Ascher is based strictly on intended sponsor content, meaning here representation, usage, instructions for use and manufacturing process identifying four categories: Repräsentationsfilm, Anwendungsfilm, Gebrauchsanweisungsfilm, and Fabrikationsfilm. Curt Ascher, "Der Industriefiml, seine Anwendung und Verbreitung," in *Das Kulturfilmbuch*, ed. E. Beyfuss and A. Kossowsky (Berlin: Carl P. Chryselius'scher Verlag, 1924), 160–65.

Classical studies of visual education / instruction distinguish between teaching film (used in schools for instruction) and educational film (used beyond school for child and adult education). Furthermore, catalogues for teaching and educational film (e.g., Ohio State, Kentucky State, Kansas State, or University of Missouri) distinguish purely instructional films (sponsored by state or educational boards) and industrial advertisement films with educational value. J. Benoit-Lévy, *L'instruction visuelle aux Etats-Unis* (Paris: Cinéopse, 1936). In the case of health-related and medical films, the latter can be assimilated with *Scientific advertisement/teaching film* (Wissenschaftlicher Werbefilm/Lehrfilm) since the pictures address adult audiences (physicians) and are classified as SA/T in the table.

Following the historical approach of an "archaeology of practices," this table refers to the categories used by Bayer in its early film catalogues to classify film: (1) Popular advertisement films (*Populäre Werbefilm*), (2) Scientific demonstration films (*Wissenschaftlicher Demonstrationsfilm*), (3) *Kulturfilm*, (4) Image-building films (*Wert-Werbungsfilm*), and finally (5) Special films (*Sonderfilm*). Image-building films analyzed here belong in classical industry film classifications to the category of representational film. Our essay argues that image-building films nevertheless represent a coherent subcategory of these. Furthermore, boundaries between categories are fluent. Bayer representational image-building films analyzed here include scenes of manufacturing processes and instruct physicians about drug use and dosage combining thus elements from training, scientific advertisement, representation, manufacturing, and popular advertisement. This table is incomplete due to lack of information for popular advertisement films produced after 1928.

Appendix 2.2: Bayer Wertwerbungs Film Corpus 1934–42 in coproduction with UFA

Title	Year	Director	Production team	Adapted / shortened versions	Length and technical details
Stored sun energy / Gespeicherte Sonnenenergie	1934	Ulrich Kayser	Script: Karl Spielmann Camera: Gerhard Müller Music: Rudolf Perak	Languages: German, Spanish, Portuguese, Italian, French, English, and Dutch	B&W, NF and SF, sound, 1036m (NF)
			Micro-cinematography: ND Animation: ND	2B: *From the workshop of modern medicaments / Aus der Werkstatt moderner Arzneimittel, Kulturfilm.*	B&W, NF, sound 382m (NF)
	1935		Narrator: Fritz Alberti Sound operator: Heinz Orlich	2C: *Under the Bayer Cross/ Unter dem Bayerkreuz.* Languages: German, Spanish, Portuguese, Romanian, French, English, Dutch, and Greek	Shortened popular advertisement film NF and SF, sound, 100m (NF)
Malaria	1934	Ulrich Kayser	Script: Karl Spielmann Camera: Erich Menzel[1] Music: Walter Schütze	Languages: German, Spanish, Portuguese, Italian, French, English, and Dutch	B&W, NF and SF, sound, 772m (NF)
			Micro-cinematography: ND Animation: Bernhard Huth	Stock shots integrated into *Plasmochin* (1934) and *Malaria. Experimental research and clinical results (Experimentelle Forschung und klinische Ergebnisse* (1934)	980m (NF)

Creeping Poison – Burden of Humanity / Schleichendes Gift – Geissel der Menschheit[2]	1936	Ulrich Kayser	Script: Karl Spielmann Camera: Gerhard Müller, W. Rahn Music: Rudolf Perak	Languages: German, Spanish, Portuguese, French, English, and Italian.	B&W, NF and SF, sound, 827m (NF) 328m (SF)
Under the banner of trust / Im Zeichen des Vertrauen	1937	Walter Ruttmann	Script: Walter Ruttmann and Emil Endres Camera: Gerhard Müller Music: Walter Zeller	Languages: German and English Shortened version: *Im Dienste der Menschheit/In the Service of Humanity*	B&W, NF, sound
Enemy Malaria / Feind Malaria[3]	1942	Militärärtzliche Akademie	Micro-cinematography: Sergius Koncek Animation: VEPRO, Denmark	Language: German	B&W, NF, sound, 1207m (NF)

Table 2: Bayer Wertwerbungsfilm corpus 1934–42

NF = Normal Film (35 mm). SF = Small Film (16mm).

Films are characterized in length in meters when possible in order to possibly distinguish different versions of a film with identical title. To translate these into spectator time, the Normalfilm (NF) projected at 24 images per second takes 3.66 minutes per 100m. The small film (SF) at the same rate takes 9.09 minutes per 100m. All versions mentioned in the following refer to films held at the Bayer Archives.

1. Erich Menzel is known for his artistic and "filmic film" framing of images and for his use of mobile camera. *Jeanpaul Goergen, "Städtebilder zwischen Heimattümelei und Urbanität," in Geschichte des dokumentarischen Films in Deutschland: Band 3, Drittes Reich 1933–1945*, ed. Peter Zimmermann and Kay Hoffman (Stuttgart: Reclam, 2005), 320–32, esp. 327.

2. The film is not mentioned in Zimmermann and Hoffmann, *Geschichte des dokumentarischen Films in Deutschland: Band 3.* Two films with partially identical title and similar subject frame the Bayer version: on the one side, *Die Geißel der Menschheit*, produced during World War I by Wiener Kunstfilm on hereditary diseases, and on the other side *Schleichendes Gift* (1946), directed by Hermann Wallbrück from a script by Stefan Wolfram. Produced in Austria, the film was released in Sweden in 1947. This production is characterized in 1968 in a correspondence between Sonderfilm-

(continued)

Verleih Zwicker and the BZGA as follows: “Wir beabsichtigen, da wir vor 15 Jahren einen Schwarz-Weiss-Film herausbrachten unter dem Titel *‘Schleichendes Gift’* einen zweiten Teil herzustellen, und zwar modern, der heutigen Zeit entsprechend.” See B310 Bundeszentrale für gesundheitliche Aufklärung: Verwaltung—Film Akten: 29, Brief von Sonderfilm-Verleih Zwicker, Rudolf Zwicker an die BZgA, Dr. Schulze-Rohnhoff 12. February 1968. I thank Anja Lauköter for directing me to this source.

3. A copy of the film exists at the BundesArchiv-Filmarchiv under the signature BAB :MNR :18107 and is dated as produced in 1940 there.

Notes

1. Stuart Ewen, *PR! A Social History of Spin* (New York: Basic Books, 1996).

2. Edward L. Bernays, *Propaganda* (New York: H. Liveright, 1928); Walter Lippmann, *Public Opinion* (New York: Harcourt, Brace and Co, 1922); and Harold D. Lasswell, Ralph D. Casey, and Bruce Lannes Smith, *Propaganda and Promotional Activities: An Annotated Bibliography* (Minneapolis: University of Minnesota Press, 1935). For an overview of these essential texts, see Ewen, *PR!*, 174–232; and Roland Marchand, *Creating the Corporate Soul: The Rise of Public Relations and Corporate Imagery in American Big Business* (Berkeley: University of California Press, 1998).

3. Marchand, *Creating the Corporate Soul*, 131.

4. Ewen, *PR!*, 207–12.

5. For the general history of the therapeutic revolution and the pharmaceutical industry, see Jeremy Greene, Flurin Condrau, and Elizabeth Siegel Watkins, eds., *Therapeutic Revolutions: Pharmaceuticals and Social Change in the Twentieth Century* (Chicago: University of Chicago Press, 2016); Jeremy Greene and Elizabeth Siegel Watkins, eds., *Prescribed: Writing, Filling, Using, and Abusing the Prescription in Modern America* (Baltimore: Johns Hopkins University Press, 2012); Jean-Paul Gaudillière and Volker Hess, eds., *Ways of Regulating Drugs in the 19th and 20th Centuries* (Basingstoke, UK: Palgrave Macmillan, 2012); Viviane Quirke and Judy Slinn, eds., *Perspectives on Twentieth-Century Pharmaceuticals* (Bern, Switzerland: Peter Lang AG, 2009); John Lesch, *The First Miracle Drugs: How the Sulfa Drugs Transformed Medicine* (Oxford: Oxford University Press, 2007); Viviane Quirke, *Collaboration in the Pharmaceutical Drug Industry: Changing Relationships in Britain and France 1933–1965* (New York: Routledge, 2007); Wolfgang Wimmer, "Innovation in the German Pharmaceutical Industry," in *The Chemical Industry in Europe, 1850–1914: Industrial Growth, Pollution, and Professionalization*, ed. Ernst Homburg, Anthony S. Travis, and Harm G. Schröter (Dordrecht, Netherlands: Kluwer, 1998), 287–88; Wolfgang Wimmer, *Wir haben fast immer was Neues: Gesundheitswesen und Innovationen der Pharma-Industrie in Deutschland, 1880–1935* (Berlin: Duncker & Humblot, 1994); Ernst Bäumler, *Farben, Formeln, Forscher: Hoechst und die Geschichte der industriellen Chemie in Deutschland* (Munich: Piper, 1989); John P. Swann, *Academic Scientists and the Pharmaceutical Industry: Cooperative Research in Twentieth Century America* (Baltimore: Johns Hopkins University Press, 1988); Jonathan Liebenau, "Industrial R&D in Pharmaceutical Firms in the Early Twentieth Century," *Business History Review* 26, no. 3 (1984): 329–46; and Jonathan Liebenau, "Scientific Ambitions: The Pharmaceutical Industry 1900–1920," *Pharmacy in History* 27 (1985): 3–11.

6. Joseph M. Gabriel, *Medical Monopoly: Intellectual Property Rights and the Origins of the Modern Pharmaceutical Industry* (Chicago: University of Chicago Press, 2014).

7. Ewen, *PR!*, 146–232.

8. Charles Mann and Mark L. Plummer, *The Aspirin Wars: Money, Medicine and 100 Years of Rampant Competition* (New York: Knopf, 1991).

9. For a corporate history of Bayer, see Erik Verg, *Milestones: The Bayer Story 1863–1988* (Leverkusen, Germany: Bayer AG, 1988); Tobias Cramer, *Die Rückkehr ins Pharmageschäft: Marktstrategien der Farbenfabriken vorm. Friedr. Bayer &Co. in Lateinamerika nach dem Ersten Weltkrieg* (Berlin: Wissenschaftlicher Verlag, 2010); Georg Meyer-Thurow, "The Industrialization of Invention: A Case Study from the

German Chemical Industry," *ISIS* 73 (1982): 363–81; John Beer, *The Emergence of the German Dye Industry* (Urbana: University of Illinois Press, 1959); and Thomas Martin Reimer, "Bayer &Company in the United States: German Dyes, Drugs, and Cartels in the Progressive Era" (PhD diss., Syracuse University, 1996). Since 1925 the three corporations Hoechst, Bayer, and BASF were associated in the IG Farben AG. On IG Farben, see Stephan Lindner, *Inside I.G. Farben: Hoechst during the Third Reich* (Cambridge: Cambridge University Press, 2008); Gottfried Plumpe, *Die I.G. Farbenindustrie AG: Wirtschaft, Technik und Politik 1904–1945* (Berlin: Duncker & Humblot, 1990); Peter Hayes, *Industry and Ideology: The IG Farben in the Nazi Era* (Cambridge: Cambridge University Press, 1987); and Helmuth Tammen, *Die I.G. Farbenindustrie Aktiengesellschaft (1925–1933): Ein Chemiekonzern in der Weimarer Republik* (Berlin: Selbstverlag, 1978).

10. Gabriel, *Medical Monopoly*, 142.

11. Jean-Paul Gaudillière and Ulrike Thoms, eds., *The Development of Scientific Marketing in the Twentieth Century: Research for Sales in the Pharmaceutical Industry* (London: Pickering & Chato, 2015).

12. Ewen, *PR!*, 3–18, 146–73.

13. Bernays, *Propaganda*, 93. Cited here after the 2005 reedition.

14. Vinzenz Hediger and Patrick Vonderau, eds., *Films That Work: Industrial Film and the Productivity of Media* (Amsterdam: Amsterdam University Press, 2009), 11.

15. Marchand, *Corporate Soul*, 174–81.

16. Anonymous, "The Ninth Imperial Power," *Zepro-Nachrichten* 1 (1934): 2–4.

17. In a general sense, *Wertwerbung* aligns with terminology of the pharmaceutical industry research and development such as *Wertbestimmung*, a term used for the experimental and clinical evaluation of the value and use of specific drugs. For analysis of the terminology, see Christian Bonah, "'We Need for Digitalis Preparations What the State Has Established for Serumtherapy . . .' From Collecting Plants to International Standardization: The Strophanthin Case, 1900–1938," in *Evaluating and Standardizing Therapeutic Agents 1890–1950*, ed. Christoph Gradmann and Jonathan Simon (London: Palgrave, 2010), 202–28. The idea of *Wertwerbung* was imported in 1922 as a principle from America, where Bayer had lost its patents and engaged court trials against American Bayer production plants that were independent subsidiaries representing the brand independently. Cramer, *Die Rückkehr ins Pharmageschäft*, 2010.

18. Gaudillière, *Development of Scientific Marketing*, 1–14.

19. *Consumer* and *consumption* are understood here as twentieth-century constructions in capitalist societies. Frank Trentmann, ed., *The Making of the Consumer: Knowledge, Power and Identity in the Modern World* (Oxford: Berg, 2006); Lizabeth Cohen, *A Consumers' Republic: The Politics of Mass Consumption in Postwar America* (New York: Alfred A. Knopf, 2003); and Heinz-Gerhard Haupt and Claudius Torp, *Die Konsumgesellschaft in Deutschland 1890–1990: Ein Handbuch* (Frankfurt am Main: Campus Verlag, 2009).

20. Gabriel, *Medical Monopoly*, 195–236.

21. Cramer, *Die Rückkehr ins Pharmageschäft*.

22. For the figure of four hundred thousand films for the United States, see Patrick Vonderau, "Vernacular Archiving: An interview with Rick Prelinger," in

Hediger and Vondeau, *Films That Work*, 53. It is estimated as well that one-third to one-half of the films have been lost, the result of neglect.

23. Many sponsored, or ephemeral, films are also orphan works, since they lack copyright owners and active custodians to guarantee their long-term preservation. Hediger and Vonderau, *Films That Work*. Also see the earlier, differing German version: Vinzenz Hediger and Patrick Vonderau, eds., *Filmische Mittel, industrielle Zwecke: Das Werk des Industriefilms* (Berlin: Vorwerk 8, 2007); and Klaus Kreimeier, Antje Ehmann, and Jeanpaul Goergen, eds., *Geschichte des dokumentarischen Films in Deutschland: Band 2, Weimarer Republik 1918–1933* (Stuttgart, Germany: Reclam, 2005).

24. My gratitude and recognition to Michael Frings and the Bayer Archives Corporate History Service for the considerable work he is achieving in conservation and restoration of films that oftentimes are designated as ephemeral due to the limited validity of their central message and thus simply disappear once they have accomplished (or not) their initial purpose. And especially for the extreme efficacy and diligence of Michael Frings in assisting my research in this domain.

25. Utility film may be defined as documentary film produced under contract from industrial, corporate, teaching or educational bodies. These films were produced under commission as purpose oriented audio-visual communication tools with clearly established objectives addressed to specific audiences that accomplish their job when messages are received by specified spectators whose behavior is influenced according to commissioner's interests. At the heart of Yvonne Zimmermann's reconceptualization of utility films lies a pragmatic analytical approach to study these films in context of film use (utility) arguing that intention and use define the meanings of the films. Yvonne Zimmermann, "'What Hollywood Is to America, the Corporate Film Is to Switzerland': Remarks on Industrial Film as Utility Film," in Hediger and Vonderau, *Films That Work*, 101–17.

26. Hediger and Vonderau, *Films That Work*; Hediger and Vonderau, *Filmische Mittel, industrielle Zwecke*; and Yvonne Zimmermann, *Schaufenster Schweiz: Dokumentarische Gebrauchsfilme 1896–1964* (Zurich, Switzerland: Limmat Verlag 2011). See as well the introduction.

27. Thomas Elsaesser, "Archives and Archaeologies: The Place of Non-fiction Film in Contemporary Media," in Hediger and Vonderau, *Films That Work*, 22.

28. For a seminal essay on the film corpus approach, see Michèle Lagny, "Film History: or History Expropriated," *Film History* 6, no. 1 (1994): 26–44.

29. For reflections on the film categories used here see the legend of appendix 2.1.

30. As an illustration, see, for example, volumes 2 and 3 of the recent history of documentary films in Germany, which has sections on cars, roads, and construction but overall pay little attention to pharmaceutical and chemical industrial films. Kreimeier, Ehmann, and Goergen, *Geschichte des dokumentarischen Films in Deutschland: Band 2*. Peter Zimmermann and Kay Hoffmann, eds., *Geschichte des dokumentarischen Films in Deutschland: Band 3, 'Drittes Reich' 1933–1945* (Stuttgart, Germany: Reclam, 2005).

31. Jonathan Auerbach and Russ Castronovo, *The Oxford Handbook of Propaganda Studies* (New York: Oxford University Press, 2013).

32. Peter Zimmermann and Kay Hoffmann, "Filmforschung im Zeichen von Totalitarismustheorie, Faschismuskritik und Propagandaanalyse," in Zimmermann and Hoffmann, *Geschichte des dokumentarischen Films in Deutschland: Band 3*, 33–37.

33. This criticism implies especially that fascism prevention and coming to terms with the NS past ultimately led to warnings about persuasion directly suggesting the exculpation of large parts of German society supposed to have been misled by a restricted number of NS propaganda activists. This interpretation has been widely revised since the 1980s.

34. Peter Zimmermann and Kay Hoffmann, "Vom, Nazi-Kino zum Film im Dritten Reich: Perspektivenwechsel in der Filmwissenschaft," in Zimmermann and Hoffmann, *Geschichte des dokumentarischen Films in Deutschland: Band 3*, 38–44.

35. Peter Zimmermann and Kay Hoffmann, "Von der Gleichschaltungs- und Propaganda-These zur differenzierten Erforschung dokumentarischer Genres, in Zimmermann and Hoffmann, *Geschichte des dokumentarischen Films in Deutschland: Band 3*, 45–56.

36. Jeanpaul Goergen, "Industrie und Werbefilme," in Kreimeier, Ehmann, and Goergen, *Geschichte des dokumentarischen Films in Deutschland: Band 2*, 33–38; and Jeanpaul Goergen,"In filmo veritas! Inhaltlich vollkommen wahr; Werbefilme und ihre Produzenten," in Kreimeier, Ehmann, and Goergen, *Geschichte des dokumentarischen Films in Deutschland: Band 2*, 348–63. Marchand, *Corporate Soul*, 2.

37. The Krupp steel corporation was one of the first German corporations to create an in-house film department. Renate Köhne-Lindenlaub, "Filme von Krupp: Anmerkungen zu ihrer Entstehung, Nutzung und Überlieferung," in *Industriefilm—Medium und Quelle: Beispiele aus der Eisen und Stahlindustrie*, ed. Manfred Raasch, Karl-Peter Ellerbrock, and Renate Köhne-Lindenlaub (Essen, Germany: Klartext Verlag, 1997), 41–58.

38. After the scenario written by the director of the educational department, Dr. Caspari. Bayer Archives, Dr. Weintraud, "Chronologische Darstellung der Entwicklung der Bayer-Filmstelle," unpublished typescript, forty-six pp. (Leverkusen, Germany: Bayer Corporate Archives).

39. Weintraud, *Chronologische Darstellung*, 2; Alexander Friedland, "'. . . doch erscheint in seiner Denkschrift die Bedeutung des klinischen Films für den Unterricht allzustark betont': Vom Scheitern des Medizinisch-kinematographischen Instituts der Charité 1923–1931," *Medizinhistorisches Journal* 52 (2017): 148–79.

40. Oskar Wagner, "The Cinematograph in the Service of Medical and Biological Research in Medicine in Its Chemical Aspects," *Reports from the Medico-Chemical Research Laboratories of the IG Farbenindustrie Aktiengesellschaft* (1934), 391–404.

41. Wilhelm Rahn was a former sales director of the pharmaceutical company Casella, which merged in 1926 with Hoechst, where he integrated the pharmaceutical department.

42. *Rats and fighting them* and *Images from German wine growing* (see appendix 2.1).

43. Martin Loiperdinger, *Julius Pinschewer: Klassiker des Werbefilms* (Berlin: Absolut Medien, 2010); and André Amsler, "*Wer dem Werbefilm verfällt ist verloren für die Welt*": *Das Werk von Julius Pinschewer 1883–1961* (Zurich, Switzerland: Chronos, 1997). For further indications, see the bibliography in Amsler.

44. Weintraud, *Chronologische Darstellung*, 6.

45. *Schlafkrankheit der Menschen* (1931; Sleeping sickness) was mounted with film material from Fernando Po gathered by the director of the Bayer scientific department, Dr. Zschuke. Further films along this line include *Beri-Beri* (16mm, silent, 1932) and *Typhoral* (1934) on typhus prevention. See appendix 2.1.

46. *Three noblemen/Die drei Kavaliere* (1932). The production was commissioned and directed on the Bayer side by Eggert, who the same year became director of the DRUGOFA in Berlin.

47. Popular advertisement film production by Bayer between 1932 and 1938 included twelve further sound shorts (120m on 35mm film) for Aspirin promotion as well as New York-produced promotionals including Disney cartoons. The Bayer film department continued to produce a variety of teaching/scientific advertisement films with time leap images of streptococci and phagocytes produced by the physician and filmmaker Sergius Koncek. Weintraud, *Chronologische Darstellung*, 23.

48. Bayer employee Dr. Schamoni, responsible for the film catalogue, finalized the film *Stammhirn und Psyche* (1938), produced by the Studio Gebrüder Epkens (Cologne) in scientific collaboration with Professor de Crinis in Cologne, before Dr. Schamoni left the film department in 1938.

49. For example, *Abenteur auf dem Meeresgrund, Ein alter Seebär erzählt, Der Wunschring* and *Taverne* (incomplete). Furthermore, VEPRO produced animated films for DEGETO (Tobis-Berlin) and for Danish industry.

50. The Bayer collaborator Dr. Gönnert initiated in 1941 the production of a color film on trachoma produced for the clinical part in Cracow under Prof. Lauber, and Dr. Keil initiated the production of a new color film on syphilis. In the Bayer production, this was the third major film on Lues (syphilis) after *Salvarsan* (1929) and *Schleichendes Gift—Geissel der Menschheit* (1934 through 1936). Images were shot on 16mm Agfa-Color-Umkehrfilm. Clinical shots were filmed by Leonid Dörner in collaboration with Oberstabsarzt Dittrich at the Reserve-Lazarett in Cologne; both films were completed in 1942. A final film production before the collapse of activities under "total war" and Germany's surrender concerned a black-and-white movie on handicapped veterans' sports activities under the direction of Dr. Remberg that interfered with the Goebbels-supported Wien-Film/UFA film *Der Wille zum Leben* (1944) and received severe screening restrictions limited to corporate internal use. The film had a wider reception after 1945, especially in circles of veteran associations and physicians of accident and rehabilitation hospitals (Unfallkrankenhäusern). The film is designated as UFA production by Weintraud, whereas Elisabeth Büttner indicates that this was the next-to-last film produced by the Austrian Wien-Film production company that monopolized film production in Austria and had been integrated into the German NS film industry. The film was directed by Ulrich Kayser and Georg Wittuhn, Kayser having directed the first two Bayer Wert-Werbungsfilme in 1934. Elisabeth Büttner, "Exkurs: 'Über allem steht der grosse Befehl': Dokumentarischer Film in Österreich," in Zimmermann and Hoffmann, *Geschichte des dokumentarischen Films in Deutschland: Band 3*, 439–49. Kay Hoffmann, "Mobilisierung der Heimatfront," in Zimmermann and Hoffmann, *Geschichte des dokumentarischen Films in Deutschland: Band 3*, 634–44. A new version of *Chemotherapie bakterieller Infektionen* was completed in the first days of 1944.

51. Gottschalk was as well the cameraman for the film *Kieferchirurgie* (1938). He worked after the 1938 crisis as an independent cameraman for Bayer.

52. Weintraud, *Chronologische Darstellung*, 8.

53. Ibid., 9.

54. Bayer Archives, A.3 Filmverzeichnisse, 92/1.1 Film Bayer Filmverzeichnis 1935/36–1974 (Leverkusen, Germany: Bayer Corporate Archives). *Bayer-Filme Aufstellung Jahreswende 1935–36* (Leverkusen, Germany: Bayer Corporate Archives, 1936). This film inventory and catalogue established the five Bayer film categories presented below.

55. Bernays, *Propaganda*; Marchand, *Corporate Soul*; and Ewen, *PR!*

56. Anonymous, "The Ninth Imperial Power," *Zepro-Nachrichten* 1 (1934): 2–4.

57. *Bayer-Filme Aufstellung 1935–36.*

58. "Zentralpropaganda Nachrichten," in-house journal for modern advertisement by Bayer, 1934.

59. The Bayer Cross is the image and value symbol invented by the corporation in 1930. It displays the corporation's name twice in the form of a cross. Bayer Archives, A.3.Filmverzeichnisse, 92/1.1 Film Bayer Filmverzeichnis 1935/36–1974. *Richtlinien für Film-Veranstaltungen 1935–36*, 4.

60. Harold D. Lasswell, *Propaganda Technique in the World War* (New York: Knopf, 1927); Oliver Thomson, *Mass Persuasion in History: An Historical Analysis of the Development of Propaganda Techniques* (Edinburgh: Harris, 1977); Garth S. Jowett and Victoria O'Donnell, *Propaganda and Persuasion* (London: Sage, 1986); and Noam Chomsky, *Media Control: The Spectacular Achievements of Propaganda* (New York: Seven Stories Press, 1991).

61. *Bayer-Filme Aufstellung 1935–36*, 1.

62. Ibid.

63. Ibid.

64. *Richtlinien für Film-Veranstaltungen 1935–36*, n.p.

65. For a contemporary definition of Kulturfilm, see Edgar Beyfuss and Arthur Kossowsky, eds., *Das Kulturfilmbuch* (Berlin: Carl P. Chryselius'scher Verlag, 1924). The second volume of the *Deutsche Geschichte des dokumentarischen Films in Deutschland* analyzes in depth the contingencies and differences between documentary film and Kulturfilm: Klaus Kreimeier, "Ein deutsches Paradigma: Die Kulturabteilung der Ufa," in Kreimeier, Ehmann, and Goergen, *Geschichte des dokumentarischen Films in Deutschland: Band 2*, 67–86, esp. 68–69. One-third of the volume is dedicated to Kulturfilm genres and Kulturfilm and film culture.

66. Film categories (Gattung) are defined by their mode of representation, e.g., fiction, documentary, animation or by their objective as in the case of promotional film or experimental film. Utility film in this sense is a pragmatic category and not a category of mode of presentation. Genres are defined by their content and structural characteristics including typical social or geographical location, specific environments or conflict constellations, subjects or emotional constellations. For the distinction between film categories (Gattung) and genres of films, see Zimmermann, *Schaufenster Schweiz*, 37.

67. Elsaesser, "Archives and Archaeologies," 19–34. Zimmermann, "'What Hollywood Is to America,'" 101–17.

68. Zimmermann, *Schaufenster Schweiz.*

69. Zimmermann, "'What Hollywood Is to America,'" 110.

70. For a history of UFA documentary film, see Hans-Michael Bock and Michael Töteberg, eds., *Das Ufa-Buch: Kunst und Krisen, Stars und Regisseure, Wirtschaft und Politik* (Frankfurt: Zweitausendeins, 1992); Klaus Kreimeier, *The Ufa Story: A History of Germany's Greatest Film Company: 1918–1945* (Berkeley: University of California Press, 1999); and Klaus Kreimeier, "Die Gründung der Ufa-Kulturabteilung," in Kreimeier, Ehmann, and Goergen, *Geschichte des dokumentarischen Films in Deutschland: Band 2,* 70–74.

71. *Richtlinien für Film-Veranstaltungen 1935–36,* n.p.

72. In 1927 Kayser directed for Deulig one of the early and aggressive agitation films, *Land unterm Kreuz* (1927), pathetically arguing for the German annexation of Oberschlesien against Poland. Later, Kayser directed for UFA films promoting modern agriculture as *Kampf um Brot* (1936). His last film direction under NS concerned one of the Wehrmacht-supported war cripple reintegration films, *Der Wille zum Leben* (1944).

73. *Bayer-Filme Aufstellung Jahreswende 1935–36,* no. 58.

74. Zimmermann, *Schaufenster Schweiz,* 69–72.

75. Christian Bonah, "'Health Crusades': Environmental Approaches as Public Health Strategies against Infections in Sanitary Propaganda Films, 1930–1960," in *Environment, Health and History,* ed. Virginia Berridge and Martin Gorsky (London: Palgrave Macmillan, 2011), 152–75; and Marianne Fedunkiw, "Malaria Films: Motion Pictures as Public Health Tool," *American Journal of Public Health* 93, no. 7 (2003): 1046–57.

76. Plasmochin was invented in 1924, marketed in 1927; Chinoplasmin's invention dates to 1930, marketing to 1932; Atebrin was invented in 1934 and marketed from 1937.

77. *Bayer-Filme Aufstellung Jahreswende 1935–36,* no. 44, *Schleichendes Gift.* This is the only film of our corpus not preserved in the Bayer Archives. A copy has been located in the Bundesarchiv-Filmarchiv in Berlin. My gratitude to Jutta Albert for her assistance in archival research.

78. Jeanpaul Goergen, ed., *Walter Ruttmann: Eine Dokumentation: Mit Beiträgen von Paul Falkenberg, William Uricchio, Barry A. Fulks* (Berlin: Freunde der Deutschen Kinemathek, 1989); and Peter Zimmermann, "Neusachlicher Technikkult und 'stählerne Romantik': Walter Ruttmans Symphonien der Industriearbeit," in Zimmermann and Hoffmann, *Geschichte des dokumentarischen Films in Deutschland: Band 3,* 231–41.

79. Goergen, *Walter Ruttmann;* Peter Zimmermann and Kay Hoffmann, "Bekannte Regisseure zwischen Avantgarde, Sachlichkeit, Idyllik und Propaganda," in Zimmermann and Hoffmann, *Geschichte des dokumentarischen Films in Deutschland: Band 3,* 110–32, esp. 112–14; Michael Cowan, *Walter Ruttmann and the Cinema of Multiplicity: Avant-Garde—Advertising—Modernity* (Chicago: University of Chicago Press, 2014); and Andreas Killen, *Berlin Electropolis: Shock, Nerves, and German Modernity* (Berekely: University of California Press, 2006).

80. Where film scholars like Leonardo Quaresima and Barry Fulks interpret Ruttmann's activity under NS as emblematic illustrations of Detlev Peukert's and Jeffrey Herf's thesis of "reactionary modernism," Martin Loiperdinger and Jeanpaul Goergen rather consider his work during this time as a private retreat into the "attics of industry." Zimmermann, "Bekannte Regisseure," 110–32, esp. 112–14; and

Heinz-B. Heller, "Avantgarde—Sozialkritik—Didaktik—Propaganda: Tendenzen der internationalen Entwicklung," in Zimmermann and Hoffmann, *Geschichte des dokumentarischen Films in Deutschland: Band 3*, 61.

81. Note that on August 1, 1940, in the context of war propaganda, the Deutsche Kulturfilm Zentrale was created as a central organ for the coordination, control, and direction of all German Kulturfilm, requiring from then on that projects needed to be approved prior to their realization.

82. The Weintraud memo omits mentioning that this film was coproduced by the Wehrmacht and the Military Academy in Berlin. This explains the stationing of Koncek in Elberfeld for the direction of microcinematography. At the same time, it sheds some light on the positioning of the Weintraud historical sketch of the Bayer film department concerning its relationships with the NS regime. Further archival research including Wehrmacht, Military Academy, and film censorship boards would be needed to clarify this point but are beyond the scope of this essay.

83. The film is credited for direction to Friedrich Luft (171) or A. Stoger (794) in the third volume of the *Geschichte des Dokumentarischen Films in Deutschland*. Christian Bonah, "'A Word from Man to Man': Interwar Venereal Disease Education Films for Military Audiences in France," *Gesnerus* 72, no. 1 (2015): 15–39.

84. Citation *Feind Malaria*, 1 minute 30 seconds.

85. See note 61 above.

86. Following the chronology of Bayer film production, three pre-1934 productions have not been taken into consideration in our corpus. *Beri-Beri* (1932) was not produced as a 35mm film and thus does not fit from its format the prestige film orientation portrayed by our image-building film corpus. *Typhoral* (1934), as the title indicates, is a more product-oriented film and has not been coproduced by UFA but, rather, by the film company Kinomat, Limberg & Peters in Wuppertal. *Allmacht Schlaf* (1934), despite its coproduction with UFA, remains apparently a product-dominated film. Neither *Typhoral* nor *Allmacht Schlaf* are preserved in the Bayer film archives today, and thus a close analysis is difficult. Most importantly, the three films were not classified by the Bayer film catalogue as *Wertwerbungsfilm* and thus have not been included in the corpus studied here. It might be that more detailed analysis of the last two films would have provided comparative information illuminating Bayer's definition of a *Wertwerbungsfilm* and its links to other categories of film—but such an analysis will have to await their rediscovery, should that ever happen.

87. For an overview, see Bonah and Laukötter, "Moving Pictures and Medicine"; Kirsten Ostherr, *Cinematic Prophylaxis: Globalization and Contagion in the Discourse of World Health* (Durham, NC: Duke University Press, 2005); Timothy Boon, "Films and the Contestation of Public Health in Interwar Britain" (PhD diss., University of London, 1999); Martin S. Pernick, *The Black Stork: Eugenics and the Death of "Defective" Babies in American Medicine and Motion Pictures since 1915* (New York: Oxford University Press, 1996); Martin S. Pernick, "Thomas Edison's Tuberculosis Films: Mass Media and Health Propaganda," *Hasting Center Report* 8 (1978): 21–27; and David Cantor, "Uncertain Enthusiasm: The American Cancer Society, Public Education, and the Problems of Movies, 1921–1960," *Bulletin of the History of Medicine* 81 (2007): 39–69. For an unpublished overview, see A. Nichtenhauser "A History of Medical Film" (1954), unpublished manuscript, National Library of Medicine, Nichtenhauser Papers, Washington DC.

88. Lucien Viborel, *La Technique moderne de propagande d'hygiène sociale* (Paris: Editions La Vie saine, 1930), 5.

89. Martin Loiperdinger, "Early Industrial Moving Pictures in Germany," in Hediger and Vonderau, *Films That Work*, 65–73; and Martin Loiperdinger, "Industriebilder," in *Geschichte des dokumentarischen Films in Deutschland: Band 1, Kaiserreich 1895–1918*, ed. Uli Jung and Martin Loiperdinger (Stuttgart, Germany: Reclam, 2005), 324–32. Jay E. Gordon, *Motion-Picture Production for Industry* (New York: Macmillan, 1961).

90. Devin Orgeron, Marsha Orgeron, and Dan Streible, eds., *Learning with the Lights Off: Educational Film in the United States* (New York: Oxford University Press, 2011). See esp. the introduction: "A History of Learning with the Lights off," 15–66. Oskar Kalbus, *Der Deutsche Lehrfilm in der Wissenschaft und im Unterricht* (Berlin: Carl Heymann, 1922); Uli Jung, "Filme für Lehre und Bildung," in Jung and Loiperdinger, *Geschichte des dokumentarischen Films in Deutschland: Band 1*, 333–56; Ursula Keitz, "Wissen als Film: Zur Entwicklung des Lehr-und Unterrichtsfilms," in Kreimeier, Ehmann, and Goergen, *Geschichte des dokumentarischen Films in Deutschland: Band 2*, 120–50; and Ursula Keitz, "Die Kinematographie in der Schule: Zur politischen Pädagogik des Unterrichtsfilms von RfdU und RWU," in Zimmermann and Hoffmann, *Geschichte des dokumentarischen Films in Deutschland: Band 3*, 463–88.

91. Timothy Boon, *Films of Fact: A History of Science in Documentary Films and Television* (London: Wallflower Press, 2008).

92. For the factory tour motive, see Marchand, *Corporate Soul*, 259–62.

93. Zimmermann, "What Hollywood is to America," 110.

94. Friedländer, "1000 Worte Werbefilm," *Die Epoche: Das Magazin des Werbefilms*, March 1, 1929, 2–4.

95. *Richtlinien für Film-Veranstaltungen 1935–36.*

96. Wagner, "The Cinematograph," 391–404.

97. Bonah, "Health Crusades," 152–75.

98. Friedländer, "1000 Worte Werbefilm," 2–4.

99. Bayer Archives, *Zepro-Nachrichten*, July 1, 1937, 12–13.

100. *Kriegsstunden am afrikanischen Himmel.*

101. Bayer Archives, *Zepro-Nachrichten*, July 1, 1937, 13.

102. MariaTortajada and François Albera, eds., *Cinema Beyond Film: Media Epistemology in the Modern Era* (Amsterdam: Amsterdam University Press, 2010).

103. *Richtlinien für Film-Veranstaltungen 1935–36*, n.p.

104. *Stored Sun Energy*, 1934, minutes 3'48" to 4'08.

105. *Feind Malaria*, 1942/43, minutes 1'50".

106. Hediger and Vonderau, *Films That Work*, especially "Introduction," 10. Hediger and Vonderau, *Filmische Mittel, industrielle Zwecke.* The special issues of the periodical *AV Montage* dedicated to "industrial film in 2005 and 2006 *Montage AV Zeitschrift für Theorie & Geschichte audiovisueller Kommunikation*, special issue *Gebrauchsfilm* 14, no. 2 (2005) and 15, no. 1 (2006) and the annotated international bibliography: Anna Heymer and Patrick Vonderau, "Industrial Films: An Analytical Bibliography," in Hediger and Vonderau, *Films That Work*, 404–61.

107. Hediger and Vonderau, *Films That Work*, 10.

108. Actors of systems of medical and health economies genuinely try to set medicaments apart from common consumption goods in that they are defined as tools of

promoting the public health. Thus, pharmaceutical objects promoted by Bayer carry with them from the very beginning a basic inherent ambiguity exploited symmetrically in their promotional films.

109. *Brücken der Hilfe,* 1952.

110. UNESCO put forward a world work plan for the mass media—films, radio, and press—in 1947 that would coordinate all the film work of the UN's special agencies and shape the postwar health information campaigns of a variety of national and international organizations. The program produced a survey of films and other direct services in 1947, eventually becoming the United Nations Film Board, responsible for coordinating all the film work of the UN's special agencies, especially the Food and Agriculture Organization (FAO) and the World Health Organization (WHO). John Taylor and Basil Wright, "UNESCO's World Plans," *Documentary News Letter* 6, no. 55 (1947): 67.

111. For example, the United Nations Film Board produced a series of motion pictures under the heading "Great Hope. The Changing Face of Europe."

Chapter Three

Conversion Narratives, Health Films, and Hollywood Filmmakers of the 1930s and 1940s

Vincent Lowy and David Cantor

Introduction

During the 1930s and 1940s, the narrative trajectories of Hollywood movies began to change. Where once gangsters, outlaws, and rebels could get away with their crimes on screen, from the late 1930s their fate was somewhat different. The gangster, outlaw, or rebel who did not reform now either died or was brought to justice, as did many of those who saw the errors of their ways after committing some unforgivable crime. By contrast, those who saw the errors of their ways in time often turned into respectable citizens and even law enforcers. Through such conversion stories, Hollywood producers both sought to counter criticisms that motion pictures contributed to moral decline and participated in efforts to transform a society suffering from the economic crisis, organized crime, and social and interracial conflict.[1] As America joined the world war, Hollywood increasing also turned the conversion narrative to wartime goals. Individuals in such stories were often persuaded to subordinate their interests to the broader goals of a nation at war. This chapter is about the relationships between the Hollywood conversion narratives of the 1930s and 1940s and those found in health education films.

This is not the first publication to acknowledge the presence of conversion narratives in health education films.[2] One of us (DC) has identified the conversion narrative as a key component of educational films produced between 1921 and 1960 for the American Society for the Control of Cancer (ASCC) and its successor, the American Cancer Society (ACS). The argument goes that the ASCC not only saw movies as transforming attitudes and behaviors by means of their visual impact, but that they also did so by telling stories. Thus, the ASCC/ACS commissioned motion pictures that told tales about the routes by which people facing the possibility of cancer got to the doctor, the obstacles that hindered them from reaching this goal, and the events that helped them take the right path as defined by the cancer organization. And, so much could hinder someone facing cancer from getting to the doctor. People might procrastinate out of fear of the disease or its treatments, because of shame about the disease, false modesty, or because they were waylaid along the way by folk healers, quacks, and the mistaken advice of family and friends. The stories told in the ASCC/ACS's films suggested that those who fell by the wayside faced a bleak prospect of death, debility and pain while those who adopted the recommendations of the cancer organizations (and, crucially, adopted them in time), were saved. Thus, in these films, whoever converted to the recommendations of the cancer organization was likely to be cured of cancer, while those who did not or converted too late often died.

This chapter expands the focus of this earlier paper in two ways. In the first place, it suggests that conversion narratives were a characteristic of health education films more generally, beyond cancer. They could be found in films made for campaigns against tuberculosis, mental health, diabetes, venereal diseases, alcoholism, and many other health issues. The recommendations in these films about what individuals had to do to combat each disease or health issue varied depending on the subject of the campaign and the approaches of the sponsor. However, the films often told conversion stories about how individuals came to adopt such recommendations (whatever they might be), the problems they encountered along the way, and the consequences both for them and for those who did not convert. Thus, the narrative forms that characterized the cancer education film could be found in many other health education films, and they all served a similar purpose of persuading audiences to adopt the sponsors' recommendations by showing the rewards for those who adopted them and the penalties for those who failed to do so.

In the second place, this essay also seeks to highlight the relations between the conversion narratives found in health education films and those in entertainment films of the 1930s and 1940s. Such relations were not new. They can be traced back to the beginnings of the public health film in the 1910s. The earliest films had often included a conversion narrative in which an individual abandoned his or her unhealthy, antisocial or immoral ways and was saved, or failed to do so, or converted too late, and suffered the consequence—ill-health, debility, pain, social isolation, or death. Such narratives provided a template for those that came later, but they were often screened in very different places to those of the 1930s and 1940s. Many were shown in movie theaters as part of the regular cinema schedule as well as in the sorts of places that would become familiar to later nontheatrical films—classrooms, factories, women's and social clubs, and many other informal film venues. At a time when the distinctions between educational and entertainment, theatrical and nontheatrical were still fluid, these early public health films also demonstrated the willingness of the film industry to reform itself, and so distance itself from accusations that it was a source of moral and social degeneration. Stories of moral, health, and social reform became emblematic of the industry's own efforts to reform and to stave off the threat of outside intervention.[3]

Part of what distinguishes the public health conversion narratives of the 1930s and 1940s is that they were shown in very different places to those of the 1910s. Most public health films were classified as nontheatricals and were no longer shown in the cinema as part of the regular schedule. The rule was not inviolate, as the discussion of Ulmer below makes clear, and Hollywood corporations sometimes made or distributed such films.[4] However, the lines between theatrical and nontheatrical films had hardened since the 1910s, and health education films were generally not a major part of Hollywood's efforts to signal its willingness to reform. As important for our argument, the sorts of conversion narratives shown in movie theaters in the 1930s were often different from those shown in health education films. The distinction between the two would blur in the 1940s, after the United States entered the war, when conversion became a mark of patriotic duty in both entertainments and educationals, and a failure to convert was often portrayed as undermining the war effort. This chapter thus focuses on a corpus of entertainments and educationals that allows us to elaborate the relationship between the conversion narratives in the public health film and those in Hollywood in the 1930s and 1940s. How did the forces that promoted the commercial use of conversion narratives influence the health education film? And how did this change with America's entry into the world war?

We will approach these questions through the work of three Hollywood directors who also made educational films: Edgar George Ulmer (1904–72), John Huston (1906–87), and John Ford (1894–1973). Ulmer is best known today as a B-list director of movies such as *The Black Cat* (1934) and *Detour* (1945), often regarded as a prototypical film noir production and a model for independent filmmaking to come. Ford by contrast was an established director, best known both for Westerns such as *Stagecoach* (1939) and adaptations of classic twentieth-century novels such as *The Grapes of Wrath* (1940) and *How Green Was My Valley* (1941). He had already won three Academy Awards for Best Director (in 1935, 1940, 1941) and was to win another in 1952. Finally, Huston, already known as a scriptwriter, was an emerging figure in Hollywood: his directorial debut, *The Maltese Falcon* (1941), was given a B-movie budget by Warner's, which was surprised to find the film praised by critics as a classic, not least because two earlier versions of the story had failed at the box office.

The three filmmakers thus had very different statuses: Ulmer was an independent filmmaker who specialized in B-movies but who spent much of his career as an exile from Hollywood because he had an affair with the wife of Max Alexander, nephew of Universal studio head Carl Laemmle, and was earning a modest income for films that have largely been forgotten; Ford was a veteran, an Oscar laureate and an A-list filmmaker at Fox; and Huston was a promising beginner at Warner's, whose early successes foreshadowed a brilliant future. All, however, made health education films. Ulmer directed a half-dozen public health films on tuberculosis for the National Tuberculosis Association (NTA) between 1938 and 1941; John Ford directed *Sex Hygiene* (1941), on behalf of the Office of the Coordinator of Information; and Huston directed *Let There Be Light* (1946) for the US Army Signal Corps to report on advances in the treatment of psychological trauma sustained by GI's during the war. Together, they allow us to compare the conversion narratives in their Hollywood films and those in their health education ones.

Commercial Cinema and Educational Film

First, it is necessary to trace the changing relations between health education films and commercial cinema after World War I, when public health films were shown less and less as part of the regular cinema schedule and tended to be shown elsewhere in schools, workplaces, women's clubs, community centers, libraries, and other informal venues. Advocates of health education films continued to suggest that they might be included in cinemas as part of the regular schedule.[5] However, such suggestions often did not succeed, and where health education films were shown in the cinema, it was generally as a special event organized by a sponsor or as a paid advertisement in the regular schedule. Claims that a well-made educational film could attract a paying audience generally did not persuade cinema owners. Increasingly, films began to be divided into theatrical and nontheatrical categories, the former including comedies, dramas, action movies, and other commercial entertainments, the latter including educationals and other special interest films, such as health education films.

The separation of commercial and educational films into theatrical and nontheatrical forms, however, did not mean that Hollywood had no influence on the health educational film. Many film techniques developed in Hollywood entertainment movies came to be used to build audience support and participation for health education campaigns, and filmmakers struggled with questions about how much entertainment should be part of an educational film and whether it distracted from or enhanced the educational message. However, because budgets for educational films were generally much smaller than their Hollywood equivalents, sponsors and their filmmakers were often frustrated in their hopes of using the technologies and techniques employed in big budget entertainment films. Long after the introduction of sound into commercial talkies, many health education films remained silent, or were silent films with a canned score and voiceover added later. A few educational films were more elaborate, sometimes competing with the best shorts produced by Hollywood; but many were not.

Health education films not only took film techniques and practices from Hollywood; they also occasionally took personnel, who brought with them ideas and practices developed in the entertainment film world and applied them to educationals. Such movements of personnel had a long history that went back to the 1910s, with directors such as D. W. Griffith making educational films that also doubled as commercial entertainments, and other personnel—scenarists, camera operators, lighting technicians, carpenters, and others—sometimes working on entertainments and sometimes educationals. Even as educational and entertainment films separated out in the 1920s and 1930s, personnel in commercial cinema continued to move into educationals, and corporations such as the Eastern Film Corporation moved from entertainment to educational films.[6] The result was that personnel themselves took techniques and ideas developed in one arena into the other.

Such interchanges of personnel and practices increased dramatically during World War II. Hollywood personnel poured into educationals to mobilize the nation for war and to instruct military and civilian audiences about issues crucial to the war effort, including public health.[7] Even before the United States entered the war, the War Department had taken over the Astoria Studios in New York, and the Army Air Force had taken over the Hal Roach Studio in Culver City, California. There followed in 1942, after Pearl Harbor, the formation of an Office of War Information (OWI), which aimed to explore the most effective use of the media, including motion pictures, to mobilize and inform the public to support the war effort. At about the same time, the US Army established an Information and Education Division, which created a filmmaking unit under the Hollywood director Frank Capra, who in turn created an animation unit headed by Theodore Geisel (known popularly as Dr. Seuss) and manned by personnel from Warner Brothers and other top studios. The navy, marines, army air force, and coast guard also created their own organizations, employing filmmakers and actors, often working in consultation with educators, psychologists, and sociologists. In the course of the war, the US military made thousands of films. Although most of these had nothing to do with public health, many films did include material on medicine and public health, and some were wholly devoted to health concerns. Among the Hollywood directors who began to make educational films at this time were John Huston and John Ford who, along with Edgar Ulmer, constitute the focus of this essay.

The Hollywood Conversion Narrative in the 1930s and 1940s

In the 1930s, the conversion narrative reemerged as one of the ways in which the film industry sought to fend off the threat of government intervention. By telling stories of reform and conversion, the industry signaled once again its own efforts to reform itself and to promote moral and social reform in its audiences. The best-known effort by the industry to reform itself was the Motion Picture Production Code (a series of moral and social strictures as to what could and could not be included in films), sometimes known as the Hays Code after Will H. Hays, president of the Motion Picture Producers and Distributors of America (MPPDA) from 1922 to 1945.[8] In 1930 the MPPDA adopted the

Production Code and began strictly enforcing it in 1934. One of the effects of this was that reform or conversion narratives, which told tales of individuals who eventually adopted norms promoted by the Production Code, came to be rewarded in Hollywood.

But films not only illustrated conversions to Production Code norms; they also used conversion narratives to tell a new tale of American identity in which stories of assimilation were displaced by ones that validated the experiences of immigrants and minority groups.[9] The roots of this lay in the growing influence of liberal or left filmmakers within Hollywood, who revitalized populist themes, empathized with minorities and the working class, and were critical of unfettered monopoly capitalism. Even films that focused on traditional white elites often took the side of the little man as he worked against the odds.[10] In these movies, as historian Lary May has argued, the successful resolution occurred when characters from the elite convert to the values of the people; this applied to about 20 percent of the decade's film plots, according to May.[11] Conversion narratives thus often aligned the middle or upper class politically with the lower class.

In other films, such an alignment could be created by the elevation of the masses. An emblematic conversion narrative here was *The Hunchback of Notre-Dame* (1939), a production of the German émigré filmmaker William Dieterle. Based on the novel by Victor Hugo, the film portrays the conflict between, on the one hand, nascent humanism represented by the invention of the printing press, the French King Louis XI's support for the latest scientific discoveries, and young Gringoire's pamphlets of liberal thinking, and on the other hand, obscure forces that that wanted to keep fifteenth-century France in a medieval world characterized by superstition, bigotry, and censorship. The pivotal scene of the film occurs when the gypsy, Esmeralda, gives the hunchback, Quasimodo, something to drink while he is pilloried by the unruly Paris crowd. Esmeralda's virtuous act changes the attitude of the crowd toward Quasimodo, its conversion moment, when the people come to empathize with the hunchback. Symbolizing a people in its stage of "infancy" being transformed, elevated, and edified, the good deed at the same time signifies the redemption of the monstrous Quasimodo.

When the United States entered the Second World War, Hollywood's conversion narratives began to change.[12] Increasingly, stories about patriotic assimilation gained greater prominence, a point emphasized by the Office for War Information's *Manual for the Motion Picture Industry* (1942), which argued that people had to put aside "national class or race war" to create for the common man a "new world free of fear and want."[13] For May, this resulted in a reversal of the 1930s conversion narrative in that the stories of the elite adopting the values of the people began be displaced by ones in which individuals who initially defined themselves by class or ethnicity abandoned such identities and came to support hierarchical, often military, institutions devoted to saving the world. (Some 30 percent of Hollywood films portrayed such stories, according to May.)[14] What this meant was that those who continued to urge class or ethnic identity could be defined as traitors. Thus, John Ford's documentary *December 7th* (1943) blamed those in Hawaii who identified themselves as ethnically Japanese for the bombing of Pearl Harbor. As the movie put it, "Citizens can still be Asian racially, but now must become 100% American culturally."

However, this trajectory from top-down conversion stories in the 1930s to down-up narratives in the 1940s does not fit the trajectory of the public health conversion narrative, which often had more in common with the wartime Hollywood conversion stories than those of the 1930s. Like wartime movies, public health films also tried to enroll people in hierarchically organized campaigns or wars against disease, and this meant encouraging audiences to follow the recommendations of the sponsoring agencies. The consequence was that public health films, like those produced during the Second World War, often told conversion stories in which individuals put aside their fears and concerns, or the false hopes offered by quacks and the ignorant, and came to accept the recommendations of the physicians and public health officials devoted to preserving their health and intervening against disease. And if they did not convert, the penalty was often death or debility. Thus, when a director such as Edgar G. Ulmer, who had worked in ethnic entertainment cinema validating the experiences of minorities and immigrants, turned to educational films, he changed his approach. While the experiences of minorities and immigrants were still validated, such validation tended to be subordinated to the medical views of disease and illness. Ethnically diverse characters in these films were saved only by turning to medical organizations and had to abandon the folk medicine and wisdom of their ethnic group where it clashed with orthodox medicine.

Ulmer and the National Tuberculosis Association

As the foregoing suggests, Ulmer's films highlight the problematic relationship between public health conversion narratives of the 1930s and 1940s and the top-down conversion narratives found in Hollywood. Ulmer had been recruited in 1937 to make several films for the National Tuberculosis Association that were to target different ethnic and social groups: African American, Mexicans, and Native Americans as well as white audiences. Formerly an assistant art director for German filmmaker F. W. Murnau, Ulmer worked briefly in Hollywood, directing a string of B-movies such as *The Black Cat* (1934) and *Damaged Lives* (1933).[15] Yet despite the success of these films, both in artistic terms and at the box office, his ill-chosen affair with the wife of Max Alexander forced him to leave Hollywood and to move to the East Coast, where he went on to make "ethnic" films: medium-length films aimed at minority groups, poorly distributed and shown on alternative circuits.[16]

These New York works are characterized by a great deal of inventiveness despite their extremely low budgets, and it was Ulmer's ability to relate to ethnic audiences that prompted the National Tuberculosis Association—concerned about the differential incidence of TB in different "racial" groups—to commission him to direct six films on tuberculosis and its treatments: *Let My People Live* (1938) for African-American audiences, *Cloud In The Sky* (1939) for Hispanics; *They Do Come Back* (1940) for young white couples (the only film in the series of which two versions exist); *Diagnostic Procedures in Tuberculosis* (1940) for the medical community, *Goodbye, Mr. Germ* (1940) for white children, and *Another To Conquer* (1941) for Native Americans.[17] In the ethnic TB the films in particular, Ulmer brought his approach to ethnic entertainments to the public health film, adopting the culture of each ethnic group and turning it to his own purposes and that of his sponsors: in all these films, he tries to align orthodox medical knowledge with the cultures of the ethnic groups portrayed, suggesting that the knowledge and wisdom of both could be used to tackle tuberculosis. These films remained paternalistic in many ways, and they often elevated medical knowledge over that of ethnic cultures. However, compared with many other contemporary health education films there is an attempt, at least on the surface, to acknowledge wisdom or knowledge on both sides and to bring these forms of wisdom together.[18]

As other historians have noted, these films—with the exception of the *Diagnostic Procedures in Tuberculosis*—urged their audiences to learn the early warning signs of the disease, to go for regular checkups from a recognized physician, to avoid quacks and folk healers, and to seek early, medically sanctioned treatment the moment the disease was identified. Often they used conversion accounts to teach these lessons.[19] However, such conversion narratives highlight a difference with the top-down models of many Hollywood conversion stories of the 1930s in which the elite adopted the values of the people. In encouraging people to seek care from a regular physician, they told stories of individuals who defined themselves by class or ethnicity eventually converting to support medical institutions devoted to saving their lives, abandoning those aspects of their culture that were at odds with medical values, and elevating those aspects that meshed with the medical. Thus, while the films validate many ethnic institutions, notably religious ones (Catholicism for Hispanics, pastors for African Americans, and traditional leaders for Native Americans), these institutions served in the films to promote a medical conversion that simultaneously validated the proselytizer. In those targeted at African Americans, Hispanics, and Native Americans, the proselytizer is a pastor, padre, or someone who represents traditional beliefs and who seeks to align such beliefs with modern medicine. At the same time, those ethnic institutions or belief systems that do not align with modern medicine are presented as dangers to ethnic audiences: folk healers, for example, are portrayed as a threat to the health of the people when they lead them away from a medically sanctioned path. The only films that do not include a role for religion are those that target white audiences, where the proselytizer is a physician or a scientist.

In many ways, these films, with their faith in medicine and science, represent something very different from Ulmer's most famous prewar film *The Black Cat*, a Universal production, based loosely on an Edgar Allan Poe short story that brought together Boris Karloff and Bela Lugosi for the first time.[20] The latter played Dr. Vitus Werdegast, a psychiatrist, who wants revenge against his former friend, the brilliant architect Hjalmar Poelzig (Karloff), a Satanist and necrophiliac whose actions apparently led to Werdegast's imprisonment for fifteen years and who then married Werdegast's wife and, after she died of pneumonia, his daughter. While traveling to meet Poelzig, a ticketing error means that Werdegast has to share a private train compartment with a honeymooning couple, Joan and Peter Allison, with whom he also shares a bus ride after disembarking from the train. When their vehicle crashes in a storm and Joan is injured, the travelers seek refuge in Poelzig's house. There, Werdegast who has a phobia of cats, learns his wife's fate, grieves for his lost daughter, and must play a game of chess for Allison's life since Poelzig plans to sacrifice her in a satanic rite. He is a sort of Faust to Poelzig's devil.

If, in Ulmer's TB films, physicians and (medical) technology are sources of salvation, they have a more ambiguous role in *The Black Cat*. Early in the film, while Joan is asleep in the train compartment, Werdegast strokes her hair, perhaps with sexual interest, because she reminds him of his wife. Later, after the crash, it is Werdegast who treats Joan's injuries, and his role in the rest of the film oscillates between longing husband, medical doctor, ill-defined threat, and paternal carer. Werdegast is not entirely stable psychologically. Poelzig calls him mad, and his terror of cats leads him to attempt to kill (offscreen) a black cat by throwing a knife at it, at which point Joan appears in a sort of daze, under the influence of a narcotic prescribed by Werdegast, asking in a dreamy manner if the doctor was frightened. Drugs in fact render Joan "mediumistic," as Werdegast puts it, a conduit for all the intangible forces around her. Her husband regards such views as supernatural baloney, but Joan has correctly divined that Werdegast is fearful; the drugs have given her insight into the strange forces around her and Poelzig's satanic plans for her.

If the physician has an ambiguous role in the figure of Werdegast, so does the anatomist in the figures of Werdegast and Poelzig. The latter has preserved the corpse of his/Werdegast's wife, along with those of other women, in the basement of his house, like a series of anatomic specimens. After saving Joan, however, Werdegast becomes the anatomist, employing his skills on Poelzig, to anatomize the anatomist. He skins him alive in the basement of the house. Peter, a mystery writer, thinks Poelzig's house is "tricky" and that Poelzig would be ideal to design an insane asylum. The climatic scenes in the former castle dungeons below the house seem to bring this comment to fulfilment. The *Black Cat* thus shows an ambiguous attitude toward medicine in the figures of Werdegast and Poelzig in which the former's medical skills intersect with his madness, threat, and sexual longing, and the latter forges a link between the anatomical museum, satanic rituals, and perverted love. There is no conversion on the part of Joan or Peter to these views of medicine, except that Joan comes to realize in the end that Werdegast is helping her.

The Black Cat thus did not provide a model for physicians in the TB films, nor does it provide the sort of conversion narratives that would characterize them. The same, however, cannot be said for another Ulmer film, *Damaged Lives* (1933), a conversion story about a couple nearly destroyed by venereal disease.[21] It tells the tale of Donny, the son of a wealthy shipping magnate, who is about to inherit the business. His girlfriend Joan wants desperately to get married and have a baby, but Donny is so busy that he has not had time to consider it fully. One day Donny breaks a date with Joan to entertain a business client, Nat, at a jazz club, together with Nat's girlfriend, Elise. Later that evening, Donny and Elise want to go home, but Nat takes them to a whorehouse. Nat goes off with one of the prostitutes, leaving Donny and Elise together. They have one last drink in a nearby illegal rundown gambling place and eventually end up offscreen in bed together. The following day, Donny overcome with guilt, agrees to Joan's pleas that he marry her, and they immediately get married in the town hall.

It is now that the trouble really begins. Elise calls him at work, asking him to see her urgently, and she persuades him that she in in real trouble. When Donny arrives at her apartment, he finds that Elise has tried to commit suicide and is told that she has to be watched. It turns out that Nat has "something terribly wrong" with him, and Elise informs him that she has it and may have passed it on to Donny. Donny does not believe her and leaves. A gunshot is heard off screen: Elise has committed suicide, but her words are prophetic. When Joan gets pregnant by Donny, she goes for a checkup and finds that she has syphilis. Donny is forced to confess his affair, and the doctor informs him that both Joan and he are infected.

If Donny's first efforts to seek redemption begin with his decision to marry Joan in the mistaken belief that he could atone for straying, it is in the clinic that his true conversion begins. Donny's doctor takes him around the clinic, where he sees what happens when syphilis is not treated in time. In echoes of scenes in earlier VD films, such as *The End of the Road* (1919), or eugenic films such as *The Black Stork* (1916)/*Are You Fit to Marry?* (1927), we are shown a man with a rash on his leg and a wheelchair-bound woman, whose six children are blind, crippled, mentally retarded, and infected with the disease.[22] Donny worries about what will happen to Joan and their baby. However, the doctor tells him that the disease has been caught in time and can be cured with medication. Joan, however, is in despair, and like Elise tries to commit suicide, unaware that the disease can be cured. She turns on the gas and lays down beside a sleeping Donny, who wakes just in time to switch off the gas. He tells Joan the good medical news, and both they and the baby are saved.

The echoes of earlier films was not an accident. *Damaged Lives* was the idea of film distributor J. J. Allen, who distributed and exhibited Columbia Pictures' movies in Canada. Allen and the Canadian Health Council wanted to make a mass-market film about venereal disease, and proposed a $100,000 movie—later slashed to $18,000—based on *Damaged Goods*, a popular play and later film about venereal disease.[23] *Damaged Lives* and its conversion narrative thus modeled itself on earlier social hygiene films. However, the fact that it crossed the boundary between and educational and entertainment meant that it did not play in some US cities until four years after it was made and when it did, it was accompanied by a film of a twenty-nine-minute lecture on the dangers of VD to raise the educational value. Despite this controversy, or perhaps because of it, *Damaged Lives* made a huge profit when it was finally shown. It was subsequently rereleased under many other names and managed to stay in circulation until the 1950s.

Damaged Lives thus highlights an unexpected source of the conversion narrative in Ulmer's mainstream work. Although the National Tuberculosis Association likely wanted Ulmer for his ability to appeal to ethnic audiences, they may also have been influenced by *Damaged Lives*, which echoed a conversion theme that had been part of TB films since the 1910s and educational programs even before then.[24] There were, of course, risks in any comparison to *Damaged Lives*, given its subject matter and the anxieties about screening it in commercial cinemas. But Ulmer's ability to make a popular film about a medical subject, and his more general interest in social estrangement—whether by disease, war, or banishment from home—and depictions of outsiders and what drew them to the margins, meant that Ulmer could be seen as someone who could lay the groundwork for a conversion story. To understand what drove people to the margins was to be a precondition for stories that also explored what brought them back to the light.[25]

Damaged Lives was thus unlike many conversion narratives found in the Hollywood films of the 1930s: it was a down-up conversion in which the protagonists are saved by adopting the recommendations of a physician, a point that would be repeated in Ulmer's TB films. To do this, Ulmer not only asked his viewers to abandon those elements of their culture that conflicted with medical recommendations, he also appropriated the mythologies of that culture to make his point. When Ulmer filmed a culture in his ethnic entertainments, he took its traditions and turned them to his own purposes, just as he appropriated the symbolic universe of Poe in *The Black Cat*. In *Damaged Lives* and his TB films he would do the same, but not solely for his own filmic purposes, but to serve the needs of his sponsors. In *Another to Conquer*, for example, the white doctor explains that he can tell if a lung is sick by listening to it, and his young Indian patient observes that "warriors put their ear to the ground to hear the footsteps of their enemy." The warrior code is thus used to enlist the tribe in a war with tuberculosis and an alliance with modern medicine. It is Ulmer's use of traditional and religious cultures that structures the NTA's search for a mutual acknowledgment of each party's "wisdom" to forge an alliance against a common enemy. This is precisely why Ulmer's ethnic sensitivities appealed to his sponsors, even though as an auteur he still had the power to subvert the medical message he was asked to deliver and to focus on the representation of a community.[26]

Ulmer's films have been described as portrayals of "infinite despair," and several of his TB films are no exception.[27] The most powerful scenes in this corpus (the conclusion of *Let My People Live*, the presentation of the Navajo reservation at the beginning of *Another to Conquer*) are examples of how Ulmer can introduce moments of poignant emotional resonance into minimal narratives without weakening the film's message on medical prevention. Other aspects of

Ulmer's film style can be detected in other TB movies. *Goodbye Mr. Germ*, for example, tells the tale of an eccentric doctor—an old, sarcastic man wearing a top hat—who invents a means of communicating with the tuberculosis germ. The naiveté of the caricature is reinforced by the backdrop of the joyfully messy laboratory where he conducts his experiments, details that are reminiscent of Ulmer's fantasy films, which are characterized by an unbalanced mix of solemnity and naiveté.[28] This film is the one in which the stylistic attributes that commonly define Ulmer's films are most visible, such as tilted framing, stylized decor, or neo-expressionist lighting.

John Ford and *Sex Hygiene*

If Ulmer's films highlight the problematic relationship between public health conversion narratives of the 1930s and 1940s and Hollywood's top-down conversion narratives, so too do John Ford's films.[29] But whereas Ulmer's were commissioned at a time when Hollywood top-down conversion narratives were at a peak (albeit declining over the period he made the films), John Ford's (and later John Huston's, the other director that is the subject of this essay) were made as down-up conversion narratives were rising and as narratives of subversion (in which an agent who intends to harm the social order or the state) were also rising.[30] Indeed, Hollywood's wartime narratives of conversion, in which an individual abandons his selfish, class, or ethnic interests in favor of hierarchical patriotic organizations, were often set against stories of subversion, which could give urgency to the need for conversion. This mix of conversion and subversion was often also incorporated into health education films, where the agent was the disease or its cause (sometimes portrayed as enemy No. 2 after the Japanese or Germans) and set the stage for stories of conversion to a hierarchical medical organization.

Before the war, Ford himself had often been celebrated for films that championed the outsider or the working class. The point can be illustrated by one of his best-known movies, *Stagecoach* (1939), often portrayed as the movie that ushered in a renaissance of the Western, which had been relegated to B-unit production for much of the decade before its release.[31] The film tells the story of a diverse group of people who travel on a stagecoach and are attacked by Apache Indians. They include the alcoholic Doc Boone (Thomas Mitchell) and the prostitute Dallas (Claire Trevor), both being run out of town by the Ladies Law and Order League, prompting the inebriated physician to tell Dallas that they are "the victims of a foul disease called social prejudice, my child." Doc and Dallas are accompanied by Lucy Mallory (Louise Platt), traveling to meet her soldier husband; a whisky salesman, Samuel Peacock (Donald Meek); and a professional southern gambler named Hatfield (John Carradine). They are joined later by the president of the local bank, Henry Gatewood (Berton Churchill), who is making away with some of the bank's funds, and still later by the Ringo Kid (John Wayne, in his breakout role), who has just escaped from prison to hunt down the man who killed his brother. A cavalry platoon offers protection for part of the route. However, the cavalry leaves them and, after a democratic vote, the stagecoach travels on alone.

Stagecoach is a story of how an assorted group of strangers are tested by danger and forced to work together, and of how those at the margins of society—the outlaw, the drunk, and the prostitute—often embody the best of qualities. For many characters, there is no conversion. The story is about how they are changed by the events on their journey, but also about how these events bring to the fore traits that were always there: Doc is at root a good physicians and despite his love of the bottle delivers Mallory's' baby safely, fights off the Indians, and stands up to the man who killed Ringo's brother; Hatfield, not quite a gentleman, reputed to shoot people in the back, is brave in the end but dies in the fight; the Ringo Kid is a rugged individualist who never varies from his goals of killing his brother's killer and marrying Dallas; Peacock, the one figure who consistently votes against traveling into danger, reveals his good nature in his farewell to Dallas where he invites her to visit him in Kansas; while Gatewood, who represents the corruption of banking/business and makes a number of conservative, Republican comments ("America for Americans," "What's good for banks is good for the country," "What this country needs is a businessman for president," and "Government mustn't interfere with business.") is revealed as not only a thief but also a coward and is eventually arrested.

Other characters, however, do change. Mallory seems to overcome her bigotry toward Dallas, whom she had previously scorned, a change brought about by Dallas's kindness toward her. However, if there is a major conversion it is that of Dallas, who after initially resisting the Kid's proposal of marriage, is finally persuaded (with Doc's encouragement) to go with him to his ranch in Mexico. Dallas is changed by Ringo, who ignores her reputation as a prostitute and sees what is there in her all the time: her inner goodness. Dallas's conversion is thus as much about bringing forth something innate to her as it is about her eventual agreement to marriage. And it is a focus on this inner self that allows Ford to elevate the outsider figures in this film, all with goodness at their core: Dallas, Doc, and the Ringo Kid. In the case of Ringo and Dallas, the two eventually leave together, out into the wilderness on their way to Ringo's Mexican ranch. As Doc says of them, "Well, they're saved from the blessings of civilization," a reference to Ringo's escape from prison, Dallas's escape from the social conventions that penalized her, and the wilds into which they are traveling.

Stagecoach was not alone among Ford's prewar films in empathizing with the marginal and powerless. *The Grapes of Wrath* (1940), Ford's adaptation of John Steinbeck's 1939 novel, was about the plight of the Joad family, sharecroppers driven from the land by drought and greedy landowners and forced to travel westward to California for jobs and survival, and of how the family slowly disintegrates under such conditions.[32] *How Green Was My Valley* (1941) covered a similar theme, showing how unfettered capitalism exploits workers and leads to a coal strike in a small Welsh mining town.[33] The strike itself, however, results in a vicious sectarianism in a once-peaceful community and (as with the Joad family, who are forced into strikebreaking) breaks up the Morgan family when the father disapproves of his sons' unionization and they leave home, and later when after the strike the sons are blacklisted and must leave for America in order to make a living. As in *Stagecoach*, it is often nature untouched by civilization that has a healing effect. Not the wilderness of the earlier film, but the Green Valley untouched by the mine, where the young protagonist literally learns to walk again after an illness.

World War II changed everything for Ford. Already in the Naval Reserve, he made films for the Navy Department's photographic unit and won two Academy Awards for best documentary for *The Battle of Midway* (1942) and *December 7th* (1943). Crucially, he abandoned his earlier empathy with the oppressed and the marginal, building instead on the themes of patriotism that had been evident in some of his prewar war films.[34] The point can be made by *December 7th*. In this film, Uncle Sam arrives in Hawaii for vacation, where he at first seems to echo attitudes espoused in Ford's earlier films: he tolerates labor strikes and Japanese Americans. Then it turns out that Japanese Americans have bilingual schools and a Shinto religion that binds them to the Japanese emperor. The Japanese spy on the American ships and Asian women tempt American sailors to give away military secrets, all of which leads to the bombing of Pearl Harbor and to Uncle Sam's conversion to a new view that Japanese Americans have to abandon the trappings of Japanese culture and become fully American.[35] Thus, conversion in this film means not only that those who initially defined themselves by ethnicity abandon such identities and come to support hierarchical, often military American institutions, but that once-tolerant people abandon toleration of class or ethnic self-identification in others, at least where it challenges the nation's military preparedness.

Such a change in perspective is also reflected in different ways in Ford's health education film, *Sex Hygiene* (1941)—one of the mostly widely screened educational films during the war—which encouraged audiences to abandon individual sexual desires and follow medical recommendations against another hidden enemy that threatened the war effort: venereal disease.[36] The film opens in a recreation hall, where two soldiers are playing pool. Another soldier, Pete, stops to greet them on his way to town. He is dressed to go out, and the two pool players seem to know what his real intentions are. The film cuts to a close-up shot of the cue ball coming up behind the eight ball. Then a close-up shows a record player, we hear jazz music, and then see a smoldering cigar resting on a banister at the top of a staircase, next to a nude statue of a woman. Other burn marks on the banister indicate that this cigar is not the first to be left there. A hand reaches down to pick up the cigar and the camera zooms out to reveal Pete. Disheveled, he does up his belt and leaves. It is clear that Pete has visited a prostitute.

The film continues with the screening of "Sex Hygiene," the film within the film, which all men at the base are required to watch. The movie they see is essentially a filmed lecture given by a military doctor (a stern, authoritative figure, quite different to the alcoholic Doc Boone), who in the film's most famous sequences discusses the various forms of venereal disease, while the camera provides graphic images of diseased penises illustrating the different types of venereal disease (the deep lesions caused by syphilis or the discharge of pus due to gonorrhea) and of open wounds and sores (on the tongue, face, etc.) along with methods of prophylaxis and treatment. We never see the consequences of Pete's decision to visit a prostitute for Pete himself, but *Sex Hygiene* indicates a likely outcome and shows how an audience responds to this. Thus, the film not only shows the film within the film, it also invites us to watch an audience of servicemen watching the film that we are ourselves watching: the reaction shots from the audience (sometimes horrified, sometimes entranced by the movie), their reactions emphasized by the close-up shots of individual audience members often filmed from below.

In such a way, Ford dramatized the conditions of reception (Our own? That of the audience within the film.), and sets the stage for conversion. However, this is not a conversion narrative in the traditional sense of the term, for we never see how the men in the film respond to *Sex Education* after leaving the screening, just as we never see the consequences for Pete himself. Are they shocked enough to follow its strictures? Ford's film has played with our expectations, for earlier social hygiene films had often included a conversation narrative to illustrate the routes to salvation and the penalties for those who did not convert, and it seems in the beginning that that is what Ford is going to do in this movie with the contrast between Pete and the "clean" pool players. Instead, what Ford does is to set out some of the conditions necessary to conversion—the knowledge deemed necessary to convert, the necessary emotional responses (shock, disgust, disquiet), the values (patriotism, and loyalty to the armed forces)—and the role of film in creating such conditions. Then he leaves it to us—the audience—to imagine the conversion, and so convert ourselves.

Ford's film echoed and amplified themes already present in earlier venereal disease films.[37] The threat posed by venereal diseases to military efficiency had been there in World War I social hygiene films, as had the idea of self-control as a patriotic act, and indeed the use of shocking images to illustrate the dangers of going with prostitutes and other women: in *The End of the Road* (1919), the shocking images focused on the insane and lesions of the leg rather than the genitals. (Nor was Ford the first to show genitals in a health education film; in *First Aid Treatment after Exposure to Syphilis* (1924), methods of early treatment of [as yet unaffected] penises are shown.) However, it is his allusion to a conversion narrative, rather than depicting it, that distinguishes his film from many of its forerunners. Many of the earlier films had incorporated a conversion narrative into the story, in which those who adopted the views of the medical profession and either abstained from sex or sought treatment early enough were saved (think here also of Ulmer's *Damaged Lives*) and those who did not suffered dire consequences. Ford, however, abandoned such explicit conversion stories but rather played with the audience, alluding to the conversion narrative without ever showing it.

Ford's reasons for doing this are not known, but he encourages a series of questions in his audiences. (What happened to Pete? Are the audience members depicted in the film persuaded by the film we/they are watching? Are you, the implied viewer of this film, persuaded? What will you/they do after leaving the screening?) Ford provides the elements of a conversion narrative: the routes to salvation (abstinence, the use of condoms, early visits to a physician, among others) and the routes to perdition (ignoring the above recommendations). However, he never shows the conversion moment itself, though there may be an implied moment of conversion as the audience members (depicted and implied) watch the film. By leaving us with the questions about the outcomes for Pete and the audiences of the film, Ford leaves us to fill in the gaps and to imagine the conversion itself. Conversion has ceased to be a narrative, but something to be enacted by the audience.

John Huston and *Let There be Light*

If Ulmer and Ford illustrate the problems with the top-down model of conversion for the public health film, so too, in a different way, does John Huston's *Let There be Light* (1946). This film about how psychotherapy can help military personnel with the trauma caused by war was banned by military censors for many years. This despite having multiple conversion points in which sick patients are made well and prepared for discharge from the military at war's end.

Huston had started in Hollywood as a screenwriter but was probably best known for *The Maltese Falcon* (1941), his directorial debut.[38] The film told the story of a private eye, Sam Spade, played by Humphrey Bogart in his breakout role, who is the cynical (almost) virtuous protagonist in a world corrupted by greed; almost virtuous, since he is having an affair with the wife of his partner in a San Francisco detective agency, Miles Archer. One day a Miss Wonderly visits the agency and there follows a night of tragedy. Miles is shot and killed, as is another man, Floyd Thursby, whom Miss Wonderly claims was involved with her sister. Miss Wonderly and Spade are then dogged by dangerous men who are all after a priceless statuette of a bird, the Maltese Falcon: Joel Cairo, a gunman who also hires Spade to find the bird; Kasper Gutman, the Fat Man who has been searching ruthlessly for it for years, and Wilmer Cook a young man with a gun in the employ of the Fat Man. Spade—also dogged by the police, who think he may have murdered Thursby—offers to help them find it, which he does after another character staggers into his office with the bird and some bullet wounds and dies. However, the falcon is revealed as a fake, as is Wonderly, whose real name is Brigid O'Shaughnessy and who was also the real killer of Miles. Spade hands her over to the police, along with some money given to him by Gutman, which could be seen as a payoff. So his credentials as an almost virtuous man are sealed.

May situates *The Maltese Falcon*—and its critique of American society implied by the story of the almost virtuous man surrounded by greed and corruption—within the context of Huston's developing interest in political and cultural reform.[39] However, with the outbreak of war, Huston, like Ford, abandoned such critiques of American society. Instead, he wrote scripts for *Sergeant York* (1941) in which the eponymous York, a Tennessee farmer, converts to the patriotic cause, seeing the war as a chance to advance the cause of liberty, and *Across the Pacific* (1942) in which Japanese farmer workers rise up against harsh plantation owners and so also align themselves with the Japanese army against American forces. However, Huston seems to have come to question unquestioning patriotism. By the end of the war some of his military films returned to a focus on socially powerless or marginal groups and were not welcomed enthusiastically by their sponsors: *The Battle of San Pietro* (1945) because it showed American soldiers mown down by Germans as a result of military incompetence by the soldiers' superiors,[40] and *Let There be Light* because, Huston believed, its portrayal of the psychologically wounded did not fit military ideals of the fighting man. Indeed, the army reshot the movie as *Shades of Gray* (1948), using a different director; removing racial minorities; using actors as patients and doctors (Huston had not used actors); and downplaying the role of combat in creating psychiatric problems, laying the blame instead on poor mothering.[41]

Let There Be Light was not the first film to illustrate the rehabilitation of patients suffering shellshock or battle fatigue.[42] However, it is quite different from the other health education films discussed in this essay, for it was never screened to its intended audience and fell under military censorship for nearly thirty-five years; paradoxically, it is the best-known and frequently discussed film in this corpus.[43] It aimed to shed light on the treatment of war neuroses (the working title of this film was *The Returning Soldier: The Psychoneurotic*) and was targeted at employers who often refused to hire veterans, whom they considered to be fragile, unpredictable and uncooperative.[44] It aimed to promote the employability of veterans and to avoid a repetition of the problems experienced by veterans of the Great War, often stigmatized and unemployable.

Let There Be Light was filmed at the Mason General Hospital in Brentwood, Long Island. This major hospital complex was used between 1944 and 1946 for the treatment of returning soldiers, and Huston chose it after visiting several other establishments. For several months the Signal Corps team, including the cinematographer Stanley Cortez, followed a group of seventy-five soldiers there.

The film begins with an explanatory text which states that about 20 percent of all battle casualties in the American army during World War II were of a neuropsychiatric nature. The goal of the film is to show that special treatments, such as hypnosis and narcosynthesis, have been particularly successful in acute cases, such as battle neurosis (though it also warns that equal success was not to be expected when dealing with peacetime neuroses, which are usually of a chronic nature). The filmmakers aimed merely to record what took place in the hospital ("No scenes were staged"), and the voiceover on the first sequence (which shows the return of veterans from abroad) expands on this more metaphorically, with an almost pacifist lyrical bent: "Here is the human salvage; the final result of all that metal and fire can do to violate mortal flesh. Some wear the badges of their pain: the crutches, the bandages, the splints. Others show no outward signs, yet they, too, are wounded."

Various cases are then presented, and we witness conversations between military doctors and patients suffering from traumatic or phobic neurosis, aphasia, amnesia, or other illnesses. The stories the soldiers tell are often moving: they are hurting, psychologically and emotionally. Some look at the psychiatrist, others avoid his gaze or look far away. Some speak clearly, others mumble, stutter, or stumble over words or seem reluctant to talk. A diagnosis is made, followed by scenes of life at the hospital, telephone calls, sleepless nights, the comfort of a nurse, physical inspections ("modern psychiatry makes no sharp distinction between the mind [and] the body"), various tests (the electroencephalograph, the Rorschach test), all of which leads up to the treatment of a form of a psychological illness labeled conversion hysteria that resulted in the paralysis of the legs. The paralyzed patient is injected with sodium amytal, which we are told induces a hypnosis-like state: a shortcut to the unconscious mind, the narrator states, that allows the psychiatrist to locate and bring to the surface the emotional conflict, which is the cause of the patient's distress, and to remove, through suggestion, those symptoms that impede recovery. The results are spectacular; the patient is able to walk after only a few minutes.

This therapeutic conversion of the patient with conversion hysteria (reconversion?) is only the start of a long period of treatment, and we are now shown other activities: art classes, occupational therapy, and sports. In group psychotherapy, patients learn the basic causes of their distress and that their inner conflicts are shared by others. None is as spectacular as the sodium amytal treatment, but their place in the film following on from the conversion hysteria sequence means that they emphasize the process of conversion from psychological and neurological sickness to health. Then we are treated to another spectacular therapeutic conversion: a patient who has amnesia, who cannot even recall his name, is hypnotized and, after reliving his experiences in Okinawa, remembers his name and begins the process of healing. Another patient who can hardly speak is administered sodium amytal and is cured of his stuttering: "I can talk. Oh God, I can talk," he is crying and is beginning to recover through further treatment. Through this mixture of dramatic and less dramatic therapeutic results, we are shown a gradual transformation of patients as they begin the process of recovery. They are converting from psychoneurotic patients into patients on their way to being well, putting the past behind them, and preparing for a civilian future in an America at peace, though they worry what the public, family, and employers will think of them.

We are watching a 1940s production: Dimitri Tiomkin's score, Stanley Cortez's photography, and Walter Huston's (father of John) voice-over are all evidence of the golden age roots of Huston's style, and particularly of the influence of productions by Warner, where Huston learned his craft as screenwriter and director. The cost of such a production was not cheap, thanks in large part to the substantial funds made available to Huston (in 1941, Ford had much less to work with, and Ulmer, of course, even less). The approach was also different from the films of the other directors: the shooting was a lengthy immersion in a health care institution, and the motion picture followed each step of the therapeutic process. Huston himself recalled that the patients came to see the cameras as part of their environment: "The cameras ran continually, one on the patient and one on the doctor. We shot thousands of feet of film . . . just to be sure of getting the extraordinary and completely unpredictable exchanges that sometimes occurred. As the men began to recover, they accepted the cameras as an integral part of their treatment."[45] Near the end, we are given something approximating a religious service: the psychiatrist quotes the bible, almost preaching, the patients listening to him like congregants, the camera lingering on their faces, mainly shot from below and to the side, light on their faces, the music rising and falling. Then, during a baseball game, we are shown—through flashbacks to when they first came to the hospital—how far patients have progressed toward recovery before they are triumphantly discharged at the movie's close. The conversion is complete: from sickness to wellness, patient to person, and armed forces personnel to civilian.

Let There Be Light was John Huston's fourth war documentary, after *Report from the Aleutians* (1943), *Tunisian Victory* (codirected with Frank Capra and George Stevens in 1944), and *The Battle of San Pietro* (1945). Generally, *Let There Be Light* is considered to the best of the four and has been described by writer James Agee as "a fine, terrible, valuable nonfiction film about psychoneurotic soldiers."[46] It was of great importance for Huston's career; he admitted to not being very familiar with psychiatric issues and to have read Freud, Jung, and Adler in order to prepare for the film.[47] The experience opened new horizons for him, and he went back to his intense exploration of the how people responded in the face of death and pain in films such as *The Red Badge of Courage* (1951), *Freud* (1962), or *Reflections in a Golden Eye* (1967).

In a 1982 interview shot by Richard Leacock for Midge MacKenzie's film *John Huston War Stories* (1999), the director explained that "documentaries have a tendency to describe rather to let the stories tell themselves. Even when they're poetic, they become epic. That's the inclination. There are some very fine documentaries, by the way, but they have a sense of detachment, as one often says." In his war films, Huston developed a naturalistic style with humanist accents that would define his later entertainments. His daughter, Anjelica Huston, further confided that during their exile in Ireland in the 1960s, his war documentaries were the only films he enjoyed watching at home.[48] In these films, he was able to express his natural empathy, his rejection of conventions, and his own faith in American democracy, which then declined until he renounced his US citizenship in the late 1960s. Ford himself explained, "Altogether, the time at Mason General affected me almost like a religious experience. It made me begin to realize that the primary ingredient in psychological health is love: the ability to give love and to receive it."[49]

Huston seems to have been convinced that he could work freely and therefore did not consider what might actually shock the public or his sponsors. The one exception concerned shock therapy, which he did not include in the film.[50] Huston noted: "In psychotic cases—schizophrenics and catatonics—shock therapy was regularly used. I knew we couldn't use it in the film; it had no place in what we were doing. But I thought it was something that should be photographed for the record. Shock therapy then was much more severe than it is today. The patient used to arch his body so violently from the shock that five people were needed to hold him so he wouldn't break his back. At the same moment he would utter a sound—a kind of primal scream—that was absolutely unnerving."[51]

The banning of the film hit him particularly hard. His earlier documentary, *The Battle of San Pietro*, had already raised eyebrows among the executives of the US Army Pictorial Services. Upon seeing the all too realistic depiction of battle confrontations, some high-ranked officers left the room during the screening, and it was only thanks to George C. Marshall's intervention that the film was released. This time, there was nothing Roosevelt's military advisor could do for *Let There Be Light*. Huston later discussed the reasons for this censorship:

> The reason given was that it violated the privacy of the patients involved. . . . As a matter of form, we had asked them to sign releases, and they were happy to do so. We pointed this out to the War Department, but when asked to produce these releases, we discovered that they had mysteriously disappeared. . . . I think it boils down to the fact that they wanted to maintain the "warrior' myth," which said that our American soldiers went to war and came back all the stronger for the experience, standing tall and proud for having served their country well. Only a few weaklings fell by the wayside. Everyone was a hero, and had medals and ribbons to prove it. They might die, or they might be wounded, but their spirit remained unbroken.[52]

The banning of *Let There Be Light* would puzzle Huston for a long time.[53] Whatever the reason, for our purposes it highlights the importance of the therapeutic conversion narrative to Huston's work, how it served as a way of framing the traumas of war, the transition to civilian life, public attitudes toward those with psychoneurotic illness, and the almost religious role of the psychiatrist as preacher, teacher, and healer. It also serves to highlight the problems with this form of conversion narrative, which was not the sort of conversion that that the military authorities wanted to project.

Conclusion

Conversion narratives have been a central part of American health education and entertainment films since at least the 1910s. However, as the foregoing has shown, the relationship between the two was complex, and it changed over time. In the 1910s and the 1930s, conversion narratives served to demonstrate the willingness of the film industry to reform and to fend off outside efforts to impose controls on its activities. They did this by telling stories of individuals who reformed in one way or another: the rewards that came to them as consequences of their conversion and the penalties for those who did not convert, or who converted too late or after committing a heinous crime that meant they could never achieve salvation without suffering some tragic event. However, as this chapter has suggested, while health education films had a role to play in the industry's efforts in the 1910s, they had only a minor role to play in the 1930s.

Part of the reason for the changing significance of the health education film was the hardening of lines between educationals and entertainments. In the 1910s, educationals, including health education films, were often screened in cinemas as part of the regular schedule. As such, a film that traced the conversion of a character to the recommendations of the National Tuberculosis Association could be screened alongside temperance movies that traced how an alcoholic achieved redemption, along with a variety of comedies and features. By making and screening these films together, the industry hoped to undermine the reputation of cinemas as dens of vice and to make them safe for the growing numbers of middle-class women and children watching films and to stave off efforts by government and voluntary groups to impose reform from outside.

By the 1930s, all this had changed. Health education films were rarely shown in movie theaters as part of the regular schedule, and their ability to demonstrate the willingness of the industry to reform had lessened. Of course, movie companies could still make educational films, and cinema owners might screen them in their theaters, and so highlight the social responsibility of the industry. However, since, in general, these films were no longer regarded as theatricals, they—and the conversion narratives embedded in them—could not demonstrate that the film industry was reforming its key product: theatrical releases. Indeed, as the discussion of *Damaged Lives* suggests, there were dangers in making films on some subjects the focus of a theatrical release. When films about venereal disease were shown to paying customers, the risk was that it might be regarded as smuggling in a sex entertainment under the guise of an educational.[54]

The conversion narratives of health education and entertainment films also diverged in other ways in the 1930s. In particular, they diverged from the 20 percent of Hollywood films that included a conversion narrative which involved the elite converting to the values of the people. Such downward conversions were highly problematic for health education films, which aimed to persuade people to accept the recommendations of their sponsors and the authority of the medical knowledge on which such recommendations were said to be based. It was thus highly unlikely that any sponsor would tolerate a story in which physicians or the sponsoring organization converted to the views of the people: how could they when the latter were often cast as ignorant and in need of emotional support? Even when a sponsor such as the National Tuberculosis Association wanted to tailor a film to particular ethnic audiences, there was no hint that medical knowledge should give up its exalted position. It is true that the Ulmer films highlight the wisdom of the ethnic groups to which they appealed and saw a marriage of folk wisdom and medical science as crucial to the success of these films and the campaigns of which they were a part. However, when folk wisdom was in conflict with medical science, the former had to give way. Individuals converted not only to medical science but also to medically sanctioned folk wisdom. Thus, these ethnic films promoted a down-up conversion narrative, as was the case with the vast majority of health education films.

If the conversion narratives in health education films diverged from those in liberal and left-wing Hollywood entertainments of the 1930s, they had much more in common with the wartime conversion stories of the 1940s. Public health organizations had long adopted the language of war and military organization in their "campaigns" and "crusades" against disease, and the narrative structure of the health education film of the 1930s anticipated many of the themes that would later characterize the wartime educational. Thus, in the 1930s, health education films tended to focus on abandoning individual selfish desires and the ignorant advice of family, friends, and the ill-informed in favor of allegiance to medical advice and interventions in a war against disease. In the 1940s, they added a patriotic element in which allegiance to medical advice and interventions was also allegiance to the wartime aims of the nation and its military. All this at the same time that entertainments told stories of abandoning class and ethnic identities and selfish individualism in favor of patriotic duty and allegiance to hierarchical military organizations.

Yet in some ways, the conversion narratives of the war were different from those of the regular public health film. Social hygiene and venereal disease movies had employed conversion narratives since the First World War, showing the benefits for those who converted to a medical (and moral) view of the disease and the penalties for those who did not convert and ignored medical advice. Moreover, such narratives can be found in many venereal disease educationals produced during the Second World War. Yet when a director such as John Ford approached the topic, he opted to play with expectations, to film the buildup to conversion but not to follow the narrative through to its end. Audiences would have been familiar with the narrative trajectory of the social hygiene film and would likely have expected to see an ending where Pete or members of the audience within the film adopted medically-militarily approved approaches to the risk of disease. Instead, the viewer is left without such an ending. Ford leaves audience members—those not shown in the film itself—to imagine the ending, and so to begin to converting themselves.

The focus on the three directors also highlights the complexity of the relationship between health education conversion narratives and entertainments films. In the case of Ulmer, we have seen how his tuberculosis films adopted a narrative structure very similar to the crossover *Damaged Lives*: part educational, part entertainment. Yet the view of medicine produced in this film and his tuberculosis movies was quite different to that in, for example, *The Black Cat*, where the doctor is a much more ambiguous, almost Faustian figure. In the case of Ford, the view of medicine in *Sex Hygiene* is very different from the colorful, inebriated, but competent Doc Boone in *Stagecoach*. Neither Boone nor Werdegast in the *The Black Cat* are the sorts of serious, authoritative figures that tend to populate the health education conversion narrative. They might be good physicians, and they might at times have honorable intentions, but they are too colorful, too entertaining, and full of too many ambiguities and complexities to promote the sorts of messages found in health education films.

Ford and Huston also highlight the complex relations between their prewar entertainments and their educationals. Before the war, both had directed feature films that were critiques of aspects of American society: Ford with his attacks on social conventions and unregulated capitalism; Huston with his portrayal of an almost virtuous man in a world corrupted by greed. These critiques were not characteristic of all films directed (or in the case of Huston, written) before the war. However, both men abandoned critiques of American society during the war and turned to films with a more patriotic tone. Thus, Ford's wartime movies discarded the progressive causes he had espoused before the war, suggesting instead that people needed to forsake ethnic, class, and individual identities and become fully American: *Sex Hygiene* fitted well into this transition, marrying allegiance to medical advice with allegiance to patriotic wartime goals of the nation. Huston too abandoned his prewar critique of American society and adopted a more patriotic tone, tempered toward the end of the war with his concerns about the impact of war on the men who served. *Let There Be Light* is an example of this later transition, with its humanistic focus on the rehabilitation of men psychologically harmed by war. Huston was by no means the first to demonstrate in film the power of medical interventions to rehabilitate men with shellshock or battle fatigue. However, the response of his sponsors to the film highlights a final point about the function of conversion in health education films. Directors had to not only convert an audience to the goals of a sponsor, but also convert that sponsor to the goals of the director.

Notes

1. On gangsters and gangster films, see Robert Sklar, *City Boys: Cagney, Bogart, Garfield* (Princeton, NJ: Princeton University Press, 1992); David E. Ruth, *Inventing the Public Enemy: The Gangster in American Culture, 1918–1934* (Chicago: University of Chicago Press, 1996); Jonathan Munby, *Public Enemies, Public Heroes: Screening the Gangster from Little Caesar to Touch of Evil* (Chicago: University of Chicago Press, 1999); and Iain Silver and James Ursini, eds., *The Gangster Film Reader* (Pompton Plains, NJ: Limelight, 2007). More generally, see Lary May, *The Big Tomorrow: Hollywood and the Politics of the American Way* (Chicago: University of Chicago Press, 2002).

2. David Cantor, "Choosing to Live: Cancer Education, Movies, and the Conversion Narrative in America, 1921–1960," *Literature and Medicine* 28, no. 2 (2009): 279. See also David Cantor, "Uncertain Enthusiasm: The American Cancer Society, Public Education, and the Problems of the Movie, 1921–1960," *Bulletin of the History of Medicine* 81, no. 1 (2007): 39–69.

3. Tom Gunning, "From the Opium Den to the Theater of Morality: Moral Discourse and the Film Process in Early American Cinema," in *The Silent Cinema Reader*, ed. Lee Grieveson and Peter Krämer (London: Routledge, 2004), 145–54; Lee Grieveson, "'A Kind of Recreative School for the Whole Family': Making Cinema Respectable, 1907–09," *Screen* 42 (2001): 64–76; Martin S. Pernick, "Thomas Edison's

Tuberculosis Films: Mass Media and Health Propaganda," *Hastings Center Report* 8, no. 3 (1978): 21–27; Martin S. Pernick, "More than Illustrations: Early Twentieth-Century Health Films as Contributors to the Histories of Medicine and of Motion Pictures," in *Medicine's Moving Pictures: Medicine, Health, and Bodies in American Film and Television*, ed. Leslie J. Reagan, Nancy Tomes, and Paul A. Treichler (Rochester, NY: University of Rochester Press, 2007), 19–35; and Miriam Posner, "Communicating Disease: Tuberculosis, Narrative, and Social Order in Thomas Edison's Red Cross Seal Films," in *Learning with the Lights Off: Educational Film in the United States*, ed. Devin Orgeron, Marsha Orgeron, and Dan Streible (Oxford: Oxford University Press, 2012), 90–106.

4. For another exception of a health education movie that made it into the regular cinema schedule, see David Cantor, *Man Alive! (1952): Cartoon Fun with Cancer, Cars and Companionate Marriage in Suburban America* (Bethesda, MD: National Library of Medicine, 2014).

5. David Cantor, "Between Movies, Markets, and Medicine: The Eastern Film Corporation, Frank A. Tichenor, and Medical and Health Films in the 1920s," chap. 1 in this volume; and Miriam Posner, "Prostitutes, Charity Girls, and *The End of the Road*: Hostile Worlds of Sex and Commerce in an Early Sexual Hygiene Film," chap. 4 in this volume.

6. Cantor, "Between Movies, Markets, and Medicine."

7. Michael Sappol, "The Public Health Film Goes to War," ed. Paul Theerman and David Cantor, US National Library of Medicine, first published January 31, 2011, http://www.nlm.nih.gov/hmd/digicolls/phfgtw/; Christie Milliken, "Continence of the Continent: The Ideology of Disease and Hygiene in World War II Training Films," in *Cultural Sutures: Medicine and Media*, ed. Lester D. Friedman (Durham, NC: Duke University Press, 2004), 280–314; John Parascandola, "VD at the Movies: PHS Films of the 1930s and 1940s," *Public Health Service Reports* 111 (1996): 173–75; and Marianne Fedunkiw, "Malaria Films: Motion Pictures as a Public Health Tool," *American Journal of Public Health* 93 (2003): 1046–57. More generally, on Hollywood during the war see Clayton R. Koppes and Gregory D. Black, *Hollywood Goes to War: Patriotism, Movies and the Second World War from Ninotchka to Mrs Miniver* (London: Tauris Parke, 2000).

8. Gregory D. Black, *Hollywood Censored: Morality Codes, Catholics, and the Movies* (Cambridge: Cambridge University Press, 2001); and Thomas Patrick Doherty, *Hollywood's Censor: Joseph I. Breen & the Production Code Administration* (New York: Columbia University Press, 2007). See also Lee Grieveson, *Policing Cinema: Movies and Censorship in Early-Twentieth-Century America* (Berkeley: University of California Press, 2004).

9. Paul Buhle and Dave Warner, *Radical Hollywood: The Untold Story behind America's Favorite Movies* (New York: New Press, 2002); and May, *The Big Tomorrow*.

10. For example, *It Happened One Night* (1934), *Lost Horizons* (1937), *You Can't Take It with You* (1938), or *Mr Smith Goes to Washington* (1939).

11. May, *Big Tomorrow*, 277–78.

12. Dana Polan, *Power and Paranoia: History, Narrative and the American Cinema, 1940–1950* (New York: Columbia University Press, 1986), 45–99; Thomas Schatz, "World War II and the Hollywood 'War Film,'" in *Refiguring American Film Genres: History and Theory*, ed. Nick Browne (Berkeley: University of California Press, 1998), 89–128; and May, *Big Tomorrow*.

13. Quoted in May, *Big Tomorrow*, 142.

14. May, *Big Tomorrow*, 156.

15. For biographical details on Ulmer, see Noah Isenberg, *Edgar G. Ulmer: A Filmmaker at the Margins* (Berkeley: University of California Press, 2014). See also Gary Don Rhodes, ed., *Edgar G. Ulmer: Detour on Poverty Row* (Lanham, MD: Lexington Books, 2008); Bernd Herzogenrath, ed., *Edgar G. Ulmer: Essays on the King of the B's* (Jefferson, NC: McFarland, 2009); and Bernd Herzogenrath, ed., *The Films of Edgar G. Ulmer* (Lanham, MD: The Scarecrow Press, 2009).

16. Ulmer turned to small production companies that targeted distinct ethnic communities: the Avramenko Film Company addressed the Russian-speaking community (*Natalka Poltavka*, 1937; *Cossacks in Exile*, 1939), the Collective Film Producers Inc. for the Yiddish-speaking Jewish community (*Green Fields* [*Greene felde*, 1937]; *The Singing Blacksmith* [*Yankel der Shmid*, 1938]; *The Light Ahead* [*Die Klatsche*, 1939]) and Meteor Productions Inc. for the Afro-American community (*Moon over Harlem* [1939]).

17. Devin Orgeron, "Spreading the Word: Race, Religion, and the Rhetoric of Contagion in Edgar G. Ulmer's TB Films," in *Learning with the Lights Off*, ed. Devin Orgeron, Marsha Orgeron, and Dan Streible, 295–315; and Christian Bonah and Vincent Lowy, "Lorsque le regard l'emporte sur le message: Les courts-métrages de lutte contre la tuberculose d'Edgar G. Ulmer," *Alliage* 71 (2012): 46–56. See also Gregg Mitman, "The Color of Money: Campaigning for Health in Black and White America," in *Imagining Illness: Public Health and Visual Culture*, ed. David Serlin (Minneapolis: University of Minnesota Press, 2011), 40–61. On the history of the tuberculosis association, see Richard Harrison Shyrock, *National Tuberculosis Association, 1904–1954: A Study of the Voluntary Health Movement in the United States* (New York: Ayer Publishing, 1977).

18. Bonah and Lowy, "Lorsque le regard l'emporte sur le message."

19. Orgeron, "Spreading the Word"; Cantor, "Choosing to Live."

20. On *The Black Cat*, see the three essays on this film in Rhodes, *Edgar G. Ulmer*.

21. On *Damaged Lives*, see esp. Isenberg, *Edgar G. Ulmer*, esp. 44–53.

22. Martin S. Pernick, *The Black Stork: Eugenics and the Death of "Defective" Babies in American Medicine and Motion Pictures since 1915* (New York: Oxford University Press, 1996); Stacie A. Colwell, "The End of the Road: Gender, the Dissemination of Knowledge, and the American Campaign against Venereal Disease during World War I," *Camera Obscura* 29 (May 1992): 91–129; and Allan M. Brandt, *No Magic Bullet: A Social History of Venereal Disease in the United States since 1880* (New York: Oxford University Press, 1985), chap. 2, 52–95. Also, Miriam Posner, "Prostitutes, Charity Girls."

23. Annette Kuhn, *Cinema, Censorship, and Sexuality, 1909–1925* (London: Routledge, 1988), chap. 4, 49–74. Also Posner, "Prostitutes, Charity Girls."

24. Nancy Tomes, *The Gospel of Germs: Men, Women and the Microbe in American Life* (Cambridge, MA: Harvard University Press, 1998), esp. 113–34. Also on TB, see Barron Lerner, *Contagion and Confinement: Controlling Tuberculosis along the Skid Road* (Baltimore: Johns Hopkins University Press, 1998); Samuel Roberts, *Infectious Fear: Politics, Disease, and the Health Effects of Segregation* (Chapel Hill: University of North Carolina Press, 2009); Georgina Feldberg, *Disease and Class: Tuberculosis and*

the Shaping of Modern North American Society (New Brunswick, NJ: Rutgers University Press, 1995); and Posner. "Communicating Disease."

25. Isenberg, *Edgar G. Ulmer*, 44–53.

26. Bonah and Lowy, "Lorsque le regard l'emporte sur le message."

27. Jean-Pierre Coursodon and Bertrand Tavernier, *50 ans de Cinéma américain* (Paris: Nathan, 1995), 945.

28. See *The Man from Planet X* (1951).

29. On the voluminous literature on Ford, see, for example, Peter Bogdanovich, *John Ford* (Berkeley: University of California Press, 1978); Tag Gallagher, *John Ford: The Man and His Films* (Berkeley: University of California Press, 1986); Ronald L. Davis, *John Ford: Hollywood's Old Master* (Norman: University of Oklahoma Press, 1995); Brian Spittles, *John Ford* (New York: Longman, 2002); Peter Cowie, *John Ford and the American West* (New York: H. N. Abrams, 2004); Sidney A. Pearson, *Print the Legend: Politics, Culture, and Civic Virtue in the Films of John Ford* (Lanham, MD: Lexington Books, 2009); Joseph McBride, *Searching for John Ford* (Jackson: University Press of Mississippi, 2011); David Meuel, *Women in the Films of John Ford* (Jefferson, NC: McFarland, 2014); and Sue Matheson, *The Westerns and War Films of John Ford* (Lanham, MD: Rowman & Littlefield, 2016).

30. May, *Big Tomorrow*, 277–79.

31. Barry Keith Grant, *John Ford's "Stagecoach"* (Cambridge: Cambridge University Press, 2003).

32. Graham Cassano, "Radical Critique and Progressive Traditionalism in John Ford's *The Grapes of Wrath*," *Critical Sociology* 34 (2008): 99–116; Graham Cassano, "The Corporate Imaginary in John Ford's New Deal Cinema," *Rethinking Marxism* 21 (2009): 480–97; and Gabriel Sealey-Morris, "Dust Bowl Iconography: Populist Translations of *The Grapes of Wrath*," *Journal of Popular Culture* 48 (2015): 198–208. On the interconnections between the film, the novel, and Farm Security Administration photographs, see James R. Swensen, *Picturing Migrants: The Grapes of Wrath and New Deal Documentary Photography* (Norman: University of Oklahoma Press, 2015).

33. Lea Jacobs, "Making John Ford's *How Green Was My Valley*," *Film History* 28 (2016): 32–80.

34. Matheson, *The Westerns and War Films*, esp. chaps. 4 and 5.

35. See May, *Big Tomorrow*, 153–56.

36. Milliken, "Continence of the Continent."

37. John Parascandola, "Syphilis at the Cinema: Medicine and Morals in VD Films of the U.S. Public Health Service in World War II," in Reagan, Tomes, and Treichler, *Medicine's Moving Pictures*, 71–92; Christian Bonah and Anja Laukötter, eds., special issue, "Screening Sex Hygiene Films in the first Half of the 20th Century," *Gesnerus* 72, no. 1 (2015): 5–93; Alain Corbin, "Le péril vénérien au début du siècle: Prophylaxie sanitaire et prophylaxie morale," *Recherches* 16, no. 29 (1978): 245–83; and Brandt, *No Magic Bullet.*

38. Gerald Pratley, *The Cinema of John Huston* (Cranbury, NJ: A. S. Barnes, 1977); Gaylyn Studlar and David Desser, eds., *Reflections in a Male Eye: John Huston and the American Experience* (Washington, DC: Smithsonian Institution Press, 1993); William Luhr, ed., *The Maltese Falcon: John Huston, Director* (New Brunswick, NJ: Rutgers University Press, 1995); and Tony Tracy and Roddy Flynn, eds., *John Huston: Essays on a Restless Director* (Jefferson, NC: McFarland, 2010).

39. May, *Big Tomorrow*, 232–34.

40. Greg Garrett, "John Huston's *The Battle of San Pietro*," *War, Literature and the Arts* 5, no. 1 (1993): 3–12; Matthew Evangelista, "Manipulation and Memory in John Huston's *The Battle of San Pietro*," *Film & History* 46, no. 1 (2016): 4–20; Lance Bertelsen, "San Pietro and the 'Art' of War," *Southwest Review* 74, no. 2 (1989): 230–56; and Mark Harris, *Five Came Back: A Story of Hollywood and the Second World War* (New York: Penguin Press, 2014).

41. Emmett Early, *The War Veteran in Film* (Jefferson, NC: McFarland, 2003), 70–71.

42. Edgar Jones, "War Neuroses and Arthur Hurst: A Pioneering Medical Film about the Treatment of Psychiatric Battle Casualties," *Journal of the History of Medicine and Allied Sciences* 67 (2012): 345–73; Tiffany Watt Smith, *On Flinching: Theatricality and Scientific Looking from Darwin to Shell-Shock* (Oxford: Oxford University Press, 2014), 164–207; and Julie M. Powell, "Shock Troupe: Medical Film and the Performance of 'Shell Shock' for the British Nation at War," *Social History of Medicine* 30 (2017): 323–45. See also Anton Kaes, *Shell Shock Cinema: Weimar Culture and the Wounds of War* (Princeton, NJ: Princeton University Press, 2009).

43. For the film's history, see Gary Edgerton, "Revisiting the Recordings of Wars Past: Remembering the Documentary Trilogy of John Huston," in *Reflections in a Male Eye: John Huston and the American Experience*, ed. Gaylyn Studlar and David Desser (Washington, DC: Smithsonian Institution Press, 1993), 33–61; Greg Garrett, "Muffling the Bell of Liberty: Censorship and the World War II Documentary," *Journal of the American Studies Association of Texas* 22 (1991): 61–73; and Greg Garrett, "*Let There be Light* and Huston's Film Noir," *Proteus* 7, no. 2 (1990): 30–33.

44. On the problems associated with the return to civilian life, see Morse A. Cartwright, *Marching Home: Educational and Social Adjustment after the War* (New York: Publication for the Institute of Adult Education by the Bureau of Publications, Teachers College, Columbia University, 1944); Charles G. Bolte, *The New Veteran* (New York: Reynal & Hitchcock, 1945); and Illinois Society for Mental Hygiene, *Proceedings of the Institute on Readjusting with the Returning Servicemen: Held March 8–9, 1945, in The Knickerbocker Hotel, Chicago, Illinois Under the Auspices of the Illinois Society for Mental Hygiene* (Chicago: Illinois Society for Mental Hygiene, 1945). More generally, on psychiatry in the military, see Ben Shephard, *A War of Nerves: Soldiers and Psychiatrists, 1914–1994* (London: Cape, 2000); Peter Leese, *Shell Shock: Traumatic Neurosis and the British Soldiers of the First World War* (Basingstoke, UK: Palgrave, 2002); Allan Young, *The Harmony of Illusions: Inventing Post-traumatic Stress Disorder* (Princeton, NJ: Princeton University Press, 1995); and Edgar Jones and Simon Wessely, *Shell Shock to PTSD: Military Psychiatry from 1900 to the Gulf War* (New York: Psychology Press, 2005).

45. John Huston, *An Open Book* (Cambridge, MA: Da Capo Press, 1994), 123.

46. See James Agee, *Agee on Film: Criticism and Comment on the Movies* (New York: Modern Library, 2000).

47. See Robert Hughes, ed., *Film: Book 2: Films of Peace and War* (New York: Grove Press, 1962); and Axel Madsen, *John Huston* (London: Robson Books, 1979).

48. See Tracy and Flynn, *John Huston.*

49. Huston, *An Open Book*, 125.

50. On this controversial therapy, see Edward Shorter and David Healy, *Shock Therapy: A History of Electroconvulsive Treatment in Mental Illness* (Toronto: University of Toronto Press, 2007).

51. Huston, *An Open Book*, 123.

52. Ibid., 125.

53. Bertrand Tavernier, *Amis américains: Entretiens avec les grands auteurs d'Hollywood* (Lyon, France: Actes Sud/Institut Lumière, 2008), 457.

54. See also Posner. "Prostitutes, Charity Girls."

Part Two

Campaigns

Chapter Four

Prostitutes, Charity Girls, and The End of the Road

Hostile Worlds of Sex and Commerce in an Early Sexual Hygiene Film

Miriam Posner

During World War I, an unusual group of watchwomen patrolled the streets around soldiers' training camps: middle-class matrons on the lookout for young women on the verge of committing sin.[1] Once identified, these young women could be grouped into two categories: the charity girl, who might exchange sexual favors for goods, but not cash; and the prostitute, who exchanged sex for money. The first was redeemable, the second a lost cause. As the World War I–era film *The End of the Road* demonstrates, this seemingly arbitrary distinction applied not just to sex but also to films about sex.

In the United States, World War I helped to usher in large-scale demographic and cultural changes, and social reformers of the era responded by policing gender roles ever more closely. *The End of the Road*, a 1919 sexual health film designed for women, is an artifact of this fraught wartime moment. A morality tale for working women, *The End of the Road* offers strict guidance on how to draw boundaries between the world of commerce and the world of sexual love. An artifact of anxiety about changing sexual mores, *The End of the* Road demonstrates how that anxiety centered on the intertwining of sex and commerce and how this unease extended beyond the film itself and into its tumultuous exhibition history. *The End of the Road* documents discomfort about the commingling of sex and commerce, but this tension wasn't confined to the film's subject matter. The film itself became an agent of furious debate when it traveled from a closed viewing circuit into commercial exhibition. The film's rocky exhibition history shows how a film conceived as part of one corpus (in this case, the generation of social hygiene films that appeared around World War I) can, in spite of its producers' intentions, develop entirely different connotations when the context of its exhibition associates it with a different corpus (commercial use). Thus, the same film could be relatively inoffensive in one setting. But charge admission for it, and the film is thrust into a different corpus altogether.

The End of the Road was part of a complement of sexual health films that emerged around World War I.[2] The period's sexual health-related releases included *Damaged Goods* (American Film Manufacturing Company, 1914), *Open Your Eyes* (Warner Bros., 1919), *The Scarlet Trail* (John S. Lawrence, 1918), *The Spreading Evil* (James Keane, 1918), *Whatsoever a Man Soweth* (Beaverbrook, ca. 1919), *The Solitary Sin* (New Art, 1919), and *Wild Oats* (New York City Department of Health, 1919). *The End of the Road*, then, is one of a number of World War I–era films and shares with its cohort concerns about large-scale changes in sexual mores and population trends: the movement of women to urban industrial centers, for example, as well as new patterns of courtship and understandings of leisure time. It is also quite distinct, though, in that it was designed specifically for female audiences; indeed, it is the first known American sexual hygiene film intended to be shown to women.

The End of the Road is part of a set in another important way. Two US-government-sponsored films about venereal disease in fact emerged from World War I, the first conflict in which the US government had film at its disposal: *Fit to Fight*, which details the risk of venereal disease for men, and *The End of the Road*, designed as a companion film for women. Their sponsors intended both films to be shown in noncommercial wartime settings, but both films entered the commercial sphere (with fairly disastrous consequences) following the close of World War I.

So in one evident way, *The End of the Road* can be read as part of a corpus of contemporaneous public hygiene films. Yet *The End of the Road*'s exhibition history helps us to see how the notion of what constitutes a corpus depends very much on context. A film's companions and comparisons can change drastically, not just over time (as, for example, a science fiction film can enter *Mystery Science Theater* territory as it ages), but over space, even within the same cultural context. In one setting, *The End of the Road* was salubrious; in another, it was smut.

In its framework, this essay relies heavily on Thomas Elsaesser's notion of the utility film, cited by the editors in this volume's introduction. Like Elsaesser, I argue that one cannot make sense of this film unless one understands the peculiar set of historical circumstances from which it originated. It is not at all clear, for example, why a melodrama about department stores and venereal disease was a specifically *wartime* formulation unless one understands the particular shape that discourse about women's sexual propriety took during World War I in the United States. The seedy outskirts of military training camps may seem a world apart from the genteel drawing rooms in which *The End of the Road*'s heroines appear. But in fact the two settings—the gritty backstreet and the middle-class parlor room—are deeply intertwined. *The End of the Road* was specifically devised as a counterbalance to the liaisons that health reformers feared were forming in the back alleys of military boomtowns. But one can't, likewise, take *The End of the Road* as a particularly accurate reflection of the way sexuality actually operated for the women whose lives it purports to document. Working women's real-life experience of sex was infinitely more nuanced than the binary framework of vice and virtue that *The End of the Road* offers. For young women in the mid-to-late 1910s, sexuality was a matter of negotiation, pleasure, and (sometimes) commerce. These shades of gray are lost in the black-and-white world of *The End of the Road.* So while at first glance, *The End of the Road* seems to document a moment when virtue and vice were cleanly delineated, a closer look at the conditions of its production and exhibition demonstrates that it captures a moment characterized not by consensus but by disunion. Women's sexuality was, during this period as always, supremely personal, context-dependent, and multivalent.

This essay joins a number of works that have looked at public health films during this period.[3] While these works offer important context, they do not focus specifically on sexual health rhetoric addressed toward women. The scholarship on attitudes toward sex during this period is likewise extensive, but film does not receive the focused treatment I give it here.[4] In fact, I argue, the cinematic rhetoric pioneered by *The End of the Road* can shed light on aspects of the history of women's sexual health that are not illuminated in other documents from the period. Specifically, *The End of the Road*'s production history illustrates an important but little-discussed strain of discourse about public health and mass culture during this period. For public health campaigners of these years, film was an attractive mechanism of disseminating a message specifically because it acted something like a pill or an injection in its ability to be absorbed by the body, its inoculating effects, and its potential application to wide segments of the population.

Several works focus on *The End of the Road* specifically, including Stacie Colwell's work on the dissemination of knowledge and the American campaign against venereal disease during World War I,[5] but my approach, which examines *The End of the Road* through the lens of the entanglement of sex and commerce, remains distinct. *The End of the Road* is closely linked with *Fit to Fight* (later reedited and released in 1919 as *Fit to Win*). I have chosen here to focus mainly on *The End of the Road* because, while the two are linked in conception and reception, *The End of the Road* has particular lessons to teach us about the application of sexual surveillance to women's bodies specifically.

In the bare outlines of its plot, *The End of the Road* is the tale of two young women whose stories serve as opposing examples of education and conduct. Mary Lee is the fortunate daughter of a modern-minded mother who educates her daughter in human reproduction. In contrast, Mary's friend Vera is shielded by her mother from the facts of life. As a consequence, Mary grows up to become a virtuous, sexually abstemious nurse, while Vera, a shopgirl, falls in with a fast crowd and contracts syphilis. Many elements of *The End of the Road* mirror aspects of popular, general-release films of the period. Its melodramatic plot arc, for example, in which virtue and vice are uncomplicated by shades of grey, is typical for films of the period. Likewise its mannered, baroque acting style is a holdover from the theatrical performance style that films had yet to abandon.

The design for *The End of the Road*'s exhibition is critical to understanding how it was supposed to work. The film was very specifically written for noncommercial audiences in an educational setting, designed to be shown with the guidance of a trained (live) lecturer who could narrate the film and lead discussions afterward.[6] The Commission on Training Camp Activities (CTCA), the government agency that sponsored the film, imagined that it would be shown in closely supervised settings, such as the Young Women's Christian Association, women's clubs, or benevolent societies, where lecturers would first screen the film and then conduct discussions afterward with the young women who were thought to be its primary audience. *The End of the Road*, then, was explicitly designed for young women and their mothers, while *Fit to Fight* was specifically designed for an audience of military-aged men. The film's personnel, reflecting its mix of sentimental appeal and uplifting message, were drawn both from the mainstream motion-picture world and from the growing ranks of professional social workers. *The End of the Road* was directed by Edward H. Griffith, director of motion pictures for the CTCA, who had also had a prewar career as a writer and actor with the Edison Company. Richard Bennett, the film's leading man, had also appeared as George Dupont, the young college graduate infected with VD, in *Damaged Goods*. The writer of *The End of the Road*, Katharine Bement Davis, was a prominent sociologist and director of the War Department's Committee on Protective Work for Girls. The film featured acting by soldiers and was filmed by cameramen from the Medical Department of the army. Shot at the Rockefeller estate in Pocantico Hills, New York, the film stars the professional actors Bennett (as the physician) and Claire Adams (as Mary Lee).

Prostitutes and Charity Girls: Sexual Mores at War

Though war makes no explicit appearance in the film, *The End of the Road* is very much a wartime film. It reflects a brand of anxiety that stems directly from the domestic training camps preparing soldiers for World War I. In fact, these camps had long been a source of embarrassment to the military. In prior engagements, prostitution, alcohol, and all manner of vice had been permitted to take place unchecked in ad hoc shantytowns surrounding the training camps.[7]

In response, Secretary of War Newton D. Baker authorized the formation of the Commission on Training Camp Activities (CTCA) in 1917. Baker charged CTCA officials with replicating the wholesome influence of the domestic environment, the absence of which had been identified as a key factor in solders' turn to prostitution and vice in prior engagements. The CTCA promulgated a four-point American Plan to prevent venereal disease: education, medical treatment for infected soldiers, recreation, and discipline. Groups such as the Young Men's Christian Association, the Jewish Welfare Board, the American Library Association, and the Salvation Army worked under the CTCA to sponsor activities and clubhouses designed to provide soldiers with the domestic settings that would give them the strength they needed to combat temptation. The Section on Women and Girls, created in 1918, was responsible for keeping an eye on women in the towns surrounding encampments through patrols, reporting, alternative recreation, and punishment of offenders.

The CTCA, like many social reform organizations of the time, embraced a view of sexual relations that saw the desires of men and women very differently. While women were generally victims of their own sexual impulses, men could exercise a rugged mastery over their desires. Men who succumbed to sexual desire could be recuperated, returning to wholesome American masculinity. Women, on the other hand, were forever soiled by sexual experimentation. Their adolescence, when these desires were most pronounced, was a period of great danger for women. Adolescent girls, then, needed protection from their own destructive wills.[8]

CTCA officials attacked prostitution with a vengeance, eradicating red-light districts through unstinting vigilance and constant patrols. Yet the goal of these efforts, the abolishment of prostitution, remained elusive. One public-health officer complained that ad hoc red-light districts had been found as far as one hundred miles away from the camps themselves.[9] Worse, prostitutes showed an infuriating canniness when it came to evading the law. "The single clandestine prostitute, moving secretly from city to city and even changing her residence with significant frequency in each city, is now the main source of infection," reported one CTCA official in 1918. "Hotel appointments, made through the agency of porters and bell-boys, and automobile excursions into the countryside with the chauffeur acting as go-between, now represent the bulk of her business."[10] In spite of the CTCA's best efforts to occupy soldiers with healthy diversions, training camps were in fact teeming with prostitution, venereal disease, and all manner of louche behavior.

Despairing of their ability to track down and imprison every prostitute, CTCA officials resolved to go after vice at an earlier manifestation: that of vulnerable young women who teetered on the brink of accepting money for sex. They paid particular attention to women whom they identified as on the verge of prostitution. "These are the 'charity girls,'" one official explained, "the runaway or incorrigible girls, or girls of low mentality who are a menace and a responsibility to the community." The "charity girl" was in fact a specific, and noteworthy, wartime formulation. She was the young woman—frequently away from her family, in an urban environment—who accepted gifts, meals, and entertainment from men in exchange for sexual favors. These women were not, in reformers' minds, technically prostitutes, because they had not taken the step of accepting cash for sex. They were, however, stepping alarmingly close to a line that hygienists saw as quite bright: the division between the ordinary woman and the prostitute.

> But all of our sex offenders are not prostitutes, as that term is generally understood. There is the so-called "charity girl"—the girl who goes with the soldier in return for dinners, automobile rides, or any present he may give her. She receives no money. In some cases she is the daughter of a well-to-do family. In many others she is the wife of a man who works at night, or is often away from home. She is usually promiscuous and, therefore, usually diseased.[11]

The charity girl, contemporary social workers emphasized, was distinctly *not* a prostitute; she was just in thrall to "an atmosphere of romantic glamor around the man in uniform." It was, however, a slippery slope from charity girl to prostitute. "From her own lover who has gone over seas, perhaps never to return, to other lovers in quick succession, becomes an easy step."[12]

To the frustration of social reformers, cities were newly bursting with just the kind of young, single women who might be susceptible to crossing the line. The advent of industrial capitalism brought an abundance of wage-labor jobs in urban centers. Young women moved to the city in unprecedented numbers, taking up residence in tenements and rooming houses, often in crowded conditions. An industry of leisure, including dance halls, amusement parks, nightclubs, and theaters awaited them outside the workplace. Unlike the late nineteenth century, when the ideology of separate spheres prescribed the social separation of men and women, this new urban environment was a heterosocial space where men and women were expected to mix freely. These women stood between two worlds: the expectations for feminine behavior lingering from the Old World and the new patterns of labor and leisure that characterized the new economy.[13]

In fact, as public health reformers sensed to their dismay, mores among working-class women *were* changing, reflecting the reality of women's everyday lived experience. During their leisure time, women navigated a new array of dance halls, theaters, and other commercial amusements. They also faced economic inequities. These women worked long hours for less pay than their male counterparts, which gave them an implicit incentive to take part in the culture of "treating," in which men paid for their dates' gifts and entertainment. So on the one hand, middle-class reformers frowned upon treating behaviors as markers of depraved promiscuity; but on the other hand, the financial pressures created by the suppression of women's wages worked on women from the opposite direction, encouraging them to derive financial benefit from male companionship. It was a double-bind that had everything to do with socioeconomic forces, a state of affairs nowhere reflected in *The End of the Road*. To navigate this heterosocial landscape of desire, entertainment, and consumption was to negotiate "subtle and flexible standards of personal conduct."[14]

So young working-class women did have moral codes by which they gauged their behavior, but these codes often differed significantly from those of middle-class reformers. For many social workers, a slide into bad behavior was irreversible. A woman could be rehabilitated, but she could never fully remove the stain of her sexual transgression. Premarital sex was a "dead line" from which there was no return. For many young women, on the other hand, sexual behavior was not so much like flipping a switch from bad to good as it was a series of nuanced, contextualized decisions. Furthermore, bad behavior for young working-class women of the period was not a matter of engaging in a particular activity; it was a question of self-respect. A woman who freely chose to court and treat had nothing to be ashamed of; a woman who was driven to sexual favors by desperation, on the other hand, was an object of pity or derision. As Elizabeth Lunbeck has shown, working women of the period tended to classify a woman as having "gone wrong" not by her engagement in sexual activity but by an attitude of despair.[15]

Reformers, however, tended not to make these subtle distinctions; to the social hygienists of the CTCA, sex was sex. And the training camps, to their supervisors' horror, seemed to act as magnets for footloose young women. "Young girls are flocking to our camp towns," lamented one social worker, "attracted by the khaki as well as by stories of the need for workers and the fabulous salaries paid them."[16] The Committee on Protective Work for Girls, formed in 1917, was a subgroup of the CTCA charged with identifying and diverting the young, sexually active women who surrounded military encampments. Committee members were assigned to act as "protective officers," patrolling amusement parks, dance halls, and streets in search of vulnerable women, who would then be returned to their homes. Patrollers were "drawn from women's clubs, business women, and paid workers in organizations for girls" and "taught how to observe and interpret the details of evidence which are constantly coming to their attention."[17] *The End of the Road* might most usefully be seen as an extension of this activity: simply a more efficient way for reform-minded matrons to reach vulnerable women—with the added benefit of melodrama to make the message more palatable. In this respect, *The End of the Road* demonstrates a curious fact about public health films: their tendency in practice to surveil women's behavior even as they purport to model it. Indeed, the setting for the film's intended screening, the club screening room, supervised by a trained lecturer, offered ample opportunities to observe and police women's behavior.

Neither charity girls nor prostitutes were respectable by middle-class standards. But reformers like those of the CTCA did draw a clear line between the two types of women. The one, who accepted gifts, meals, and entertainment, was vulnerable but could be rescued. An attentive benevolent worker could identify these at-risk women, help them to recover through wholesome activities and lectures, and return them to the fold of virtuous womanhood. The other kind of woman, on the other hand, who took money in exchange for sex, had "crossed the line." She "was deemed dangerous, not only to the young men she allures, but, earning money easily, dressing more showily, furnishes a dangerous example to girls of weak will and unsatisfied desires."[18]

Reformers' beliefs about the difference between the charity girl and the prostitute were not simply theoretical. They had real and profound repercussions for the women so designated. Charity girls found circulating military training encampments could be simply sent home (perhaps with supervision).

Prostitutes, on the other hand, were incarcerated without trial and sent to reformatory institutions, often in remote country locations.[19] So while young women made decisions about sex according to a complicated calculus that reflected the changing world around them, sexual health reformers hewed to a bright line that acknowledged no such complexity.

Hostile Worlds: End of the Road *and Monetized Sex*

Reformers, then, were quite sensitive to young women's contact with money, particularly when that money might be construed as a payment for sexual favors. Treating, as I've explained, was one thing; money in exchange for sex was a very different proposition. Viviana Zelizer offers a convincing explanation for this curious sensitivity to the contact of sex with money, arguing that in monetized economies, rhetoric stringently polices the separation between money and intimacy. Zelizer calls this rhetorical insistence on the separation of money and intimacy the "hostile worlds" view. Americans have piously declared the incommensurability of, for example, money and sex, even as they mount furious court battles about alimony and child support or negotiate household finances in divorce court.[20] This fastidious rejection of a relationship between love and money is very much in evidence in *The End of the Road*'s content, in its conception of its audience, and in the conditions of its exhibition (and ultimate suppression).

Zelizer traces anxiety about the intermingling of intimacy and commerce to the competing virtues, originating in nineteenth-century social analysis, of Gemeinschaft and Gesellschaft: loosely, community-oriented sentiment on the one hand and rational self-interest on the other.[21] The two values, in this view, must never become confused for fear of contamination. The efficient operation of industrial capitalism required its evacuation of sentimentality. Likewise, the sphere of sentiment needed protection from the ruthless machinery of the rational market. As Eva Illouz has pointed out, this rhetorical separation of love and commerce is ironic, given the central role of the market in creating the imagery and language we associate with romantic love.[22]

The End of the Road conforms to this rhetoric of hostile worlds in its themes, characterization, and imagery. Vera—the character who contracts venereal disease—is led to her downfall specifically through a series of contacts with the marketplace. From the outset of the film, on the other hand, Mary (the future nurse) is situated well within a circle of feminine domesticity, carefully isolated from contact with the workings of the marketplace. Early in the film, for example, Mary and her mother, both dressed in white, begin their discussion of reproduction with a mother hen and her baby chicks, a sweetly sentimental marker of maternal care. When Mrs. Lee describes her pregnancy, the film cuts to another scene of maternal domesticity: Mrs. Lee is sewing before the fireplace. Vera Wagner's mother, on the other hand, is consistently associated, thematically and visually, with commerce and consumerism. Mrs. Wagner is pictured reading a popular romantic novel, too preoccupied to give Vera her attention. While Mrs. Lee wears simple clothing, Mrs. Wagner is given to feathers, lace, and other such frippery. When Mrs. Wagner rejects Arthur, Vera's young suitor, it is not because of his personal qualities but because Arthur's bank balance does not meet Mrs. Lynch's expectations.

As Vera and Mary grow older, they follow their mothers' examples: Mary distances herself from any connection with commerce, while Vera takes the opposite path. At the girls' graduation, Mary, the valedictorian, appears in a simple, girlish dress, while Vera, fussily adjusting her hair and gown, wears an ornate ensemble. Tellingly, Mary chooses nursing as her profession—depicted here as an extension of feminine domestic care. Vera, on the other hand, is urged by her mother to become a shopgirl, the better to "find a rich man." In a superimposed image, Vera first imagines her future in a simple cottage but is chastised by her mother. Urged on by Mrs. Wagner, Vera replaces the daydream of a simple life with an image of a fast car, dapper husband, and large mansion.

While Mary blossoms into a nurse under the tutelage of the physician Philip Bell, Vera finds a situation a large New York City department store, believing it to be her best chance of meeting a rich man. Vera works behind the counter, displayed like the goods that surround her. When she makes a date with Howard Lord, the dandy she meets at the store, it is because she's besotted with Howard's car. Later, Howard and Vera negotiate Vera's fate over the shop counter, Howard promising Vera a luxurious life if she becomes his mistress. When Vera makes her fateful decision, it is amidst the opulent surroundings of the apartment where Howard promises to install her. And when Howard finally decides to leave Vera, he pays her for her time, giving her $1,000. Each decisive moment in Vera's decline into disrepute is pointedly underlined with a financial transaction.

Sexual Health and the Cinematic Marketplace

If the message of *The End of the Road* is clear, the film's postwar fate is interestingly messy, showing how a film conceived as part of one genre can take on ribald associations when it becomes attached to another. Following the war, CTCA, seeing an opportunity to expand its message, contracted with Public Health Films to release the film to general audiences. It must have seemed a reasonable decision. *The End of the Road*, after all, had been well-received in the churches and YWCAs where it had screened during the war—why not expand the reach of its message? *The End of the Road's* commercial run, however, did not go as planned. Once the film began to circulate in the commercial sphere, its message was suddenly not salutary but sensational. Just as, in *The End of the Road*, women are condemned for mixing sex with commerce, sexual hygiene films themselves became salacious when they entered the marketplace.

The film began its commercial run in the spring of 1919. Where it was permitted to be shown, *The End of the Road* was in fact a commercial success. That

May, *Variety* reported that *The End of the Road* was "playing to capacity in the fifth week" of a Brooklyn run.[23] In Chicago, screenings were "booked solid" with "every theater playing report[ing] capacity houses."[24] And it even seemed to accomplish its intended effect of raising awareness of venereal disease; the Chicago Social Hygiene League told the *Exhibitor's Herald* that *The End of the Road* "has brought more cases to their dispensary in the past three months than they had in the entire year of 1918."[25] So women, at least in broad terms, seemed to respond fairly positively to the film, apparently appreciating the discussion of women's sexuality, however oversimplified.

In many locations, *The End of the Road* also met with a positive reception from local women's clubs and reform organizations. In Atlanta, Chicago, and Los Angeles, women's civic clubs organized group screenings of the film.[26] More than five hundred Boy Scouts attended a screening (accompanied by their fathers) in Atlanta.[27] "To my mind this picture is wonderful," said the vice president of the Atlanta Woman's Club. "I urge every mother to go with her daughter to see it and every father to take his son. Every man and woman in Atlanta should see it."[28]

Despite this popular acclaim, the film lit a firestorm of debate within the motion picture industry. Film executives blanched at the film's controversial subject matter; worse, the year 1919 saw the release of a number of other sex hygiene films in addition to *Fit to Win* and *End of the Road*, including *The Spreading Evil, Open Your Eyes, The Solitary Sin, Wild Oats, A Victim of Sin*, and *The Scarlet Trail.* Faced with this barrage of VD films, movie executives—already nervous about film's low-class connotations—feared that the medium would slip from one corpus, the wholesome body of social hygiene films, and into another, the seedy ranks of the exploitation film. The fact that it was in part the government saddling the industry with these controversial films inspired incredulity, not confidence. "We have no word of criticism for Government officials who see the peril of disease and wish to warn the public of it," avowed the *Exhibitor's Trade Review.* "We cannot understand, however, why it is that these same officials persist in giving endorsements to every picture of the sort that comes along."[29]

Actually, fictionalized treatments of sexual hygiene were not entirely new to American audiences. Eugène Brieux's theater play *Damaged Goods*, about a man who passes VD on to his wife and child, presented controversial subject matter but, unlike *The End of the Road*, received general critical acclaim. Produced in New York City in 1913, *Damaged Goods* presented a stern sermon on venereal disease.[30] Critics questioned venereal disease's suitability for stage presentation but agreed that the importance of the issue and the somber tone of the play justified the explosive subject matter.[31] Soon, *Damaged Goods* also appeared on screen. Produced by the American Film Manufacturing Company from a scenario by Harry Pollard, the film version of *Damaged Goods* was released by Mutual in 1914. The film, critics noted approvingly, was "free from taint which inheres in most of the 'sex problem plays,'" according to the *Moving Picture World.* "It does not parade evil in order that good may come of it." Audiences, too, gave the film their approbation; in Detroit, three policemen were enlisted to control the crowds the film generated.[32] Aided by a landmark public-relations campaign, *Damaged Goods* succeeded in casting itself as a public-minded morality tale, appropriate for upstanding audience members.[33]

In contrast to *Damaged Goods, The End of the Road* and its like appear to have been too frank (or less cannily advertised) for movie-industry authorities. Shortly after *The End of the Road*'s release, representatives of the National Association of the Moving Picture Industry resolved "war to the bitter end on anyone making or showing salacious pictures and obligating themselves to submit every film to National Board of Review."[34] On September 20, 1919, an ad appeared in *The Moving Picture World*, signed by Surgeon General Rupert Blue, advising that "the Public Health Service has withdrawn its indorsement of the films, *Fit to Win, End of the Road*, and *Open Your Eyes*, and all other pictures dealing with venereal diseases that have been shown or are to be shown commercially."[35]

The Catholic Church condemned *Fit to Win*, arguing that the film flouted Catholic prohibitions against prophylaxis and birth control. Other groups condemned the film's representation of soldiers' sexual behavior, complaining that the film shows "a carelessness and lack of moral responsibility in sex matters which casts an unmerited reflection upon the decency of the average American home and of the Army."[36]

Why did *Fit to Win, The End of the Road*, and their cohort of sex hygiene films meet with so much controversy? Eric Schaefer identifies three reasons. First, these films—particularly *Fit to Win*—mention the use of prophylaxis (as a last resort), thus earning the ire of the Catholic Church. Second, *Fit to Win* presents a view of American soldiers that is not entirely spotless, a view that angered some observers. Finally, *Fit to Win* and *The End of the Road*, in contrast to *Damaged Goods*, posited a kind of egalitarianism, subjecting both middle- and lower-class protagonists to similar fates. In *Fit to Win*, the five soldiers come from disparate classes, ranging from college student to boxer to cigar salesman. In *The End of the Road*, venereal disease is a shared affliction of both upper-class matrons and flighty shopgirls. In Schaefer's analysis, this vision of shared fates among disparate social groups may have been acceptable during the war, when Americans were accustomed to rhetoric about the need to pull together in the national interest. But following the war, such assertions of equality among classes looked less like patriotism and more like dangerous radicalism.

Stacie Colwell argues that the outcry which greeted *The End of the Road* stemmed in part from the film's "effective orphanage by its promoters and producers in the face of the rising public censorship."[37] During the war, the CTCA represented a forceful coalition of diverse interest groups. Following the end of the conflict, however, the government disbanded the CTCA, ordering some of its member agencies absorbed into government bodies and some released into civilian life. Without the backing of a strong coalition, *The End of the Road* was defenseless against attacks by censors and critics.[38]

Schaefer and Colwell both make important points, but press reports about the exhibition of *The End of the Road* and its ilk hint at another reason for the controversy. Discourse surrounding the films suggests a distinct discomfort with VD films' entrance into the marketplace, as opposed to military encampments and chaperoned private venues. The NAMPI (National Association of the Moving Picture Industry) itself told the surgeon general that it would withdraw its complaints about the film, provided that "the film is not distributed through commercial channels for profit" and that "the financial returns from the exhibition fees be devoted to some public purpose and not to the profit of some commercial organization."[39] The NAMPI in particular appears to have been quite sensitive to the prospect of these films, which deal with exceedingly private matters, entering the commercial marketplace. Safely ensconced in women's clubs, military camps, and noncommercial venues, these films were unobjectionable. But once tickets were sold at a profit, *The End of the Road* and *Fit to Fight* were engaging in a kind of commerce and so associating themselves with a kind of film that looked alarmingly similar to other, seedier transactions.

The End of the Road and its cohort also had the misfortune of entering the marketplace at a moment when the industry was drawing lines between "educational" and "entertainment" films. In the first fifteen years of cinema's history, such distinctions did not abide; nonfiction "actualities" regularly shared bills with story films. Some films we might think of as specialty scientific films—Jean Comandon's 1909 films of microbes, for example—were mainstream fare at movie theaters. But following World War I, the designation "educational" began to describe films that circulated outside of the commercial circuit. Kay Sloan attributes this change to the increasing popularity of feature-length films, while Lee Grieveson argues that the prospect of censorship encouraged the film industry to market film as a harmless diversion.[40] The reaction to *The End of the Road* and its ilk in the trade press supports Grieveson's assertion, but it also suggests that exhibitors were alert not to inflammatory material per se, but specifically to inflammatory material that entered the marketplace. *The End of the Road* and other sexual hygiene films did not discredit film exhibitors when screened for free. It was only when theaters showed these films for a profit that these topics became scandalous.

NAMPI succeeded in its campaign to censor the two films. No theater that showed *The End of the Road* or *Fit to Win* would be permitted to lease films from NAMPI's member distributors, thus effectively cutting off a theater's supply of mainstream films. This moment in fact had important implications for the American film industry. By identifying *The End of the Road* and *Fit to Win* as illicit (albeit lucrative) materials, and by forcing theaters to choose between mainstream and marginal films, NAMPI helped to create a separate category of shadowy "exploitation" films: a genre of films distinct from the mainstream movie industry and with their own dedicated theaters, where off-limits subjects could be broached.[41] The censure brought down on *Fit to Fight* and *The End of the Road* simultaneously had the effect of evacuating teaching films on controversial subjects from the marketplace, moving them into classrooms and other noncommercial venues.[42]

The outcry over *The End of the Road* and *Fit to Win* made it abundantly clear that there were certain films for which it was not appropriate to exchange cash for tickets. But anxiety can often be traced to an undercurrent of social change, and this may well have been the case for the producers of *The End of the Road* and for the critics who decried its commercial exhibition. World War I offered a loosening of labor restrictions for women, and while these changes were often temporary, they were accompanied by changing standards of sexual behavior and evolving perceptions of what women might do with their leisure time. The imagined "new woman" of the 1920s was not truly emancipated from older restrictions on work and sexual behavior, but she did represent an altered understanding of how women might function in American society. A sophisticated consumer, the new woman moved easily through the workplace and the marketplace. As *The End of the Road* demonstrates, the intermingling of sex, labor, and money was not uncomplicated for women, but it was also, increasingly, part of their reality.

Notes

1. Jane Deeter Rippin, "Social Hygiene and the War: Work with Women and Girls," *Journal of Social Hygiene* 5, no. 1 (January 1919): 126.

2. Annette Kuhn, *Cinema, Censorship, and Sexuality, 1909–1925* (London: Routledge, 1988), 49.

3. Leslie J. Reagan, Nancy Tomes, and Paula A. Treichler, eds., *Medicine's Moving Pictures: Medicine, Health, and Bodies in American Film and Television* (Rochester, NY: University of Rochester Press, 2007); Eric Schaefer, *Bold! Daring! Shocking! True!: A History of Exploitation Films, 1919–1959* (Durham, NC: Duke University Press, 1999); Martin S. Pernick, "Sex Education Films" *Isis* 84 (1993): 766–68; and Devin Orgeron, Marsha Orgeron, and Dan Streible, eds., *Learning with the Lights Off: Educational Film in the United States* (New York: Oxford University Press, 2012).

4. See, for example, Timothy J. Gilfoyle, *City of Eros: New York City, Prostitution, and the Commercialization of Sex, 1790–1920* (New York: Norton, 1992); Kathy Peiss, *Cheap Amusements: Working Women and Leisure in Turn-of-the-Century New York* (Philadelphia: Temple University Press, 1986); Nancy K. Bristow, *Making Men Moral: Social Engineering during the Great War* (New York: New York University Press, 1996); and David Pivar, *Purity and Hygiene: Women, Prostitution, and the "American Plan," 1900–1930* (Westport, CT: Greenwood Press, 2001).

5. Stacie A. Colwell, "The End of the Road: Gender, the Dissemination of Knowledge, and the American Campaign against Venereal Disease during World War I," *Camera Obscura* 29 (May 1992): 91–129. See also Pernick, "Sex Education Films"; and Schaefer, *Bold! Daring! Shocking! True!*

6. Colwell, "The End of the Road," 92.

7. Bristow, *Making Men Moral*, 5–26.

8. Elizabeth Lunbeck, "'A New Generation of Women': Progressive Psychiatrists and the Hypersexual Female," *Feminist Studies* 13 (1987): 513–43.

9. George J. Anderson, "Making the Camps Safe for the Army," *Annals of the American Academy of Political and Social Science* 79 (1918): 143–51, 149.

10. Anderson, "Making the Camps Safe."

11. Henrietta S. Additon, "Work among Delinquent Women and Girls," *Annals of the American Academy of Political and Social Science* 79 (1918): 155.

12. Rippin, "Social Hygiene and the War: Work with Women and Girls," 126.

13. Peiss, *Cheap Amusements*, 110–79.

14. Ibid., 112.

15. Lunbeck, "A New Generation of Women," 532.

16. Additon, "Work among Delinquent Women and Girls," 155.

17. Rippin, "Social Hygiene and the War: Work with Women and Girls," 133.

18. Katharine Bement Davis, "Social Hygiene and the War, Part II: Woman's Part in Social Hygiene," *Journal of Social Hygiene* 4, no. 4 (October 1918): 533.

19. Martha P. Falconer, "The Segregation of Delinquent Women and Girls as a War Problem," *Annals of the American Academy of Political and Social Science* 79 (1918): 160–66.

20. Viviana Zelizer, *The Purchase of Intimacy* (Princeton, NJ: Princeton University Press, 2005).

21. Zelizer, *Purchase of Intimacy*, 24.

22. Eva Illouz, *Consuming the Romantic Utopia Love and the Cultural Contradictions of Capitalism* (Berkeley: University of California Press, 1997).

23. Colwell, "The End of the Road."

24. "End of the Road Booked Solidly in Chicago District," *Exhibitor's Herald and Motography* 9, no. 4 (July 19, 1919): 34.

25. "End of the Road Booked Solidly."

26. "Health Lecture to Women," *Chicago Daily Tribune*, May 12, 1919; "Attend Film Showing: Women's City Club Members Hear Startling Statistics," *Los Angeles Times*, August 26, 1919; "Amusements," *Atlanta Constitution*, March 31, 1919, 16.

27. "Boy Scouts to See 'End of the Road,'" *Atlanta Constitution*, March 29, 1919, 9.

28. "Amusements," *Atlanta Constitution*, April 2, 1919, 16.

29. "The Decision in the Fit to Win Case," *Exhibitor's Trade Review* (July 26, 1919): 607.

30. Schaefer, *Bold! Daring! Shocking! True!*, 22.

31. Ibid.

32. Ibid.

33. On the public relations campaign that helped cast *Damaged Goods* as respectable entertainment, see Ewen Stuart, *PR! A Social History of Spin* (New York: Basic Books, 1996), 159–64.

34. "National Association Wins Fight to Bar 'Fit to Win' in New York," *Exhibitor's Herald and Motography* 9, no. 5 (July 26, 1919): 72.

35. Quoted in Schaefer, *Bold! Daring! Shocking! True!*, 37.

36. Karl S. Lashley and John B. Watson, *A Psychological Study of Motion Pictures in Relation to Venereal Disease Campaigns* (Washington, DC: United States Interdepartmental Social Hygiene Board, 1922).

37. Colwell, "The End of the Road," 111.

38. Ibid., 112.

39. "Association Goes After Fit to Win," *Moving Picture World* 40 (May 24, 1919): 1141.

40. Kay Sloan, *The Loud Silents: Origins of the Social Problem Film* (Urbana: University of Illinois Press, 1988); Lee Grieveson, *Policing Cinema: Movies and Censorship in Early-Twentieth-Century America* (Berkeley: University of California Press, 2004).

41. Schaefer, *Bold! Daring! Shocking! True!*, 31.

42. Martin S. Pernick, "More than Illustrations: Early Twentieth-Century Health Films as Contributors to the Histories of Medicine and of Motion Pictures," in Reagan, Tomes, and Treichler, *Medicine's Moving Pictures*, 19–35.

Chapter Five

Film and Anti-alcohol Campaigns in the Soviet Union of the 1920s

Alexandre Sumpf

In the early twentieth century, movies came to play an important role in Russian and later in Soviet campaigns against alcoholism. To physicians and public health officials, alcohol was the oldest and deepest social problem, an evil greater than syphilis or tuberculosis, and movies had a unique power to challenge it. From small beginnings before the revolution,[1] Russian and Soviet anti-alcohol films took off during the 1920s as part of a broader effort by the central state to intervene in citizens' lives and shape "the new man,"[2] free from the flaws of the former regime. The promoters of this campaign argued that social diseases had to be eradicated in order to cleanse the new society, and alcoholism was a key target.

Russian and Soviet anti-alcohol films were thus not stand-alone productions. They must be understood as part of broader campaigns against alcohol and to promote "the new man," and this means that we must take a different approach to these films than many historians of cinema in the USSR. In general, the latter have tended to concentrate on one film, generally one that is fairly well-known, in order to elaborate theories on the history of cinema, on propaganda, and on social realities reflected or transformed on the screen. However, such an approach has limitations for the campaign film: not only does it fail to situate the film within the broader set of educational media productions employed by such campaigns, it also does not allow us to consider the porous nature of different genres among films within (and without) a campaign, the mutual influences between films, the relations between different types of films shown at a screening, and the various ways in which they attempted to elicit a reaction from the viewer. To explore such issues, one has to look at the corpus of films produced by a campaign and their relations to other educational media produced by it. In short, it might be argued that one also has to look at the corpus of other media productions—the pamphlets, posters, lectures, and other educational media of the campaign—and how aesthetic, scientific, and moral discourses weave their way through all these media, including film.

My focus is on the corpus of films of different genres that formed part of anti-alcohol campaigns in Russia and later the Soviet Union, and with three categories of viewers: the general public, the sick, and (medical and film) experts. I will give particular attention to anti-alcohol specialists who believed in the didactic and civic powers of cinema: who they were; how they came to be involved in this undertaking; how they came to form a community of common interest in film; and how, between the end of the Tsarist era and the beginning of the Soviet period, these doctors convinced—each in a different manner—their partners in the studios to produce these films. This period—the late Tsarist and early Soviet period—was marked by considerable change in the relations between the film and medical communities. The rise of the social hygiene movement combined with the Bolshevik regime's emphasis on film production, mobilization through propaganda, and the shaping of the "new man" by education, meant that doctors went from being film consultants to key participants in a field which was just opening up.

Given the Soviet enthusiasm for both film and anti-alcohol campaigns, the paradox is that only a few anti-alcohol films were made. While the USSR invested unprecedented resources in the production of nonfiction propaganda (in the neutral sense of the term) and in education films, of the 112 health and sanitary education films approved for screening in the Soviet Union in 1928, only 5 addressed the alcohol issue.[3] Admittedly, some films are missing from this figure, including Iu. E. Genik's *Alcohol* (1927) and three fascinating 1929 productions: *Saba, To Your Health,* and *Tanka the Innkeeper.*[4] But the corpus of Soviet anti-alcohol films remains small, even though mortality from alcohol consumption was rising: it killed fifteen times more people in 1928 than in 1923. Part of the reason had to do with health and studio priorities. Studios generally privileged the theme of prostitution, since syphilis was designated public enemy number one, with infection rising exponentially, the direct consequence of eight years of war as well as problems with its diagnosis in Russia.[5] Moreover, this was a "hot" topic that leaned toward erotic film and romantic dramas that Soviet authorities violently condemned but that attracted (male) audiences. Alcohol could not compete against such forces, and it was also complicated by contradictions in state policy toward alcohol that this essay will document.

This essay seeks to explore this contradiction over state policy toward alcohol and how it affected policy toward educational films on alcoholism. It also seeks to document the debates over the types of film most likely to persuade the public to change its behavior, debates which had kept film scholars busy since the industrial and commercial revival of Soviet cinema in 1924. Filmmakers and sponsors alike were unsure what type of films would work best. Should films—and in particular the *kulturfilm*—be purely scientific or involve a plot; should they appeal to reason alone, or also to emotion? What genre should dominate? In this chapter, I consider the corpus of anti-alcohol films not only as a subcorpus of the broader corpus of health education films, but also as a hybrid corpus comprising fiction, documentary, and edifying films as well as newsreels, which shared some of the same political objectives and used similar aesthetic techniques. This hybrid nature emerged from these debates over what types of films worked best in anti-alcohol movies and indeed, I suggest, in health education films more generally. As such, a focus on the hybrid nature of anti-alcohol films more generally provides a window onto the hybrid, shape-shifting nature of the health education film.

Moral, Medical, and Political Hybrids

These motion pictures were not only hybrids of different types of film; they were also hybrids in that they mixed medical, moral, and political perspectives. Doctors, pharmacists, and psychiatrists had first defined alcoholism as a disease in the 1860s, and the word *alkogolizm*, synonymous to the English term *alcoholism*, began to be used alongside the word *pianstvo*, the existing vernacular term for drunkenness. Research conducted in the 1890s by the Swiss physician E. F. Erisman further sought to medicalize alcoholism by focusing on treatment as key to modernizing Russia and improving the status of laborers.[6] Yet the medical explanations did not do away with moral ones. Just before World War I, nearly eight thousand temperance societies with five hundred thousand members were dedicated to the fight against alcohol on mostly moral grounds. And physicians rarely argued for medical approach alone, but tended to mix the moral and the medical, something that would eventually also shape their approaches to film.[7]

The moral dimensions of the fight against alcohol were particularly common among prerevolutionary private practitioners. They tended to blame alcohol for preventing the emergence of the citizen as an autonomous, responsible, hardworking, and morally irreproachable person and argued in favor of either reducing individual consumption or finding medical treatments. But even on the left a moral argument of sorts can be detected, but one that shifted the blame for moral decline onto social and economic conditions. Thus, socialist medical professionals who criticized urbanization and industrialization tended to stress the role of social and environmental causes. They argued that alcoholism did not lead to poverty but resulted from it; it did not cause street crime but was another symptom of capitalist exploitation.

The mix of medical and moral also found its way into Soviet anti-alcohol campaigns that sought to promote the "new man." For example, in 1922 the Soviet view of alcoholism as both a social and a health issue was the subject of a poster distributed by the Ministry of Internal Affairs.[8] The poster depicted two contrasting worlds on both sides of the silhouette of an inebriated worker: that of alcoholism and that of socialism, which in the words of Lenin "are incompatible." This represented the Soviet worker confronting a choice: a dissolute lifestyle of domestic violence, poverty, crime, heightened risk of work-related accidents, hedonism, and venereal disease, all leading to death; or a respectable lifestyle in a healthy environment, with a thriving family, good work productivity, spare time, and health. This binary view was not unique to Russia; it also characterized other Western European and North American policies and campaigns at that time.

Soviet movies also reflected this tendency to see the world in black and white rather than in shades of gray. Astonishingly, and this is a central point of this chapter, the strict moral condemnation of alcoholism as one of the worst social diseases resulted not in restrictions on the sale of alcohol, but the *cancellation* in 1929 of a prohibition on strong alcohol and the replacement of a bootlegging economy around homemade brandy or moonshine (*samogon*) with a state monopoly on vodka. In other words, the moral condemnation of alcohol paved the way to a marginalization of private producers and retailers and the rise of state-produced and sold alcohol.

There is a further paradox to highlight here. Cinema was a symbolically modern means of promoting Party and State objectives, and in particular the "new way of life" (*novyi byt*). The New Economic Policy (1921–28) consisted in a return to capitalism under state control and imposed strict financial constraints on private and state companies (*samookupaemost*). The chronic underfunding of film studios forced them to take into consideration both state control and commercial imperatives. The paradox of this story is that the return to capitalism under state control in the film industry led to a reassertion of state control of the alcohol industry.

Beginnings

The first public education films about alcohol were released in the 1910s, part of a broader set of anti-alcohol campaigns in Russia that were influenced by philanthropic temperance in the provincial administrative centers and in the two capitals and by social hygiene promoted by the *zemstvos* (elected councils in tsarist Russia, created to administer local affairs after the abolition of serfdom).[9] At the turn of the century, these campaigns increasingly promoted their message through thousands of lectures, which combined a mix of medical and moral discourse depending on the leanings of the organizers and speakers and on their purpose—popular edification or fund-raising. These public talks—expressions of the civil society (*obschestvennost*) that all cities were expected to have following the Great Reforms ushered in by Tsar Alexander II in the 1860s—were accompanied by slideshows, which included some medical content but often verged on traveling picture shows, and paved the way for the use of film. The people's educators (*vneshkolniki*), who worked in the "people's houses" network funded by the *zemstvos*, believed that film was likely to attract the public as it was a new and alternative means of conveying educational messages.[10] It would, they argued, not only improve the quality of hygienist propaganda, but also increase the number of people reached, especially peasants, who would consequently be quicker to renounce traditional evils including illiteracy, superstitions, alcoholism, and petty crime (*khuliganstvo*).[11]

The stage was set for anti-alcohol films by the production in 1908 of the first scientific films in Russia, particularly by Scientific Cinematography in Odessa.[12] Shortly after, in 1912, at the same time that the Congress of Popular Instruction recommended the extensive use of film for educational purposes, its subcommission in Moscow organized educational film sessions in schools that reached fifty thousand children and adolescents that year. Health and medical film were also institutionalized at that time. For example, in Nizhny-Novgorod, K. A. Gratsianov created the Educational Cinematography Company for the Hygiene and Education section of the local chapter of the Society for the Protection of National Health. Unique in its kind, this company's activity was funded by private patrons and public funds; a two thousand ruble grant from the Ministry of Instruction allowed their collection to quickly expand and include fifty thousand meters of film.

At this stage, most anti-alcohol films were little more than vehicles for a medical discourse and did not conform to any of the cinematographic types that would later dominate such films: *kulturfilmy*, fictions or newsreels. The most famous prewar film against alcoholism, *Pianstvo i ego posledstviia* (Drunkenness and its consequences), was released in 1913 by the Khanzhonkov studio, the largest film company in Russia·[13] As the only professional producer of Russian documentary film, Khanzhonkov had in 1911 created a department for scientific film, which released its first film in March 1912. Yet the department was only a tiny part of the company (its 50,000 ruble budget represented only 2 percent of Khanzhonkov's annual budget)[14] and the hope was that *Pianstvo i ego posledstviia* might change this by popularizing the new genre of scientific educational documentary film for which Khanzhonkov had high commercial expectations. The company recruited four eminent medical/scientific specialists who acted as consultants, and the 850 meters of film show frontal views of different organs being attacked by alcohol, alongside numerous diagrams designed by the Anti-alcoholism Museum of the Muscovite Association for the Patronage of Popular Temperance—all designed to emphasize the dangers of alcohol.[15] *Pianstvo i ego posledstviia* was and still is renowned for an interlude created by the animator Ladislas Starevich in which a devil emerges from a bottle of vodka and haunts a drunkard played by Ivan Moszhukhin, the most popular actor of the time.

The film met with extraordinary success in the capitals and provinces, acclaimed by both the general and specialized press, and was widely distributed and seen by large numbers of people, including the Tsar, to whom it was presented in April 1914.[16] Not only was it a great commercial triumph, but the enormous promotional resources put into it, combined with a popular hygienist theme, meant that it was credited with contributing to the total prohibition of alcohol in August 1914 (although the war and mobilization riots also played their part).

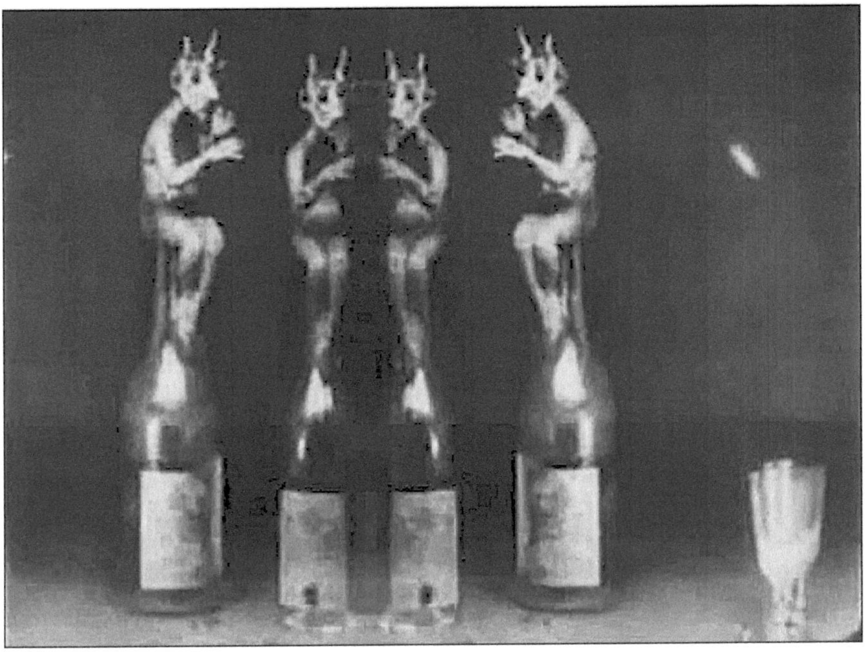

Figure 5.1. Ivan Moszhukhin, a drunkard, is haunted by the alcoholic Devil in Khanzhonkov's *Drunkenness and Its Consequences* (1913).

In Russia, film and the fight against alcoholism thus intersected before the October Revolution. Yet as *Pianstvo i ego posledstviia* illustrates, it was a protean combination in which medical demonstrations and moral themes, fiction and reality, all struggled for effective articulation on the screen.

War, Revolution, and After

The Great War and the Revolution changed everything for those interested in making anti-alcohol films. In the first place, during the war a theme of rehabilitation began to creep into filmmaking. For the first time, films not only showed damaged human bodies, but also the ways in which they could be rehabilitated. A case in point is the film *Reborn to Life* (1916), which followed war invalids and their wounds through to their rehabilitation. More broadly, a focus on rehabilitation raised the possibility not only of physical repair, but also of behavioral change: a notion that had appeal to those interested in making films which demonstrated the possibility of recovery from alcoholism. Moreover, because anti-alcohol films were often tied to broader concerns about social order, the new focus on rehabilitation opened a door to the emergence of a new, orderly society where all excess was banished.[17]

The beginning of the Bolshevik era saw four major changes that would affect the production and distribution of anti-alcohol films. The first was the growing prominence of the hygienist vision promoted by *zemstvos* doctors through People's Commissar of Public Health Nikolai Semashko and the State Institute of Social Hygiene (established in 1923). In the newly opened specialized dispensaries, the social dimension of alcoholism was treated by taking into account the inebriate's environment. The scales tipped toward prevention, at least until 1930, when psychiatrists took the lead after persuading officials of the high efficacy of the psychiatric treatments they offered to drunkards. Social hygiene was influenced by the translation of important German studies into Russian, as well as the arrival of the first German films. Commentators in both nations argued that their countries were faced with the threat of anomie in the postwar period. While the Great War and the prevailing anti-German sentiment had temporarily curbed this influence, the two countries soon rekindled their scientific, technical, and commercial collaboration.

The second change was attempts by the Soviet state to control the film industry, a difficult task that took a long time and was never entirely achieved. Thus, following a first (failed) attempt to nationalize the industry in 1919 and the exile of the majority of cinema producers during the civil war, the Soviet state took several years to impose a legal framework on film studios, creating a series of monopolies in the film industry as part of a broader effort to create a market economy under state control known as the New Economic Policy.

Before its reorganization, the film industry in the early 1920s was a complex mix of production and distribution companies. Private studios (such as Rus') coexisted alongside parastatal regional (Sevzapkino), national (Goskinprom Gruzii in Soviet Georgia) ones; studios created by the formerly independent republics (Nemkino, Tatkino, Chuvashkino) were forced to merge in 1926 into Vostokkino; film production facilities run by associations (Proletkino) or by the army (Gosvoenkino); and the state-run Goskino. Goskino was thus only one of many film production and distribution companies, and not the leader even if it counted amongst its directors Sergei Eisenstein.

Then, on June 13, 1924, the Sovnarkom decree established Sovkino, a new state-run film production trust intended to replace Goskino (which remained in existence until 1926) and sought to control film distribution in order reduce resources and revenues for studios other than Sovkino. There followed, in March 1928, a conference on cinematographic affairs, which led to the takeover by the Communist Party of anything related to motion pictures. Rus (now Mezhrabpom-Rus, following a merger with the Workers International Relief based in Berlin) was partly nationalized in September 1928 and transformed into Mezhrabpom-Film; the Soviet state forced its participation in the capital and held the majority of shares. By the end of the decade, this meant that with the creation in February 1930 of the film company Soyouzkino, theoretically the only film studio allowed at the time, the Soviet state had established a de facto monopoly for films, even if in practice Vostokkino and Mezhrabpom remained in existence.

The third change was the opening up of the USSR to the rest of the world, which would result in the growing influence of German Kulturfilm on Soviet cinema in the 1920s. The Treaty of Rapallo, signed on April 16, 1922, with Weimar Germany, had reopened Russia to international trade partnerships; reestablished former film circulation circuits; and allowed the Universum Film-Aktien Gesellschaf (UFA), Germany's leading motion picture production company, created in 1917, to seduce those who shaped the studios in the USSR.[18] The Soviets noted enviously that UFA medical films were screened in Paris during the 1927 Congress of Medicine.[19] Thus, in an international film market now dominated by American films, German Kulturfilms gained significant popular and critical success in the USSR.[20]

This is not to say that German Kulturfilms went without criticism in the USSR. For example, the *Der Steinach Film* (UFA, 1922), which explains the surgical method of testicular grafting for men developed by and named after the Austrian physiologist Eugen Steinach (1861–1944), was lauded by some seeking to promote the UFA model in the USSR but was widely criticized by the medical community, which sought to unmask what many saw as a scientific imposture. More generally, while the medical film expert, Lazar Moiseevich Sukharebskii, argued that imported Kulturfilms were preferable to films from the tsarist era because of their newness, he also noted that their sensationalist nature and "petty bourgeois" [*meschanskaia*] ideology meant that they did not serve the goals of health education.[21] In addition, only copies (not the original negatives) were sold, and the overused reels often broke. All this served as a stimulus to the Soviet film industry to produce its own health kulturfilmy—along with fictions and newsreels—particularly on social diseases. As I will elaborated in a moment, such demands meant that the USSR came to be one of the leading centers for the production of kulturfilmy, including those against alcohol. This style had little to do with hygienist lobbying but was a response by the studios to state demand, since increasingly, film studios came to compete for contracts and orders from different ministries and state institutions.

In 1926, the number of scientific films distributed in the Soviet Union through the Sovkino ad hoc collection was 736 units. Although medical films ranked only fifth (of six categories) in terms of the number of films available (ninety-seven according to Strashun), they exceeded agriculture and natural sciences in terms of their total length (with 61,974 meters out of a total of 313,811 meters), behind travel films and industrial films, both very popular genres worldwide.[22] Medical and health education films were the longest (638 meters on average per film), ahead of travelogue films (537 meters), which devoted much footage to scenery, and industrial films (351 meters), a specific form of advertising for Soviet business and industry, consumer products, the new lifestyle (*byt*), regions, or economic sectors. The length of medical films can be explained by the influence of foreign feature-length films that came on the market following the phenomenal success of *Der Steinach Film*. Strashun also recommended films from Pathé: *La Vie au sanatorium* (1914)[23] or *Le Dispensaire Léon Bourgeois* (1918), by Jean Comandon, and even a later series of "filmed slogans" of 30 m to 50 m released in 1924.[24]

It should not, therefore, be assumed that Soviet film production dominated the supply of motion pictures. Although the state studio Sovkino had obtained the monopoly of distribution in Soviet territory in 1924, officials could not ban films that had previously been imported and distributed. (Indeed of the 736 scientific films available in 1926, only 18 percent were Soviet productions.) However, the very few copies of Soviet films in circulation wore out quickly, especially since projectionists' demand remained high and Soviet production grew only slowly, with studios scrambling to find sources of funding to supplement the monies they got from Sovkino, which often did not provide all the funds necessary to make a movie. For example, Sovkino provided only 2526.28 rubles toward the production of *Fatigue and the Fight against It*, which cost in total 13,887.14 rubles.[25] The paucity of funding from Sovkino was thus a major concern for studios, and perhaps especially in science films. In 1926–27 the Sovkino studio dedicated 9.5 percent of its budget to so-called science films, even though it represented one-quarter of their titles and 22.8 percent of film footage.[26]

The fourth change was to do with the Soviet state's ambivalent attitude to alcohol. Alcohol might have been regarded as a threat to the "new man," but it was a huge source of income for the state, and the state was keen to reap the profits. Thus, in 1923 the Bolshevik state began marketing 30° proof vodka and then, in October 1925, after ten years of prohibition, the state alcohol monopoly was reinstated with 40° proof vodka at a price low enough to stimulate widespread demand. Trotsky had in 1923 famously proposed to "replace vodka with cinema"[27]—the expected cinema profits were to replace the colossal profits from the vodka monopoly, and the hope was that entertainment and education were to replace social and physical decay as a consequence. After Trotsky's political defeat, his plan was revived to promote a new prohibition in 1928.[28] However, this project had to contend with the operating losses of Soviet films released since 1924. In 1926–27, "science" films brought Sovkino only 29,046 rubles, largely from theaters in Moscow (17,097 rubles) and Leningrad (4,156 rubles).[29] Of those addressing the theme of alcohol, on average kulturfilmy only made back half of their budget: *Alcohol* recouped 43.7 percent of expenditure and *Tanka the Innkeeper* 42.2 percent.[30] (An exception was *Anxiety*, which generated a profit of over 200 percent.) So bad was the situation that at times the revenue from alcohol sales had to be used to finance the next series of anti-alcohol films.[31] The fact that the secretary of the Muscovite section of the Association for the Fight against Alcoholism recommended *Saba* but requested that the insert title against *Tsentrospirt*, the state alcohol monopoly, be removed, articulated the paradoxical position of the state.[32]

The low cost of kulturfilmy facilitated their production, but their diffusion was problematic. One difficulty was that adequate setups for projections were not always available. In order to avoid losing the audience, an expert speaker was also ideally needed at each performance to make sure the propaganda was adequately conveyed. Yet often no expert came; the Gladiator Theatre in Moscow used a "melancholic piano" to accompany *Abortion* (1926) in order to lure viewers with music that suggested they would see a "great psychological drama."[33]

The insufficient number of films and copies of kulturfilmy was also a problem for their inclusion in daily screening schedules. An alternative recommendation consisted in creating a network in the schools and opening theaters dedicated to scientific and educational films like the Artes cinema in Moscow. Appeals were made to state regulation for aid to the studios, in order to continue making profits from the subsidized market; to projectionists, to compensate for the low profits made from these films; and to the promoters of Kulturfilm to ensure the recruitment of lecturers and musicians.

The Artes cinema opened on October 23, 1926, in the Academy of Communist Education (AKV) building.[34] On February 1, 1927, *Wege zu Kraft und Schonheit* (1925) was the first picture projected. However, while Wilhelm Praeger's film did not include any scientific images, it was received in Russia as a German model for Kulturfilm on financial and aesthetic grounds (especially its use of slow-motion techniques).[35] The situations in other cities varied. While the kulturfilmy cinema in Baku closed in early June 1928, the Soleil cinema in Leningrad changed its name to Kulturfilm on August 6, 1928. But despite being the model kulturfilmy cinema, Artes also had obstacles to overcome, including an investigation by the Worker and Peasant Inspectors into a charge of embezzlement.[36] The cinema closed for several months before Mezhrabpom, with the assistance of several voluntary associations, including the Society for the Fight against Alcoholism (OBA) created under the sponsorship of the prominent Bolshevik Nikolai Bukharin, had it reopened.

Doctors

Against this backdrop of changes in the motion picture industry, a small if growing number of doctors began turn to film as consultants, as actors playing doctors, but also as scriptwriters, directors, critics, and theorists on the relationships between film, medicine, sanitary education, and the public. The absence of personal or corporate archives makes a full account of this group quite difficult. What can be said is that there were very few barriers for medical men—especially those with practices in either of the two capital cities—who wanted to work with film, and that they came to form a small, well-connected knowledge community about anti-alcoholic campaigns on the screen, albeit one that constantly had to assert its expertise on questions that were actually very new to them, such as popularization, film aesthetics, and the effect of film on the public, and they found themselves struggling to make their opinions count. They could not entirely lean on their traditional authority on medical matters but had to reframe it in order to be listened to.

During the war, one of the main protagonists in the alcohol debate, the renowned psychiatrist V. M. Bekhterev, was particularly enthusiastic about the potential of film to contribute to anti-alcohol campaigns. In his eyes, cinema was the only art form that could fully record the disease and therefore was the best suited to serve the cause of prevention and treatment.[37] After 1917 a half-dozen leading doctors lent their support to such a view, beginning with Lazar Moiseevich Sukharebskii, a medical graduate who dedicated his life to health-related cinema. Over the course of a very long career that lasted into the 1960s, he went on to become one of the most prominent theorists on interactions with the audience, on the use of film in science, and on the use of science in film, as well as a dedicated promoter of popular science films.[38]

Among the new cohort of physicians interested in film was Boris Samoilovich Sigal, born in 1893 and professor at the Mechnikov Academy of Medicine in Leningrad until 1959. Less of a theorist and more of a popularizer, Sigal approached film from a position that was more discursive and moral than technical or medical. He was the most prominent specialist of health "agitation trials" (*agitsudy*), a theatrical genre that emphasized amateurism and that addressed the audience directly. Sigal wrote no less than thirteen "sanitary agitation trials" (*sansudy*)—on syphilis, tuberculosis, poor motherhood, smoking, and village healers. A popular theatrical genre that included at least 130 titles in the 1920s, the agitation trial drew its roots from popular education methods at the end of the tsarist era, Bolshevik political agitation during the civil war, and the spontaneous workers culture promoted by the paragovernmental association Proletkult.[39] As early as 1904, *Vodka on Trial* applied the basic principle of this genre to temperance: presenting a case taken from familiar daily life with a short format (one or two acts) and ending with a confession of guilt through which truth and good triumphed.[40]

Sigal showed a particular penchant toward the subject of alcoholism, and his plays became a model that influenced film production on the subject. *The Trial of a Drunk*, the last of his four plays on the subject, was released in 1929.[41] The story of the trial of Ivan Stepanov, a typical worker in his thirties, this play realistically portrayed the judicial process: accusations, witnesses, and judgment. The play was a melodrama that used Manichean archetypes and portrayed urban life as a life of excess—a cocktail of violence, sex, and narcomania. It was, like other agitation trials, staged by semiamateur troupes in cities, and its presentation in the countryside encountered manifold problems due to lack of transport, housing, stage set . . . and actors' competence.[42] Like other agitation trials, it provided training in citizens' conduct, just as medical films provided training in detailed experimental and therapeutic procedures. The *Trial of the Drunk* was an enactment of a trial in which the audience was supposed to react as if it were a real trial. However, with its long speeches and intricate technical papers delivered by medical experts on the stand, it had little to appeal to audience members' sense of identity and emotions.

In Sigal's anti-alcohol agitation trials, the doctor's testimony always filled the largest number of pages. The speeches were not simply "appropriate content," but aimed to serve as an "effective and affective theatrical form" of propaganda.[43] By introducing spectators to scientific logic, they were also a pedagogical means of emphasizing the idea of self-transformation. For example, in *Trial of Illegal Distillers* (1925) the country doctor demonstrates, in simple terms, that neither moonshine (*samogon*) nor any other alcohol nourishes or fortifies—on the contrary, it poisons. At Stepanov's trial, the dispensary's narcology expert pronounces a rather technical diagnosis of the drunkard, pointing to visible symptoms and evaluating who (or what) was responsible. In these instances, doctors engaged in health education were not taking any chances with their prognoses: "Of course, [Stepanov] *can* be cured, especially if he himself *wants* to stop drinking. On this condition alone, his health *can* improve significantly."[44] Sigal thought science to be less efficient in transforming audience behaviors than the "conscience" of the individual.[45] Besides being a melodrama tinged with political overtones and a preoccupation with health, the agitation trial was intended to persuade, with arguments (including medical ones) adjusted to audience members of different intellectual attainment. In effect, audiences were always more of a complex social mix than the commonly used labels such as "workers" or "peasants" suggest.

Sigal's many agitation trials mark him an influential figure of the Soviet anti-alcoholism campaign, promoting its goals through cultural action. This doctor was also an important critic of health education films and played a major role in shaping public discussion about them in his many articles in the press. In *Kino-nedelia*, "Dr. Sigal" (as he signed his significant articles) attempted to set standards for health education films (*sanprosvetfilmy*). He particularly criticized complex films that required explanations from a commentator (such as Khanzhonkov's *Drunkenness and its Consequences*) and argued for the use of impromptu shots of daily life that clearly distinguished Soviet Kulturfilm from foreign productions that were "strictly scientific."[46] Instead of expert discourse and a position of superiority, he advocated the use of fiction (especially fiction that encouraged identification with the spectator's own experience) as the best way to spread hygienist theories among the population.

Dr. Abram Solomonovich Berliand, an author of sanitary agitation trials and scenarios himself, was the third prominent critic of health education films of the 1920s. Like Sukharebskii and Sigal, he shifted from medicine to cinema, but with less success and longevity in his new profession—if we believe the very scarce documentation available on this figure (inadequate records are a major issue for the historian of Soviet health education movies). Unlike Sigal, who had similar medical training, Berliand's expertise lay in the accuracy of scientific demonstration rather than in the dramatic devices of agitation trials. In 1928 he wrote the leading manual for those involved in the anti-alcohol campaign, *Alcohol and the Fight against It*, sponsored by the People's Commission on Health and the General Committee on Political Education (Glavpolitprosvet), which made extensive use of diagrams and was sold for the relatively expensive sum of 1.30 rubles. After an initial run of ten thousand copies, a further twenty thousand were printed in 1929 for political educators and doctors. It was in part because of this background that A. N. Tiagai, the head of the Office of Scientific Educational Films of Mezhrabpom-Rus, invited him to write the screenplay for *Alcohol, Work and Health*.[47]

Berliand illustrates a further point about the changing role of physicians in film. If during the tsarist era they had been content to be film consultants, providing scientific backing to projects initiated by a studio, by the 1920s they increasingly took the role of screenwriters and even directors. This shift is also illustrated by the case of Noi I. Galkin, a doctor who directed health education films up into the 1960s and then switched careers entirely. His filmography includes *Abortion* (1926, not preserved), the Soviet health education film that spurred the most discussion and that was often cited as a model for other films on this subject. Two years earlier, he had mocked his own ambition in a pastiche autobiography: in response to the question "What will you become?," he answered, "The best producer of all doctors and inversely."[48] Although Galkin did not produce any anti-alcohol films, he gave numerous lectures on this theme and even published a lecture accompanied by twenty-five slides.[49] Throughout his career, he remained interested in the great social epidemics of his time.

Galkin's cinematic ambitions were not without problems. The film community rejected his 1929 effort, *Neurasthenia* (with Sukharebskii), although his talents as director were recognized.[50] Nor did the medical community accept him. Galkin was singled out for not being a medical specialist but a simple medical popularizer, and critics said he had no medical credentials for producing health films. He was criticized for not fully demonstrating the links between examination, diagnosis, and treatment on the screen, which was the least one could expect from a medical cinema consultant, according to his critics.[51] Generally, the medical community regarded doctors turned filmmakers with a skeptical eye and preferred the productions of its own members. For instance, cinema critics particularly praised Iu. E. Genik's production of *Alcohol* (1927, not preserved) for Sovkino, arguably because the People's Commissar of Public Health himself, Nikolai Semashko, had written the script.[52]

Within the studios, Sukharebskii's command of theory, Sigal's landmark writings, and Galkin's willful resolution made them key figures among the doctors working in film. However, the greatest authority was undoubtedly A. N. Tiagai, head of the Office of Scientific Educational Films of Mezhrabpom-Rus, though as I shall show even the greatest authority was subject to considerable criticism.[53] During his medical studies, which he completed in 1920, he enlisted in the Red Army to supervise the health education of the twelfth army in 1918, an experience that made him a firsthand witness of the civil war epidemics.[54] His knowledge of major social epidemics and his commitment to educating adults with the most modern resources facilitated his shift from medicine to cinema.

Tiagai was particularly renowned for having written the screenplay for the *Mechanics of the Brain* with Vsevolod Pudovkin in 1926. The involvement of Pudovkin and of the Academy member and Nobel Prize–winner Ivan Pavlov were widely publicized by the studio. Stills from some of the scenes were regularly used to illustrate press articles on health education films. And the *Mechanics* was often mentioned—maybe a bit less than Galkin's *Abortion*, though—in the discussion on models of films to produce. Being strictly scientific, Pudovkin's film presented clinical experiments on the screen in a pure and didactic manner. This came precisely at a time when Soviets were at work on the creation of a new genre that was halfway between educational efforts to appeal to reason and

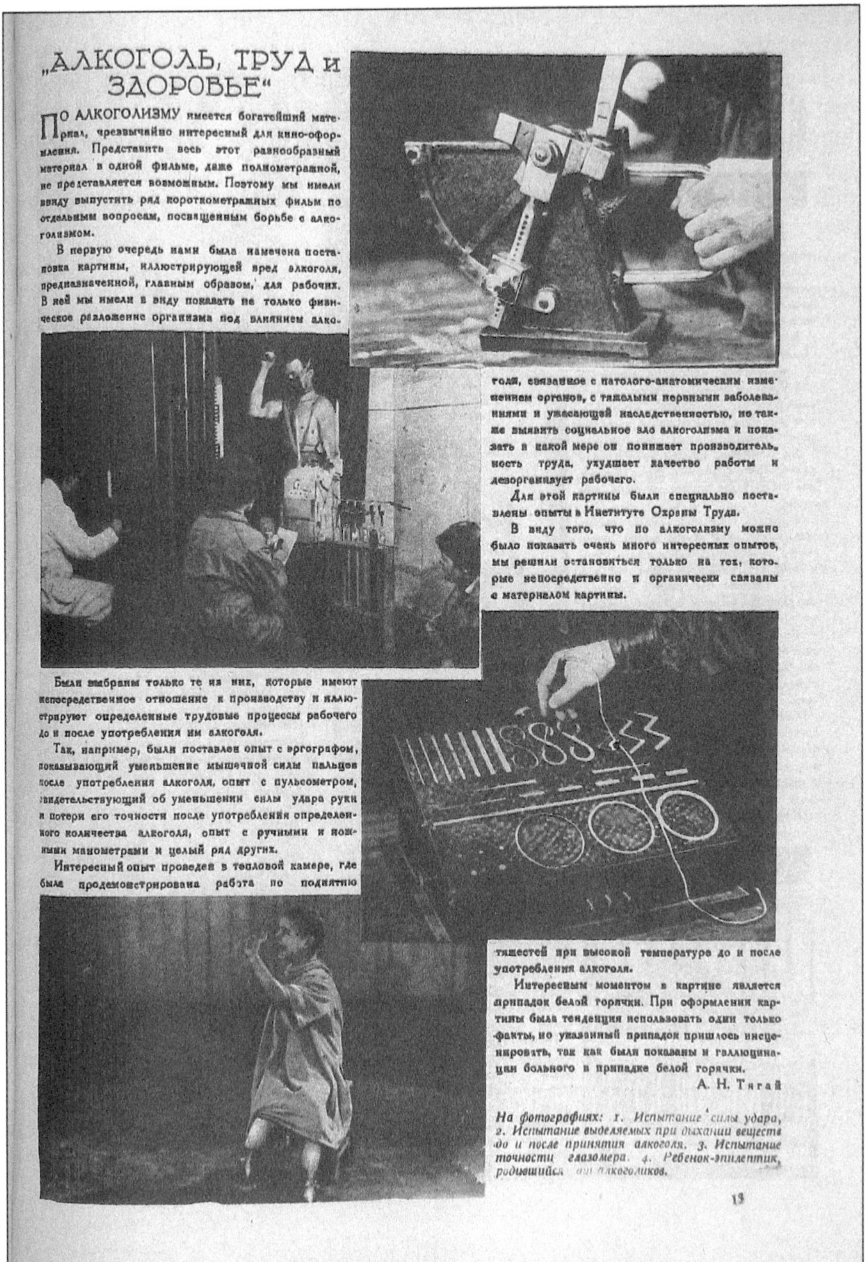

„АЛКОГОЛЬ, ТРУД и ЗДОРОВЬЕ“

ПО АЛКОГОЛИЗМУ имеется богатейший материал, чрезвычайно интересный для кино-оформления. Представить весь этот разнообразный материал в одной фильме, даже полнометражной, не представляется возможным. Поэтому мы имели ввиду выпустить ряд короткометражных фильм по отдельным вопросам, посвященным борьбе с алкоголизмом.

В первую очередь нами была намечена постановка картины, иллюстрирующей вред алкоголя, предназначенной, главным образом, для рабочих. В ней мы имели в виду показать не только физическое разложение организма под влиянием алкоголя, связанное с патолого-анатомическим изменением органов, с тяжелыми нервными заболеваниями и ужасающей наследственностью, но также выявить социальное зло алкоголизма и показать в какой мере он понижает производительность труда, ухудшает качество работы и дезорганизует рабочего.

Для этой картины были специально поставлены опыты в Институте Охраны Труда.

В виду того, что по алкоголизму можно было показать очень много интересных опытов, мы решили остановиться только на тех, которые непосредственно и органически связаны с материалом картины.

Были выбраны только те из них, которые имеют непосредственное отношение к производству и иллюстрируют определенные трудовые процессы рабочего до и после употребления им алкоголя.

Так, например, был поставлен опыт с эргографом, показывающий уменьшение мышечной силы пальцев после употребления алкоголя, опыт с пульсометром, свидетельствующий об уменьшении силы удара руки и потери его точности после употребления определенного количества алкоголя, опыт с ручными и ножными манометрами и целый ряд других.

Интересный опыт проведен в тепловой камере, где была продемонстрирована работа по поднятию тяжестей при высокой температуре до и после употребления алкоголя.

Интересным моментом в картине является припадок белой горячки. При оформлении картины была тенденция использовать одни только факты, но указанный припадок пришлось инсценировать, так как были показаны и галлюцинации больного в припадке белой горячки.

А. Н. Тягай

На фотографиях: 1. Испытание силы удара, 2. Испытание выделяемых при дыхании веществ до и после принятия алкоголя. 3. Испытание точности глазомера. 4. Ребенок-эпилептик, родившийся от алкоголиков.

13

Figure 5.2. A. N. Tiagai presents his *Alcohol, Work and Health* in the illustrated journal, the *Soviet Screen* 10 (1927): 13.

efforts to promote viewer identification with the message on the screen through an appeal to emotion.

Tiagai was greatly respected for his career (and his participation in the civil war), his key position in a leading studio, and his status as medical doctor. He shied away from fiction and limited himself to the scientific field, remaining primarily a scientist who worked behind the scenes as producer, scenarist, and art director. Tiagai not only wrote the script for *Mechanics*, but he released *Alcohol, Work and Health* the same year, 1926, with the help of Berliand as a screenwriter and a Dr. Solovev as medical consultant. The film displayed two types of medical authority on the screen, with scenes depicting scientists and detailed scientific experiments, echoing a formula developed by Khanzhonkov thirteen years earlier. The film compares a healthy heart and an alcoholic's heart in a manner akin to Khanzhonkov's earlier anti-alcohol motion picture using experiments conducted on animals, not on humans.

Tiagai, however, faced virulent criticism for this style of filmmaking. He had not anticipated contemporary Soviet documentary film developments, including Vertov's "film truth" (meaning here a quest for truthfulness deeper than a veracity seen by the human eye and cinematographically obtained with fragmentary pieces of actualities shot without planning) or Esfir Shub's "factography" (referring to a journalistic cinematography that compiles and edits footage) that had won critics' praise. For such viewers, the bare truth had to be shown not to shock or even to edify, but to establish a direct connection between the images and the viewers. That precisely was what critics complained about when they argued that the audience did not receive *Alcohol, Work and Health* favorably. For example, working-class viewers from the railroad unions who gathered for a screening organized by the Association of Revolutionary Filmmakers (ARK) complained that they were not "glued to the screen" by the evils of alcohol portrayed and called the acting "artificial."[55] Tiagai, who was present at this preview, a prerequisite for any filmmaker in search of artistic and political recognition, had to promise to revise his screenplay.

As the foregoing suggests, regardless of how doctors invested in health education films, their success was never complete. No one managed to establish a norm or to find a formula that satisfied both professionals and the public. Despite the enthusiasm of some advocates, health education films were only ever a minority interest in the film and medical communities, and it was not immediate clear how support in the two communities could be mobilized. For filmmakers this would be a real problem, since it meant that health education films, including those against alcohol, were likely to be poorly distributed, which in turn affected the profitability of the films produced and the viability of the industry that produced them.

Kulturfilmy, Fictions and Newsreels, 1924–29

Anti-alcohol films tended to fall into several different types after 1924—popular kulturfilmy, fiction films, and newsreels. I refer to these as types, but as the following account will show, types were not fixed genre categories, but, rather, blurred into one another. Indeed, I suggest that genres are less important to an understanding of the history of the anti-alcohol film than the anti-alcohol campaigns themselves. These not only determined the development of such films, but also ensured that film producers used whatever form of film worked best for them and mixed genres where necessary.

As regarded the first of these types, kulturfilmy, the state studios made three such films between 1924 and 1927 that showed the "front lines" of the fight against alcohol in Russia. The first was *The Spider and the Fly* (1924), financed by Goskino, that depicted class struggle in the countryside and a new institution for political education, the *izba-chitalnia,* rural reading houses created to combat (political) illiteracy.[56] This was a prominent topic in a year when the "worker-peasant alliance" (*smychka*) was reinitiated by the Stalin-Kamenev-Zinoviev triumvirate opposing the left-wing pro-worker fraction of the party.[57] The film shows the village's political educator (*izbach*) reading aloud a newspaper, with every act caused by alcohol excess mentioned illustrated on the screen. Sukharesbkii, the coauthor of the screenplay, had harsh words about it: "Strictly speaking, there is no health education material. The film is boring and difficult to bear."[58] The film indeed lacks pedagogic material and cinematographic pace, despite the use of flashbacks. Nevertheless, Sukharebskii recommended it for the countryside, undoubtedly because the film echoed the political circumstances. In 1925 the Proletkino Studio, tied to the leftist Proletkult movement, also released *Moonshine: Enemy of the People* to combat narcomania (alcohol, tobacco, and cocaine), a film that has not been preserved and about which there is very little information.[59]

Finally, a provincial division of the state studio Sovkino produced the film *Anxiety* in 1927. As Stalin had decided to purge the Communist Party of its Trotskyist opponents, this was a year of great political tension. Although *Anxiety* promoted discipline in factories by targeting alcoholism among workers, the censor only grudgingly authorized its distribution.[60] Sukharebskii believed that this film was the "best on this theme," artistically and educationally, with ideal, "simple, short and understandable" insert titles.[61] But in *Pravda,* S. Ermolinskii opined that, aside from the didactic intertitles, Evgeny Petrov had failed to address the issues.[62] Petrov was a filmmaker of some renown who had directed a number of documentary films and kulturfilmy. Unsurprisingly, his latest work was better received by doctors who knew of his investment in health films than by his peers in the film community who did not comprehend or approve of the developing film type.

Fiction films were the second focus of anti-alcohol productions. Between 1924 and 1929, Soviet studios produced a dozen full-length films for the fight against alcohol, which—in contrast to the didactic kulturfilmy that denounced alcohol by means of documentary images or diagrams—used an array of visual inventions to do so: for example, *Saba* (1929) or *The Devil's Wheel* (1926) did not explain the impact of the alcohol on the body, but tried to make the viewer feel them through camera effects staging blurred eyesight, dizziness, or bursts of violence. But they were a problematic intervention in part because of Soviet criticism of the prewar film *Drunkenness and Its Consequences* for depoliticizing the subject. While many critics were envious of its success, they argued that it focused on the spectacular aspects of the problem at the expense of its social aspects and on morally condemned, marginalized urban classes.

Aware of these concerns, Grigorii Kozintsev and Ilya Trauberg set *The Devil's Wheel* (1926) in Leningrad's petty crime underground.[63] Within the first two minutes of the film, there is a close-up of a man wrinkled by alcohol, drinking slowly from a bottle of vodka, facing the camera. The film is constructed like a spiral or a vortex, which is suggested with music and visual effects. The fall of Ivan Shorin, a sailor on the battle cruiser *Aurora*—a symbol of the October Revolution because it had bombed the provisory government headquarters—occurs in a Luna-park where he loses his balance and bearings and where distorting mirrors reflect the vision problems caused by alcohol. A pool game metaphor illustrates his fate, that of a ball hit by others and falling in the pocket. The loss of his social (and political) position that led to him drowning in alcoholism is shown in two cabaret scenes. The motion picture, released in March 1926, was immediately a subject of debate and the reason for a special meeting of the ARK.[64] A decision from the Glavrepertkom, the body in charge of authorizing the film's release, forced the producers to edit the film to show the sailor's punishment.[65]

Such endings were not uncommon. Most fictions did not promise a cure but rather the punishment or redemption of the alcoholic; they neglect the medical aspect to concentrate on the social and moral dimensions. In a political atmosphere that encouraged finger-pointing, such endings fit well with the trend toward depictions of agitation trials in literature and organized leisure, and the rise political trials such as the campaign against Trotskyists in 1927 or the first show trial at Shakhty in May and June 1928.

One might think that Soviet newsreels—the third type of anti-alcohol film, a half-dozen of which were produced between 1924 and 1929—would adopt a technical discourse and show scientists fighting alcohol. Since the liquidation of the cinematography division of the Skobelev Committee in 1918, newsreels were state-controlled and released weekly under the name *Sovkinozhurnal* (SKŽ) from April 1, 1925.[66] They seldom made reference to the alcohol issue: only 1 percent mentioned it between 1925 and 1930. In 1927 SKŽ showed a few images from a serialized film that criticized alcohol abuse.[67] In the same year, it broadcasted a segment showing children marching against alcoholism—images that would become commonplace in the last years of the decade.[68] And in 1928, SKŽ staged an adult demonstration in front of the Krasnoe Sormovo factory in Nizhny-Novgorod on payday, as paydays were frequently days of alcoholic excess and drama as depicted in the fictional film *Saba*.[69]

Newsreels also contrasted the alcoholic with the model of the "new man": a 1928 reel denounced a "festival of drunkenness and gluttony" by juxtaposing footage of a sports competition in an open-air stadium and of a polluted bazaar where drunkards repeatedly downed glasses of vodka.[70] In 1929 the tone became

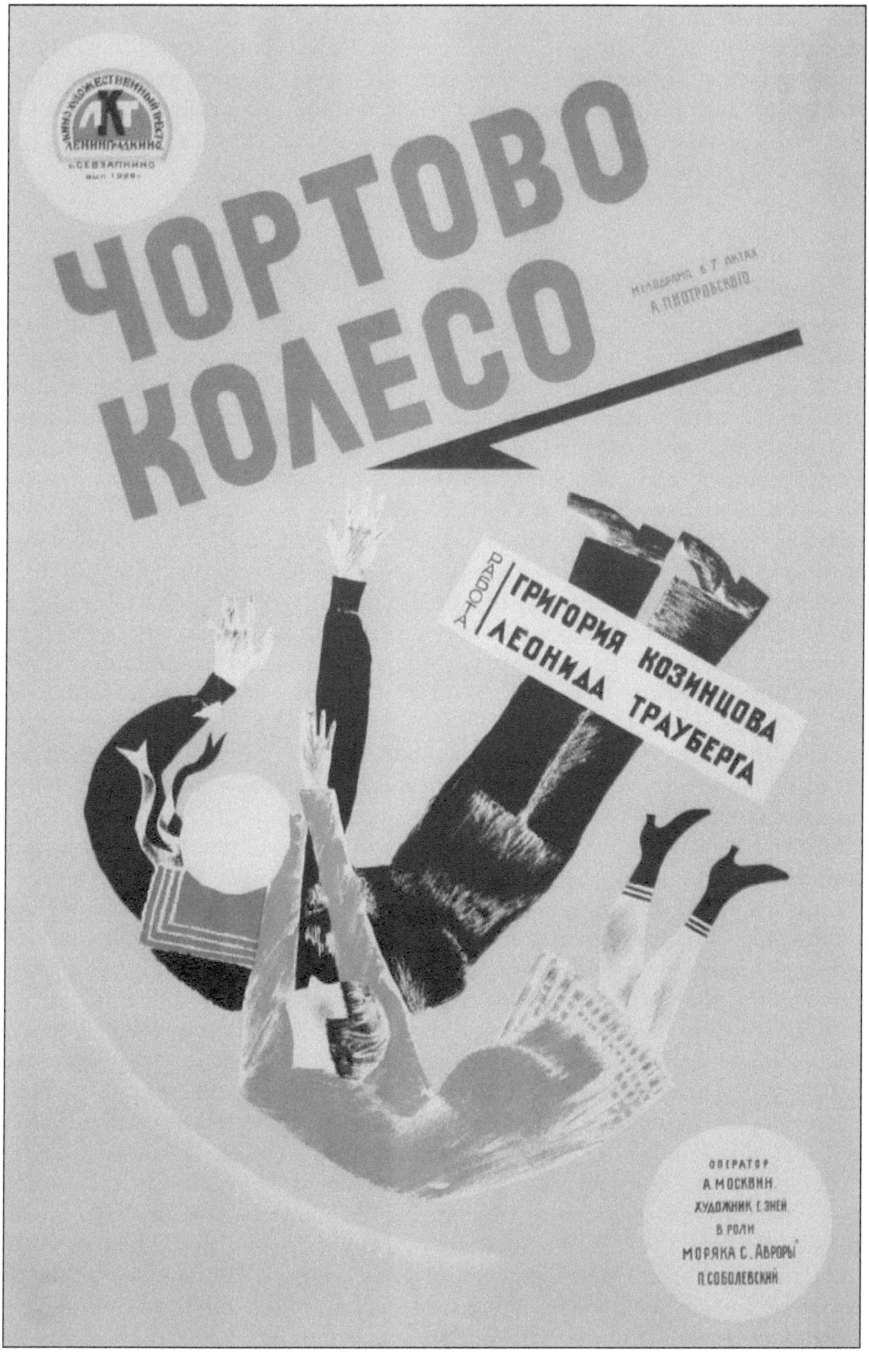

Figure 5.3. Advertizing poster for Kozintsev and Trauberg's *The Devil's Wheel* (1926).

more virulent and the target more clear, with factories leading the fight against absenteeism at the beginning of the Five-Year Plan.[71] In the Podolsk machine-building factory, for instance, a campaign was organized to denounce the time and money lost by workers waiting in line for alcohol. This involved showing the arrest of a drunken man in addition to an anti-alcohol exhibition displayed on the factory grounds.[72]

Saba (1929)

In 1929, after three years of propaganda, three new anti-alcohol films were released: one Kulturfilm (*To Your Health*) and two fictions, *Saba* and *Tanka the Innkeeper. Saba* is worth analyzing in detail because it illustrates how filmmakers not only sought apply Sigal's "agitation trial" model to film (increasingly regarded as of greater value to the hygienist cause than plays), but also to meet criticisms of the agitation trial model of storytelling. One critic, I. D. Strashun, a Soviet health film specialist, criticized the lengthy and repetitive character of this dramatic genre; he feared that the film viewer would end up confusing all the social illnesses into one "single grey stain."[73] Despite this kind of disclaiming, in *Saba* (1929) the filmmaker Mikheil Chiaureli brought his own idea of an agitation trial to the screen with additional story lines that added a further layer of narrative complexity to its tale of redemption from alcoholism. Renowned critic Khrisanf Khersonskii claimed it incited true "hatred for alcohol."[74]

The film tells the story of a streetcar conductor Saba, who spends all his wages on drink, and of his son, who finds him usually in cheap eating and drinking establishments. Saba eventually loses his job, and one day he steals the keys from a former colleague and borrows a streetcar with tragic results—he kills his own son. Saba is brought up before the workers' court, but the court decides that Saba is not the only one at fault. Instead, it finds his colleagues also guilty for not helping him with his drink problem. The court ends with a call for banning drink and providing cafeterias for the workers. Throughout the film, Chiaureli provides the audience with a guide to their emotional response by using actors to dramatize the emotions (rage, sadness, joy, etc.) prompted by Saba's story, like a Greek tragedy chorus. After an appeal for clemency from the prosecutor, Saba is spared a jail sentence; the bars are closed and he is reunited with his family in a happy ending. Saba becomes an anti-alcohol spokesperson and is filmed by Chiaureli campaigning in a real Communist Youth club.

We do not know if Chiaureli used the agitation trial because this theatrical genre was particularly suited to emphasizing the condemnation of alcoholics or because a trial is a fairly cinematographic type of drama in itself. The film's mix of literary and theatrical influences, moral and political concerns, and aesthetic inclinations lends it a hybrid character. As such, it reflects the film community's hesitations regarding the best type of film to use and the best means of diffusion and promotion.

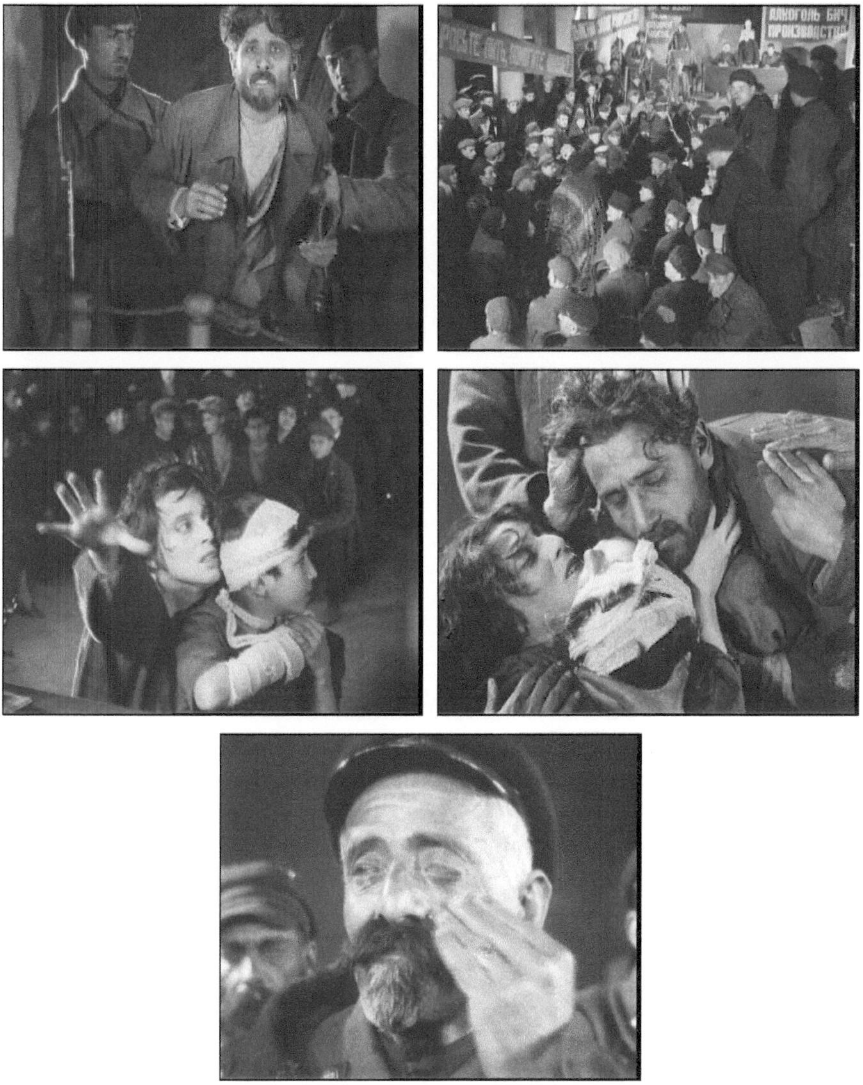

Figure 5.4a–e. The spectacle court in Chiaureli's *Saba* (1929). As he sits at the left of the stage between two guards, the accused drunkard watches his wife and son cross the room to testify.

The film was acclaimed by the public, particularly by the members of the Tiflis ODSK and the streetcar workers from the depot where it was filmed.[75] (ODSK stands for the Society of the Soviet Cinematography's Friends—a mass "volunteer organization" acting as an ideological lever for some upper Bolshevik leaders of the agitprop against the "commercial" motivations of the Sovkino

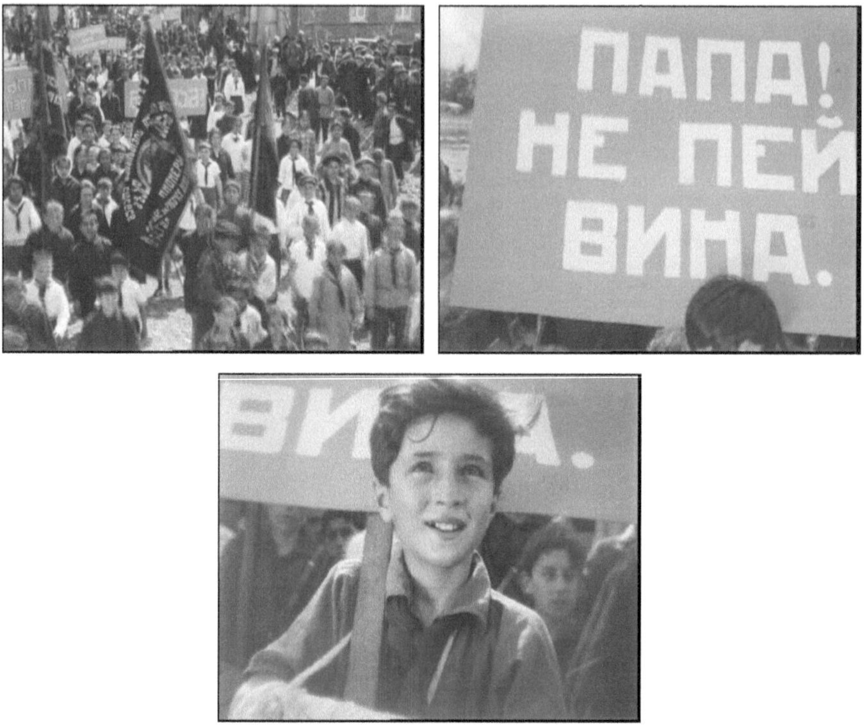

Figure 5.5a–c. Vakhtang, Saba's son, demonstrates with Tiflis' youth against alcoholism waves a placard proclaiming: "Daddy! Do not drink wine" in Chiaureli's *Saba* (1929).

state studio.) As Julie Cassiday suggests, what gave the film its power was its melodramatic format, its call for audiences to reform, and the stock character of the drunkard who embodied both villainy and innocence.[76] Thus, at the beginning of the film, the portrayal of Saba's abused wife and son suggest an indictment of the drunkard as an *individual*. But *Saba* is not only a villain but also a victim, and after his downfall the failure of Soviet society as a whole is acknowledged and resolved in the catharsis in a second trial that "exemplifies" (*pokazatelnyi*) Saba's case. The ambiguity of his status (i.e., victim or culprit) erases the boundary between reality and fiction and pushes the viewer to have faith in a redemption that is only possible if the community contributes. Here, the on-screen depiction of the agitation trial is primarily aimed not at alcoholics but at the nonalcoholics, who are called upon to organize the fight against this scourge and who are offered the chance to redeem other drunkards like Saba.

Physicians had a different reaction. Although they acknowledged that the young director had talent, they faulted him for the mishmash of genres and aesthetics crammed into his film, probably inspired by his experience as a watcher of kulturfilmy. Chiaureli, who—quite exceptionally—had written the script without a medical consultant, took a gamble in going against the expectations of viewers as well as critics and censors: the medical argument against alcoholism was not, as was customary, shown in a lengthy doctor's deposition at the trial. The only scene that featured the traditional tropes of the depiction of medicine (with surgeons working meticulously in a spotlessly clean and quiet environment) did not directly address alcoholism but showed the treatment of Vakhtang, Saba's son, who was run over when Saba was drunk at the controls of the streetcar.

Similarly, the classic scene of binge drinking at the *traktir* involves themes of carnivalesque role reversal. The guest of honor, who was forced to drink himself into unconsciousness, is revealed at the end to be a traveling anti-alcohol lecturer. The table host (*tamada*) pronounces a toast with a pseudo-history of wine that parodies the lecture that the guest could have given; filmed close up with his eyes looking straight into the camera, he openly ridicules expert authority. It is, however, worth considering that the inclusion of documentary film excerpts in the closing scenes might have been an attempt to make a connection with the viewers' real world.[77] The still shots of seven alcoholics increasingly affected by putrefaction show illness, sadness, and guilt. This sequence powerfully stimulates the viewers' imagination by *preventing* them from identifying with the diseased and pushing them to relate to Saba. His destiny, crime and redemption included, seems comparatively less shocking, more understandable and acceptable.

To Your Health (1929)

If *Saba* illustrates the transformation of the agitation play into cinematic form, *To Your Health* (1929) is a window onto the audience reception of anti-alcohol films, a difficult subject to explore given that although physicians and film experts often commented on such films, they generally did not do so in public, and during the 1920s, the national medical press rarely referred to cinema as an educational tool; in fact, it almost never even mentioned films. The documentary record of *To Your Health* provides a welcome respite from the silence on this subject.

To Your Health is undoubtedly the best example of what Soviet filmmakers sought to accomplish on the theme of anti-alcoholism. The film retraces the life and destiny of Leningrad worker A. P. Chistiakov, a drunkard who poisons the lives of those around him, loses his job, and then decides to get help. The fictional portions of the film freely reuse other directors' ideas, such as imitating blurred vision and hallucinations, as well as an ironic tone to criticize the protagonist's way of life (*byt*). Three scientific episodes play on different scientific codes: rigorous reasoning, technical precision, and medical authority. First, an experiment on an egg demonstrates the genetic influence of alcohol: the hands of a laboratory technician are filmed against a neutral background, which allows the audience to follow each step of the experiment and of the anti-alcohol

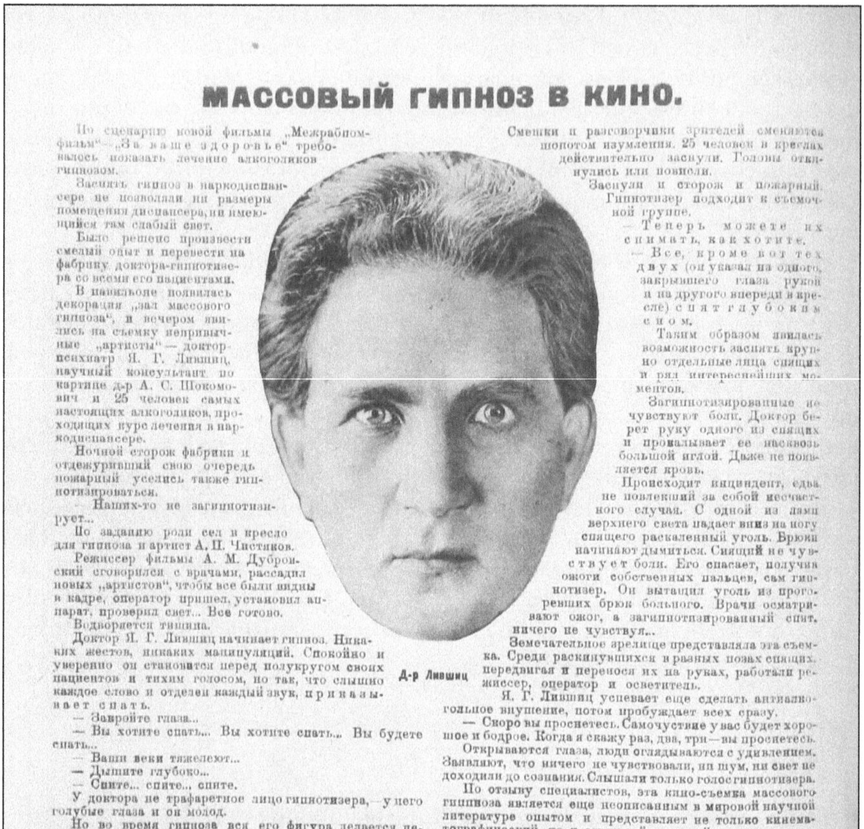

МАССОВЫЙ ГИПНОЗ В КИНО.

По сценарию новой фильмы „Межрабпом-фильм“ — „За ваше здоровье“ требовалось показать лечение алкоголиков гипнозом.

Заснять гипноз в наркодиспансере не позволяли ни размеры помещения диспансера, ни имеющийся там слабый свет.

Было решено произвести смелый опыт и перевести на фабрику доктора-гипнотизера со всеми его пациентами.

В павильоне появилась декорация „зал массового гипноза“, и вечером явились на съемку непривычные „артисты“ — доктор-психиатр Я. Г. Лившиц, научный консультант по картине д-р А. С. Шокомович и 25 человек самых настоящих алкоголиков, проходящих курс лечения в наркодиспансере.

Ночной сторож фабрики и отдежуривший свою очередь пожарный уселись также гипнотизироваться.

— Наших-то не загипнотизирует...

По заданию роли сел в кресло для гипноза и артист А. П. Чистяков.

Режиссер фильмы А. М. Дубровский сговорился с врачами, рассадил новых „артистов“, чтобы все были видны в кадре, оператор пришел, установил аппарат, проверил свет... Все готово.

Водворяется тишина.

Доктор Я. Г. Лившиц начинает гипноз. Никаких жестов, никаких манипуляций. Спокойно и уверенно он становится перед полукругом своих пациентов и тихим голосом, но так, что слышно каждое слово и отделен каждый звук, приказывает спать.

— Закройте глаза...

— Вы хотите спать... Вы хотите спать... Вы будете спать...

— Ваши веки тяжелеют...

— Дышите глубоко...

— Спите... спите... спите.

У доктора не трафаретное лицо гипнотизера, — у него голубые глаза и он молод.

Но во время гипноза вся его фигура делается необыкновенно властной, глаза — устремлены вперед. Лицо — концентрированная воля.

Д-р Лившиц

Смешки и разговорчики зрителей сменяются шопотом изумления. 25 человек в креслах действительно заснули. Головы откинулись или поникли.

Заснули и сторож и пожарный. Гипнотизер подходит к съемочной группе.

— Теперь можете их снимать, как хотите.

— Все, кроме вот тех двух (он указал на одного, закрывшего глаза рукой и на другого впереди в кресле) спят глубоким сном.

Таким образом явилась возможность заснять крупно отдельные лица спящих и ряд интереснейших моментов.

Загипнотизированные не чувствуют боли. Доктор берет руку одного из спящих и прокалывает ее насквозь большой иглой. Даже не появляется кровь.

Происходит инцидент, едва не повлекший за собой несчастного случая. С одной из ламп верхнего света падает вниз на ногу спящего раскаленный уголь. Брюки начинают дымиться. Спящий не чувствует боли. Его спасает, получив ожоги собственных пальцев, сам гипнотизер. Он вытащил уголь из прогоревших брюк больного. Врачи осматривают ожог, а загипнотизированный спит, ничего не чувствуя...

Замечательное зрелище представляла эта съемка. Среди раскинувшихся в разных позах спящих, передвигая и перенося их на руках, работали режиссер, оператор и осветитель.

Я. Г. Лившиц успевает еще сделать антиалкогольное внушение, потом пробуждает всех сразу.

— Скоро вы проснетесь. Самочувствие у вас будет хорошее и бодрое. Когда я скажу раз, два, три — вы проснетесь.

Открываются глаза, люди оглядываются с удивлением. Заявляют, что ничего не чувствовали, ни шум, ни свет не доходили до сознания. Слышали только голос гипнотизера.

По отзыву специалистов, эта кино-съемка массового гипноза является еще неописанным в мировой научной литературе опытом и представляет не только кинематографический, но и огромный научный интерес.

Даль

Чистяков под гипнозом

Figure 5.6. A focus on A. Dubrovskii's *To Your Health* (1927) in the article "Collective Hypnosis in Movies," *Soviet Screen* 39 (1928): 19.

argument. The technique, the instantly recognizable nature of the experiment, and the evident cleanliness of the room serve to build the audience's trust. The masterful time-lapse photography, though it accentuates the impression that we are witnessing a "magic act" in the scientific scenes, is the perfect synthesis of the experiments seen on USSR screens since 1925 and fulfills the didactic goal of the film.

Then, the third scene shows experiments on the influence of alcohol on movement and balance performed at the Central Institute for Labor Protection, which incidentally was a producer of health education films on safety measures in the workplace.[78] This rather amusing scene, depicting problems encountered in daily life, presented arguments on two levels, appealing to empiricism and common sense. Lastly, the film outlines the most spectacular treatments, such as electroconvulsive treatment and insufflation of oxygen under the skin, but these were presented as counterpoints serving to emphasize the success of Dr. Livshitz's method, demonstrated by Dr. Livshitz himself. Inspired by V. M. Bekhterev's works at the turn of the century, Dr. Livshitz's technique involved the practice of group and individual hypnosis and the learning of self-persuasion techniques. Close-up shots of his face, his eyes, and his lips articulating the hypnosis scripts are intercut with shots of the patients being hypnotized. However, the insert titles do not convey the strengths of his discourse and a full cure seems quickly achieved; the demonstration almost feels like a magician's trick.

The Association of Revolutionary Cinematography meetings were a major forum for discussing what constituted Soviet films. *To Your Health* was discussed there on April 16, 1929, to the dismay of the director Aleksandr Dubrovskii, who had not been forewarned. The film had earlier been received negatively at the premiere held on March 24, 1929, at the Artes movie theater. Rejected by Sukharebskii, the film, based on a script by Tiagai, disappointed critics who attacked the mix of acting and nonacting, the lack of cinematic innovation, and the tendency to favor fiction at the expense of effective scientific anti-alcohol arguments. Furthermore, Mezhrabpom's true motives for making the film also became a matter of controversy at a time when Sovkino looked to take over the last private studio in the USSR. Although the cinematographer Lemberg backed Mezhrabpom's foray into more serious subject matter about which few screenplays had been written,[79] others only saw in the production of *To Your Health* a slick maneuver to accumulate "ideological capital" without ruining its "bankable capital."[80] It is doubtful that, in light of previous events, there was any truth in the latter assumption, but it is certain that the firm had an advantage over other producers of health education films.

Each studio looked to consolidate its position by organizing projections for select audiences. This is the focus of my second line of inquiry into the reception of these films. Lemberg described a session at the OBA headquarters where *To Your Health* was compared to Genik's *Alcohol*, and the room was divided. The workers did not reject Dubrovskii's film, finding it "good";[81] but viewers of Genik's film enjoyed its gritty quality and found it more convincing.[82] Those who preferred *To Your Health*, however, regretted its lack of educational material.

Dubrovskii obviously did not seek to shock by showing the ravages of alcoholism on the body and mind or to instruct and convince with animated diagrams. The critic of the workers' newspaper admonished the easy cure that was presented following a somewhat random overview of various other treatments.[83] However, the claim that the director was incapable "of selecting interesting facts to demonstrate scientific thought" overlooked his attempt to satisfy both the medical and the film community by striking a balance between medical discourse, didactic diagrams and experiments, and narrative.[84] As for uninvited or unwarned viewers, almost no source recorded their opinion. It is worth reminding that these projections were in the city and in custom-made venues, with a public chosen according to their class and in particular workers, who were expected to display a superior degree of conscience.[85] The situation was quite different in the far vaster and less understood countryside.

Tanka the Innkeeper (1929)

The third of the three films released in 1929, *Tanka the Innkeeper* provides a window onto a further aspect of the film component of the anti-alcohol campaigns: their focus on the countryside. In a country where 80 percent of the population lived outside the cities, the probability that the rural population might come across these health education films is an important factor to consider, as is the ability of the totalitarian state to saturate the cultural space and to influence intellectual spaces with its propaganda. How this campaigning in the countryside worked out is the focus of this section.

The director of the Social Hygiene Institute, A. V. Molkov, believed that living conditions accounted for alcoholism among laborers; peasants, he thought, drank out of habit. To the officials, it was not the state, but the individual who was responsible for his or her alcoholism. It was therefore not necessary to deny access to alcohol, but to reform the urban environment and reeducate peasants. There was also an underestimated economic dimension to the alcoholism issue. Vodka had virtually no place in a village; it was expensive and reserved for urbanites who, in any case, drank more than rural dwellers. Therefore, state and propaganda initiatives targeted the moonshine, or *samogon,* produced by clandestine and artisan distillers. The production of samogon boomed with the prohibition and the war. In 1914 this activity became profitable, playing a part in the black market between villages and cities and finding new local consumers—refugees, prisoners of war, wounded soldiers—victims directly affected by the conflict and inclined to take to drinking. The Soviet economy, built on shortages, saw the system expand: 60 percent of peasant farms produced *samogon* in 1922, while 70 percent of townspeople drank unregulated alcohol sold illicitly in the street or in restaurants as "lemonade."[86] The 1923 "scissors crisis" (a drop in agricultural prices and uncontrolled rise in industrial prices) amplified this phenomenon. Alcohol did not spoil, could be stored, and brought in several times the amount paid for grain to the state or even on the free market.

In villages, alcohol played a major role in sociability that the authorities preferred to ignore. Distillation brought neighbors together more easily than any other economic activity. It required materials that poor peasants working together could easily obtain: 8 kg of potatoes, 4 kg of flour, 3 kg of malt, and a little yeast were necessary to make 9.5 liters of moonshine. Most rural people saw alcohol as a popular remedy that provided physical strength, as witnessed by its use in village rituals. Many annual village holidays, both religious and popular, punctuated local life at set dates that closely followed the agricultural seasons.

Ritual consumption of alcohol ran deep in the roots of Russian cultural identity. In villages and cities, taverns (*traktir*) were a major site of male socialization. Taverns usually sold vodka that had been mixed with other substances in order to make a profit, at best with water, but often with noxious chemical substances. Increasingly expensive due to government taxes, yet of poor quality, it pushed levels of consumption higher. This was well known among the screenwriters who decided to set the action of *Tanka the Innkeeper* in a tavern. In this film, young Tanka dreams of joining the village Pioneer brigade, but she is turned away because she is the innkeeper's daughter. Her father, not content with just exploiting and beating his only daughter, also thwarts her desire to escape her circumstances. He fights against the influences of "cultural forces" in the village that plan to replace his tavern, which seduces villagers with vodka and gambling, with a club offering tea and "reasonable" entertainment. The attempted assassination of the Communist teacher, the innkeeper's enemy, is foiled thanks to Tanka, who is eventually saved and allowed to join the village pioneers. The final scene shows the village women cleaning the tavern of its impurities.

This forty-three-minute film about the peasant way of life, a genre of its own addressing working-class or peasant lifestyles and typical of 1920s productions, is reminiscent of the agitation trial but does not include any scientific content. The film is concerned with cultural and political education (*kulturpolitprosveitelnyi*) rather than the popularization of scientific material (*nauchno-populiarnyi*). Shot in 1928, this film coincided with the peak of social hygienism aimed at traditional or "backward" group behavior and consumption. It was released in early 1929 to a limited viewership. In Omsk, Siberia, 3,579 viewers saw *Tanka* at the Luch cinema in the third week of February. This made the film sixteenth in the city rankings (the best earner being *The Capitan's Daughter*, with 10,837 viewers in just six days), but second best in this rather small theater.[87] Among the twenty-one films that were released at the time, not a single one was scientific, much less dealt with health issues; the agitation campaigns mainly relied on fiction or semifiction films.

Tanka placed the fight against alcohol in the broader perspective of the advent of the new way of life (*novyj byt*). The choice of this theme, a prominent one in all works concerned with shaping the "new man" in the city and in the countryside, opened new horizons for the funding of films specifically about peasants like *Tanka*. The script dramatizes Manichean oppositions between superstition and science, prejudice and common sense, gullibility and critical thinking. In a key scene, the innkeeper's superstitious and illiterate henchmen set a trap for

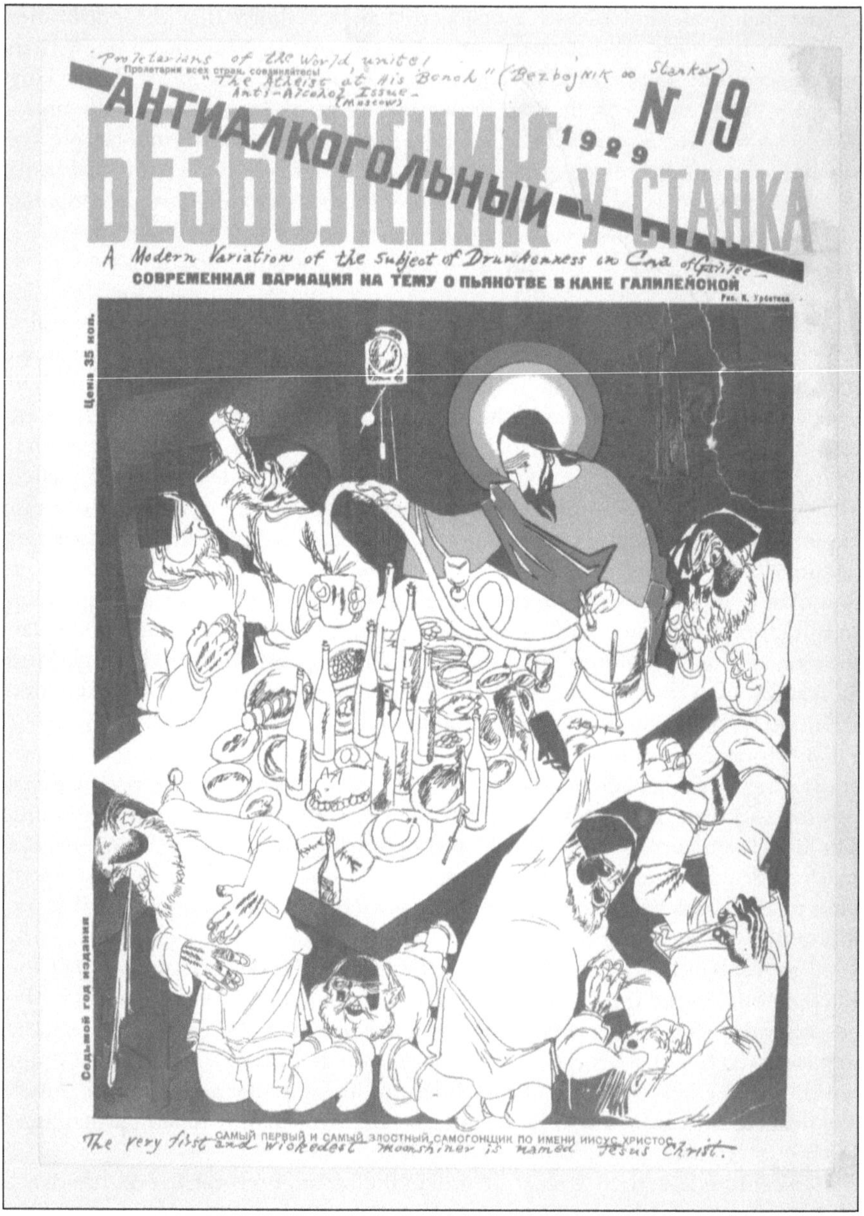

Figure 5.7. The campaign against Church's influence related moonshine, popes and kulaks. Cover for *The Godless Worker* 19 (1929), special issue against alcoholism.

the teacher at a place called the "devil's bridge," deep in a marshy forest. The sounds of nature and the cries of a pioneer caught in quicksand frighten the villagers who calm themselves by downing bottles of alcohol, which only heightens their fear. Aware of the power of superstition, the young Communist intellectual decides not to fight but to use a clever ploy. He disguises his troika as a "devil's chariot" and thereby disbands his adversaries. Despite the high expectations placed on them, the films which arrived irregularly and often out of season were not able to effectively root out rural beliefs and impose the Marxist worldview in their place.

Tanka not only sought to challenge rural religious beliefs, it also raised questions about the effects of alcohol on women and rural youth. One of concerns about alcoholism was the violent expression of desire among village men for young women liberated from old customs. Becoming actors of their own fate, these women tried to persuade the worst alcoholics to become good sober comrades. This ideal of radical social change reflected the growing autonomy of peasant women but also worsened already tense gender relationships in the village, particularly concerning alcohol consumption.[88] At Tanka's father's tavern, the few women patrons drink tea, while all the men drink moonshine concealed in teapots.

The frenetic tavern scene that stands out in an otherwise slow-paced film reflects a frenzy of consumption that apparently nothing can stop. Hands shake, eyes shine, the patrons do whatever they can to avoid falling down dead drunk and lower their heads in connivance. Alcohol twists bodies and words and annihilates the Soviet progress of women's liberation and education. The enslaved Tanka is forced to sacrifice her studies. At the tavern, she tries, in vain, to keep up with the lids flying off teapots and the hot water pouring out of the tap. Beaten for having betrayed her father, she is locked in the cellar—where barrels of alcohol are stored, symbolizing obscurity (*temnota*), that is, peasant backwardness traditionally regarded with contempt in Russia.

Anti-alcohol activists suspected the enemy of using alcohol to subvert and stupefy the weakest in the village and then maintain their narcotic, and ultimately economic, dependence. Propaganda directed to rural villages emphasized the connection between the church, the domination of the rich (*kulaks*), and alcohol, even claiming that monasteries were the principal places of alcohol production and consequently the beneficiaries of its sale. It criticized "religion and vodka at the service of the *koulak*" for ruining the health and savings of the poor with countless village festivities.[89] The church remains absent from the film, unlike in many films about peasant life.[90] But Tanka's father, the "class enemy," is repeatedly shown serving drinks but never drinking himself: he *knows*—and the audience understands it—that alcohol is harmful. His understanding of the ins and outs of politics and health issues merely serves his agenda of hijacking Communist orders. He is shown conscientiously brushing his teeth but actually does not care about hygiene. The Soviet authorities intended to use modern means such as radio and cinema, which fascinated the rural population, to promote their objectives. In the film, Tanka's father, who is otherwise uncultivated, uses the radio to lure the villagers in, thereby competing with the *izba-chitalnia*, the local "reading hut" that was a pillar of rural political education. The point implied is that modern media are worthless without proper supervision, and they could be misinterpreted by spectators since, in the absence of a commentator, these attitudes resembled a "new man" profile.

A projectionist touring in the Nizhny-Novgorod province during the last quarter of 1927 described cultural opposition witnessed at a screening: "I suggested to one of the members of Communist Youth (Komsomol) that he read the insert titles, but opposition rang out in the audience. One of the peasants declared that there should no longer be a single illiterate on the tenth anniversary of October; that everyone should read the titles themselves."[91] This ironic comment, which turned Bolshevik slogans against their promoters, singles out this peasant as an adversary of Soviet authorities. Through his discourse, using irrefutable logic, he monopolized the expression of public opinion and prevented the projectionist from carrying out his minimal duty, reading. We may thus imagine that during that screening, part of the audience was able to read the insert titles while the others simply reacted to the images, with the projectionist neither narrating nor explaining the action. It is highly surprising that the projectionist, the members of Komsomol, and the local officials followed the lead of this peasant, who was more educated that most. We might ask whether it was indifference on the part of the projectionist, ready to compromise, as long as the session would run, in his words, "smoothly" or rather a sign of this peasant's power, who, as indicated in several reports, was able to sponsor screenings by providing a venue and even selling seats to other villagers.

It might also be noted that anti-alcohol campaigns—with or without films—often found it difficult to overcome the economic problems that promoted the sale of samogon. *Samogon* bootleggers in the city were often poor women peasants with no other source of income, and many such women were among the distillers that were arrested after a law made the activity a crime punishable with three years in prison and fines up to five hundred gold rubles.[92] In the first half of 1923, the police made nearly 300,000 arrests, and 194,000 trials were organized that year. This was illustrated in 1926 in Abram Room's *Chasing the Distiller*, a police comedy inspired by American films but which elicited little enthusiasm from audiences and critics.[93] Fines, confiscations, and public work detail seem to have had very little educational effect on the poorest villagers, those who faced the harshest sentences and, probably, those most guilty of clandestine distillation. Furthermore, many sources point to cases of inebriation among local authorities in spite of their proclaimed Communist ethics. In 1928 the officials from the Ukrainian town of Ostrog tried to lead inspector Fomin into their drinking session of "fire water," vodka. But Fomin requested that Moscow punish them for having harassed the young volunteer who accompanied him and for having wandered about Ostrog dead drunk. Sources do not indicate whether this request was honored, but he did receive two hundred rubles for an impromptu campaign against alcoholism.[94]

Tanka and the Dearth of Health Film Screenings

One of the problems facing the makers of *Tanka* was a problem that bedeviled advocates of health education films in anti-alcohol campaigns in general: the dearth of films outside of the two capital cities. In places such as Omsk, one of the main Siberian cities, or in Tula, a small industrial center and satellite city of the capital, very few sanitary films were shown, and even when they were, turnout could be low as the periodical *The Omsk Spectator* reported.[95] However, the main problem was screening the films for peasant audiences.[96] Cinemas in permanent structures with their own equipment were not common and remained the exception, even in the provincial capitals. The bulk of the screenings was left to itinerant projectionists; some made a career of it, but most kept this job only for a few months. Expansion of the state-sponsored network began in 1924 under the auspices of the Main Committee for Political Education Glavpolitprosvet and reached a climax during the first Five-Year Plan (1928–32). A decree by the Council of People's Commissars (Sovnarkom) on July 12, 1928, established Gosplan objectives and gave priority to a new network supervised by Tsentrosoiuz. This Cooperatives' Union offered financial strength and solid rural connections to meet the standards that had been set. In one year, 1,569 projectors were obtained, for a total number of 1,869 units. Tsentrosoiuz, which now funded 55 percent (formerly 15 percent) of all the equipment in the Soviet countryside, was in a "dominant position."[97] The problem remained that Tsentrosoiuz was also responsible for the distribution of vodka in Soviet territory.

In addition to material difficulties, the authorities struggled to ensure that projectionists delivered the discourse that was meant to go with the film, and competition between institutional networks impeded work in the field. Rural screenings had to show films authorized for the peasant audience, but the lists were constantly changing; Sovkino's "rural" collection mainly included fiction. Although six thousand viewers along the Leningrad-Moscow rail route saw the film *Abortion*, the twenty performances were improvised without a lecturer. Sigal noted with understatement that this produced an "undesirable effect."[98] Even regardless of these problems, a corps of expert speakers was lacking anyway. In 1924 only twelve provinces had a Lecturers Office, while a mere six other provinces had organized dedicated health education sessions with films in workers' clubs.[99] The province of Leningrad created high-quality itinerant cinemas for health education, but rooms were often overcrowded and the noise from the projector drowned out the voice of the specially trained medical lecturer.

Tanka was already outdated by the time it was released (there was, for instance, no mention whatsoever of collectivization in the film), and as a consequence its commercial potential was cut short very early. Yet in the months after it had stopped being screened, the film was a subject of heated debate in public opinion, particularly in the cities: "This film, which is very mediocre both in terms of content and of artistic form, has within a few months become the banner around which the many proponents of clear and simple language in Soviet cinema have rallied. . . . For *Tanka the Innkeeper* and against obscure, convoluted works such as [Dovzhenko's] *Arsenal*—these have roughly been the terms of the debate. In the heat of the controversy, *Tanka the Innkeeper* was even declared the best film of the season, in comparison with [Pudovkin's] *Storm Over Asia, Arsenal,* etc."[100] In most cases, kulturfilmy and social hygiene films, whose production and diffusion were limited, only reached the cities at best. The diffusion of a film like *Tanka,* even though it was more likely to reach villages than other kulturfilmy, appears to have been virtually nonexistent. There is no trace, in central and local archive sources, of the ideal screenings envisioned by political educators and social hygienists—organized by a demonstrator and accompanied by an exhibition at the izba-chitalnia. The efforts of the filmmakers to address concerns about the effect of alcohol among rural peasants on class and gender relations, which I have cited, thus often did not reach its intended audience.

Conclusion

In the USSR, after the Revolution, the collective quest for a distinctively Soviet form of cinema was a matter of concern beyond the confines of the film community. Political leaders, social activists, scientific experts, and the public regularly participated in the debate, be it spontaneously or upon the invitation of actors from the film community. While they neither had decision-making powers nor the ear of those who had, the doctors involved in the production of health films largely had their say and were important contributors to the forums that influenced the studios' work. However, these committed doctors were only a handful, and those few were placed in an uncomfortable position halfway between the film and medical worlds; furthermore, their legitimacy to express themselves was sometimes contested in both.

In this very Soviet way of defining the best film model to educate and entertain, mobilize, and attract audience, foreign influences should not be underestimated: of 112 health education films approved for screening in Soviet Union in 1928, 13 were French and 16 German. Soviet films attempted to compete with models discussed by specialists and appreciated by the public, like *Der Steinach Film* or *Wege zu Kraft und Schönheit.* In particular, the German Kulturfilm produced by the UFA was admired for its cinematographic qualities, its rigor, and its commercial success. Soviet Kulturfilm stands out for its effort to strike a balance between purely scientific discourse and narrative in order to facilitate viewer identification.

In contrast with Germany, not only was there no dominant studio, but the sponsors were from different sources. Not a single series of films addressing the same issue was produced in the 1920s, and no business or institution was powerful enough to finance the promotion of solutions to the country's public health problems on the screen. The state only played a limited role as inducer, not as prescriber, and did not provide large financial support. Without the success of the Mezhrabpom-Rus studio, the other studios would probably have not made the venture. Competition was thus more of a factor than state commissions in the production of health films. Likewise, the market had a significant impact on this activity, which studios were reluctant to fund at a loss: the recourse to fictional storylines was not only an attempt to combine rational demonstration and emotional viewer participation. It was also a concession to audience tastes that made many uneasy in both the film and the medical community. In the subsequent decade, the term Kulturfilm would no longer apply to fashionable films that combined avant-garde creativity and scientific knowledge. Instead, it was used in a derogatory sense to refer to films seen as antithetical to popularization (*nauchno-populiarnye*) films, which were now produced as series and remained strictly scientific.

Under the general Kulturfilm label, there were actually as many approaches as there were films. Depending on the objective pursued, on the target audience, and on the director's background, Kulturfilms combined fiction and documentary filmmaking to various extents. Directed in 1927, the Kulturfilm *To Your Health* is rooted in didactic expertise but still includes a light plot and spectacular scenes. In contrast, the redemptive drama *Saba* proposes a reflection on the medical and legal discourse *and* the legal and cinematographic view of the experts. These variations are equally due to the degree of liberty taken by the directors and cinematographers in proposing new types of images, by the screenwriters (often doctors) in adapting medical discourse to social reasoning, and by the distributors in organizing suitable screenings.

The failure of Soviet health educational films ultimately did not have so much to do with the small amount and uneven quality of the pictures produced as with their poorly organized distribution. It was not that the public was not able to understand these films; to assess the health, social and even political issues; to love them or reject them. The problem was that these films were not shown outside a few select theaters as a network of cinemas dedicated to the genre had not been organized, and that they remained confined to Russia's main cities. More generally, the anti-alcohol theme was overall never an important issue on the screens: during the decade, the subject was only addressed in three newsreels and in two fiction films, *The Devil's Wheel* and *Saba*, which though directed by renowned filmmakers were considered a minor work in their filmography. *Tanka* did elicit some debate, but it served to reveal contradictions between political agendas within the party-state more than it efficiently promoted the cause it was meant to defend.

Anti-alcohol films could only conceivably appeal to two categories of viewers. First, the many who were invited to screenings organized by the ARK and ODSK, the studios, and the unions. They were summoned to provide their reaction and expected to give comments that added up to form a collective "opinion" on the film, which would then be used as a weapon in the raging debate between different groups in the film community. Then, those who had a stake in the anti-alcohol issue (the doctors) and in the health film medium (film professionals) were also invited and found themselves among peers. These viewers learned nothing from the films, which essentially served as vehicles of disputes between experts and possibly as mutual sources of inspiration. Films against alcoholism hardly reached any alcoholics in the USSR. Even if sources were to show that these films were screened in specialized treatment institutions, the huge masses of alcoholics with no exposure whatsoever to the health system did not see them. There is no evidence in the specialized press and in the minutes of local society meetings that medical congresses on alcohol included screenings that would have popularized the use of cinema as a preventive medium. Perhaps it is precisely because these films failed to resonate with doctors, at least in that decade, that they did not reach their intended audience.

Notes

1. Denise J. Youngblood, *The Magic Mirror: Moviemaking in Russia, 1908–1918* (Madison: University of Wisconsin Press, 1999).

2. David L. Hoffmann, *Cultivating the Masses: Modern State Practices and Soviet Socialism, 1914–1939* (Ithaca, NY: Cornell University Press, 2011).

3. Lazar M. Suharebskij, *Obzor sanprosvetitel'nyh kinofil'm* (Moscow-Leningrad: GIZ, 1928), 24–27.

4. *Saba,* Mihajl Čijaurelli, Goskinprom Gruzii, 1929, 6 parts, 2100 m. *Za vaše zdorov'e* (*pod gipnozom*), Mihajl Dubrovskij, Mežrabpom-Rus', 1929, 5 parts, 1400 m. *Tanka traktiršica,* Boris Svetozarov, Sovkino, 1929, 42 minutes and 25 seconds. These films are preserved at the national film archives (Gosfilmofond, Belye Stolby, Moscow province), where mainly fictional works are stored. However, there are no films concerning the fight against alcohol or the broader theme of alcohol as a social disease in the collections of the national archives of documentary film and photography (RGAKFD). It is probable that medical institutions—the Academy of Medicine, Military Academy of Medicine, and prominent medical schools—have retained reels, and these will be the focus of upcoming archival work.

5. This is described by Mikhail Bulgakov, *A Country Doctor's Notebook* (London: Collins-Harvill, 1995).

6. Kate Transchel, *Under the Influence: Working-Class Drinking, Temperance, and Cultural Revolution in Russia, 1895–1932* (Pittsburgh: University of Pittsburgh Press, 2006), 50–53.

7. *Trudy Vserossjskogo s"ezda po bor'be s p'janstvom,* 1909–10.

8. The poster read, "The Workers of the USSR Do Not Have the Right to Poison their Strength, Body, and Mind, Which Are Needed for the Collective Work of the Socialist Construction of the Proletarian State."

9. This was the local rural administration created in 1864 in provinces and districts, three years after the abolition of serfdom by Tsar Alexander II.

10. In particular, this was the case of the first Congress of Extra-curricular Instruction in December 1913 and January 1914, which stressed the need to organize production of scientific films and their distribution in special showings. V. K. Čarnoluskij, *S"ezdy po narodnomu obrazovaniju* (Petrograd, Russia, 1915), 12.

11. *Vestnik kinematografii* 86 (1914): 19.

12. S. V. Skovorodnikova, "Prosvetitel'nyj kinematograf v Rossii (1908–1917)," *Kinovedčeskie zapiski* 18 (1993): 38–60.

13. *P'janstvo i ego posledstvija,* Khanjonkov, 1913, 3 parts, 850 m. Not preserved.

14. Semen S. Ginzburg, *Kinematografija dorevoljucionnoj Rossii* (Moscow: Iskusstvo, 1963), 97.

15. *Vestnik kinematografii* 6 (1913): 1.

16. Under the same circumstances, Pathé had distributed a film shot in Russia, *Pasynki sudby,* in December 1912. The Tsar's decision to introduce a temporary "dry law" was followed by a proposal to make prohibition permanent in August 1915 in the Duma, which accepted the principle in June 1916. The provisional government signed the decree in March 1917.

17. *Vozroždaemye k žizni,* RGAKFD, film no. 786.

18. Nikolai Lebekev, who lived in Berlin between 1925 and 1927, appears to have been the most active promoter of the UFA *Kulturabteilung* model, admired for its "determined march towards *kulturfilm.*" Nikolaj Lebedev, "Kulturfilma na zapade i u nas," excerpts from his unpublished manuscript kept at the Moscow Museum of Cinema, *Kinovedčeskie zapiski* 58 (2002): http://www.kinozapiski.ru/ru/article/sendvalues/315/.

19. *Sovetskoe kino* 1 (1927): 6.

20. In addition to a verification of the filmed experimentation commissioned by agitprop of the Red Army (PUR) under the direction of the renowned cameraman Lemberg, Steinach's experiences were challenged by Professors Voskresenskij and Uspenskij in Tver and Professors Khalatov and Notilov in Leningrad (separately). *Kino-nedelja* 12 (1925): 10.

21. Suharebskij, *Obzor,* 8–9.

22. V. G., "Položenie i perpektivy naučno-vospitatel'nogo kino," *Sovetskoe kino* 3 (1926): 12.

23. This recommendation likely referred to *La Vie au sanatorium de Bligny,* a 1914 film made by Jean Comandon.

24. I. D. Strašun, "Nasuščnye voprosy sanprosvetèkrana," 35. This probably referred to the short films proposed by the Kino-Moskva by the *Compagnie France-Caspienne* in 1925, like *La Diffusion de l'alcool* (49 m) or *Petite cause, grands effets* (41 m). Central Archives of Moscow City (CAGM), f. 2238, op. 1, d. 24, l. 94. The RGAKFD only preserved one film of this type, *La vie des microbes* (Pathé, 1910, film n°12588). Strašun's article was illustrated with three photographs of a scene from *Alcohol, Work and Health* showing respiratory tests, which underlines the identification of Mezhrabpom and Tiagai as essential sources of health education films.

25. State Archive of the Russian Federation (GARF), f. 8326 (Sovkino), op. 2, d. 16, ll. 126–33.

26. Their subsequent project, *Alcohol,* was far from the most prolific, but the costs multiplied: 30,027.16 rubles, about double the average expense for this type of production, in addition to 5004.60 rubles for making copies. GARF, f. 8326, op. 2, d. 8, l. 148 ob. Russian State Archive for Literature and Art (RGALI), f. 645 (Glaviskusstvo), op. 1, d. 391, l. 209.

27. Lev Trotskij, "Vodka, the Church and Cinema," first published in *Pravda,* July 12, 1923. English translation in Ian Christie and Richard Taylor, eds., *The Film Factory: Russian and Soviet Cinema in Documents, 1896–1939* (London: Routledge, 1994), 94–97.

28. Sergej Syrcov, *Kino v mesto vodki* (Moscow-Leningrad: GIZ, 1928).

29. GARF, f. 8326, op. 2, d. 8, l. 115.

30. RGALI, f. 645, op. 1, d. 368, l. 53.

31. Circular of the Party's Central Committee, *Izvestia*, February 20, 1929, 5. *Kommunističheskaja revoljucija* 3 (1929): 95.

32. *Tribač*, 6/8/1929, Gosfilmofond, f. 2, op. 1, d. 805, l. 15.

33. Boris Sigal, "Novosti èkrana—Moskva," *Kino-nedelja* 6 (1925): 6.

34. Grigori M. Boltjanskij, *Kinospavročnik na 1929* (Moscow: TeaKinoPečat', 1929), 62.

35. *Sovetskoe kino* 2 (1927): 21.

36. GARF, f. 374, op. 28, d. 2305 and 2786.

37. Vladimir M. Behterev, "Kinematografija i nauka," *Vestnik kinematografii* 10 (1915): 39–40.

38. Having graduated from the Moscow medical school in 1922, he was a social hygiene propagandist from the Central Union Syndicate of Moscow, and he taught as the chair of cinema at the University of Moscow (MGU) from 1928. RGALI, f. 984, op. 1, d. 192, ll. 6-6 ob.

39. Julie A. Cassiday, *The Enemy on Trial: Early Soviet Court on Stage and Screen* (DeKalb: Northern Illinois University Press, 2000).

40. *Sud nad vodkoj*, a play written under the supervision of the A. Nevskij Society for Sobriety, 1904.

41. *Sud nad p'janicej*, 1929. This forty-eight-page *agitsud* was released with the printing of ten thousand copies, followed by twenty thousand copies of the second edition the same year, and thirty thousand copies of the third edition in 1930. Boris Sigal also published *Sud nad Stepanom Korolevym* (*posledstvija p'janstva*) (Moscow: VTsIK's Committee for the amelioration of children's life, 1924, 48 pages), *Sud nad p'janicej Ivanom Nikiforovym* (Samara, Soviet Union: Sejatel' pravdy, 1925, 14 pages) and *Sud nad Ivanom Lobačevym po obvineniju v p'janstve i huliganstve* Leningrad: Priboi, 1926). He outlined his socio-medical ideas in two popular books: *Alkogolizm i molodež* (Moscow: Molodaja Gvardija, 1925, 58 pages) reprinted in 1930; and *Pravda na spirtnyh napitkah* (Moscow: Molodaja Gvardija, 1926, 38 pages).

42. Alexandre Sumpf, *Bolcheviks en campagne: Paysans et éducation politique dans la Russie des années 1920* (Paris: Editions du CNRS, 2010), 216–17.

43. Julie A. Cassiday, "Alcohol is Our Enemy! Soviet Temperance Dramas in the 1920s," in *Imitations of Life: Two Centuries of Melodrama in Russia*, ed. Louise McReynolds and Joan Neuberger (Durham, NC: Duke University Press, 2000), 159.

44. Sigal, *Sud nad p'janicej*, 38.

45. Sigal, *Sud nad samogonšikami*, 25.

46. Boris Sigal, "*Razvitie čeloveka*," *Kino-nedelja* 8 (1925): 14.

47. *Algogol, trud i zdorov'e*, Mezhrabpom-Rus, 1927, 581 meters, not preserved.

48. RGALI, f. 2733, op. 1, d. 1131, 1 f. (1924).

49. Dr Noi I. Galkin, *Alkogolizm i bor'ba s nim* (Moscow: Kul'tkino, 1925).

50. *Bolnye nervy*, N. I. Galkin, Sovkino, 1930, 5 parts, 1635 m.

51. "Prosmotr fil'my N.I. Gal'kina *Nevrastenija*," August 1, 1929. RGALI, f. 2494 (ARK), op. 1, d. 279, 11 ff.

52. *Alkogol*, Sovkino, 1927. For this, Genik consulted a specialist of blood vessels, student of I. Pavlov, Sergei I. Chechulin (1894–1937).

53. Valérie Posener et al., *Le studio Mejrabpom ou l'aventure du cinéma privé au pays des Bolcheviks* (Paris: RMN/La Documentation française, 1996).

54. RGALI, f. 2374, op. 1, d. 87, ll 1-1 ob.

55. "Prosmotr fil'my A. N. Tjagaja *Alkogol', trud i zdorov'e*," April 23, 1926. RGALI, f. 2494 (ARK), op. 1, d. 38, ll. 11–12.

56. *Pauk i muha*, film by A. I. Ivanov-Gaj, screenplay by N. I. Galkin and L. M. Suharebskij, Goskino's 3rd studio, Moscow, 1924, 5 parts, 1500 m.

57. Sumpf, *Bolcheviks*, 45.

58. Sukharebskij, *Obzor*, 27.

59. "*Samogon—vrag naroda*," *Novyj zritel'* 11 (1925): 18.

60. *Trevoga*, film by Evgeny Petrov, screenplay by V. Beljaev, Sovkino Nizhny-Novgorod studio, 5 parts, 1927 (not preserved). Premiere on May 11, 1928. Gosfilmofond, f. 2, op. 1, d. 939, l. 2.

61. Suharebskij, *Obzor*, 26.

62. S. Ermolinskij, "Trevoga," *Pravda* 116 (1927): 6.

63. *Čertovo koleso (Morjak s Avrory)*, Kozincev & Trauberg, Leningradkino, 1926, 7 parts, 2100 m.

64. *Kino*, March 16 1926, 4.

65. Russian State Archive of Socio-Political History (RGASPI), f. 17, op. 60 (Agitprop), d. 809, l. 20.

66. RGAKFD Archive holds the complete collection. Films cited: n°1534, 1550, 2029, 2082.

67. RGAKFD, film n°12788. The original film is not clearly identified.

68. RGAKFD, film n° 7937, 239 m.

69. *Sojuzkinožurnal* n°58/167.

70. *Sojuzkinožurnal* n°68/177.

71. Krasnyi Bogatyr factory in Moscow is reported on in *Sojuzkinožurnal* n°22/201.

72. *Sojuzkinožurnal* n°61/240.

73. I. D. Strašun, "Nasuščnye voprosy sanprosvetèkrana," *Sovetskoe kino* 6 (1925): 34.

74. Hrisanf Hersonskij, "*Saba*," *Sovetskij èkran* 26 (1929): 7.

75. Rezoljucija obščego sobrania, 5/19/1929. Gosfilmofond, f. 2, op. 1, d. 805, l. 17.

76. Cassiday, "Alcohol is Our Enemy!," 165–66.

77. This is Cassiday's conclusion.

78. GARF, f. 5515, op. 4, d. 194.

79. RGALI, f. 2494, op. 1, d. 142, l. 2.

80. Iv. Astrov, *Kino*, April 23 1929.

81. RGALI, f. 2494, op. 1, d. 264, ll. 1–5.

82. RGALI, f. 2494, op. 1, d. 142, l. 2.

83. "Za vaše zdorov'e," *Rabočaja gazeta*, April 4 1929.

84. K. Fel'dman, "Budni sovetskoj kul'turfil'my," *Sovetskij èkran* 24 (1929): 11.

85. Alexandre Sumpf, "Le public soviétique et *Octobre* d'Eisenstein: Enquête sur une enquête," *1895: Revue de l'Association Française de Recherche sur l'Histoire du Cinéma* 42 (2004): 5–34.

86. Helen Stone, "The Soviet Government and Moonshine, 1917–1929," *Cahiers du monde russe et soviétique* 3–4 (1986): 359–79.

87. "Hronika," *Omskij zritel'* 2 (1929): 13.

88. Jane Burbank, *Russian Peasants Go to Court: Legal Culture in the Countryside* (Bloomington: Indiana University Press, 2004).

89. I. Alekseev and V. Šišakov, *Kulackie okopy: religija i vodka v derevenskom bytu* (Moscow: Bezbožnik, 1930).

90. Moreover, antireligion films often addressed the question of alcohol. *Opium*, a film by Vitali Zhemchuzhnyi based on a screenplay by Ossip Brik, compared religions to "poisons" such as opium and alcohol consumed at each festivity. *Opium*, Sovkino, Studio for *Kulturfilmy*, 1929, 6 parts, 1649 m. RGAKFD, film n°2762.

91. A. Okun'kov, "Kino v nižegorodskoj derevne (po pis'mam i dnevnikam)," *Kommunističeskoe Prosveščenie* 2–3 (1928): 265.

92. Transchel, *Under the Influence*, 78.

93. *Gon'ka za samogonkoj*, film by A. Room, Goskino, 4 parts, 1200 m. Gosfilmofond, f. 2, op. 1, d. 186.

94. "Zapisi inspektora Gubpolitprosveta Fomina proizvedennye pri rabote v Rostoveckoj volosti Kaširskogo uezda s 28/V po 8/VII," CGAMO, f. 966, op. 4, d. 1741, l. 100–111 ob.

95. There was also a parallel network for screenings in schools and military facilities, which has received little attention from historians as yet.

96. Alexandre Sumpf, "Le 'grand muet' à la campagne. Educateurs politiques, projectionnistes ambulants et paysans dans l'URSS des années 1920," *1895*: *Revue de l'Association Française de Recherche sur l'Histoire du Cinéma* 52 (September 2007): 57–88.

97. G. Esikov, "Potrebitel'naja kooperacija i kinofikacija SSSR," *Kino i kul'tura* 7–8 (1929): 34, 29.

98. Boris Sigal, "Naučnaja fil'ma. Sanitarnoe prosveščenie čerez kino," *Kino-nedelja* 20 (1924): 5.

99. I. D. Strašun, "Iz materialov S"ezda. Sostojanie sanitarnogo prosveščenija v Respublike," *Sanitarnoe prosveščenie* 4–5 (1924): 43.

100. Boris Alpers, "Zavoevanie ekrana," December 1929, in *Dnevnik kinokritika* (Moscow: Iskusstvo, 1971), 64–65.

Chapter Six

"Where There's Life, There's Soap"

Municipal Public Health Films and Municipal Cinema in Britain between the Wars

Elizabeth Lebas†

Introduction

In Britain, the creation of the Ministry of Health in 1919 marked a new stage in the politics of health and the role of local authorities.[1] The great infrastructural improvements in sanitation of the nineteenth century that had accompanied the creation of modern local government had largely been accomplished. Now both national government and local authorities faced a new challenge, that of persuading its electorate—soon to be universally enfranchised—that personal responsibility for one's good health was part of the postwar contract of citizenship.[2] The local state would be there to provide the ways, deliver the means, and if necessary, refine and adapt national policy. In turn, the new citizen would make him or herself receptive to engagement in a renewed and modern everyday life. It was the duty of the citizen to be healthy. Being healthy was, to use a popular expression, to be "up to the minute." There could be no more modern way to communicate this message than through the latest of media, cinema. The Ministry recognized the value of the good health of the population in actuarial terms. Commercial ideas of promotion and propaganda were at the same time gaining ground in the newly created public sphere.[3] From the outset, there was a potential market for health films. Municipalities were themselves such a market. Yet they were forbidden to compete with commercial cinema and eventually had to create their own social space for their films.

In the interwar period, British local authorities had growing responsibilities bound by legislation for the prevention of disease and the promotion of health care. This came at a time when a local parish-based charitable system of health care under the Poor Laws was being abolished.[4] The most significant aspects of public health were embedded in housing, education, and public health acts. Medical Officers of Health (MOHs) employed by the municipality had the power to designate slum areas and demolish them. Clearance was associated with the eradication of disease, tuberculosis in particular. Since the early part of the century, local educational authorities had carried responsibilities for the health and welfare of all children from nursery to the end of secondary school (aged four to fourteen). They also had responsibility for mothers and young children under Maternity and Child Welfare legislation adopted in the 1920s, along with the prevention and treatment of specific diseases such as tuberculosis and syphilis. This essay presents two case studies of the making and sponsorship of health films by the Bermondsey Borough Council and Glasgow Corporation, in the context that I call "municipal cinema."[5] These two municipalities are significant for us in that, although they were not alone in this kind of activity, they made significant numbers of films, and survival of paper records enables us to construct an account of their institutional provenance and political conjunctures, and therefore of the nature of the films and shifts in their messages.

The films produced and screened by Bermondsay and Glasgow were part of two broader corpuses. One was of health films screened by almost all of the 350 councils existing between the wars. These came from a variety of provenances, mainly voluntary health associations such as the British Hygiene Council (formerly the National Council for Combating Venereal Disease) and even the Ivory Castle League, a cover for the Gibbs toothpaste company.[6] Most interwar films were short: between ten and fifteen minutes long and on 16mm stock, making them cheap to make and easy to project. All, at least before about 1933, were mute and most were in black and white.[7]

The other, much smaller corpus, was that of films made or sponsored by local authorities. Out of about 350 councils active between the wars, 70 were involved in the film sponsorship of small numbers—no more than two or three films each. Although only a few survive and have been identified, most "municipal films" were portmanteau films depicting service provision in action, including health, but also police, fire, and sanitation services. These films were effectively visual annual reports demonstrating accountability to a new taxpaying electorate. Municipalities also made films to celebrate special events such as royal visits, charter celebrations and "holidays at home."[8] The purpose of these commemorative films was to create a collective visual history and identity that was entirely modern.[9]

With the exception of the topic of baby care, municipal health films were not strictly instructional: they illustrated such topics as the discomfort of wearing tight clothing (*Health and Clothing*, Bermondsey Borough Council, 1928). At most they reprimanded viewers against the possible dire consequence of not inoculating their children against diphtheria (*The Empty Bed*, Bermondsey and Camberwell Borough Councils, 1937).[10] Mostly they showed where services were, what they looked like, reminded users of their existence, and reassured them as to what to expect from health professionals when they and their children used them. They are essentially films of persuasion of a secular kind.

These municipal films were shown free on council premises (schools and clinics) and territory (streets, public parks and gardens) or on those of local voluntary organizations supported by the council. Compared with other health films of the same period, municipal health films differ in their local democratic emphasis; they suggest that citizenship and entitlement should be universal and introduce their audiences to what was yet to come in everyday life in a new society. They were also a means whereby a local council could distinguish itself from national policy while concurrently sharing an unassailable consensus with the central state about improving the health of the people.[11] The fact that council health films were mostly screened on council territory (and therefore could not compete with commercial cinema) had particular importance in asserting a new political relationship between citizen, local taxpayer, and access to health provision and education. In these contexts, municipal health films reduced the distance between electorate and services, thus contributing to a political process of consensus creation by showing a practice of service consumption. Municipal films illustrated how to be a citizen by showing ordinary people (mostly children)[12] using the solarium or the baths or going on municipal holiday camp. Familiarity was essential. Real places and local people were used, adding veracity to the political experience. By being on film, the audience's own collective everyday lives took on an epic quality. The municipal health film message was simple. With the help of the council, it was possible to take care of oneself and one's family and it really was free.

Nine local authorities other than Bermondsey and Glasgow are known to have produced specifically health films, but these were one-offs, each with a specific health topic. For example, Camberwell, Birmingham, Heston and Isleworth, and Holborn each produced a film in the context of the 1930s drive for immunization against diphtheria.[13] Essex County Council's Education Department also made its own films, setting up after the war its own educational film unit not only to make educational films, but also to teach teachers how to make them. Its audiences consisted exclusively of school children.

There were various ways for councils to get films made; some early examples were commissioned as newsreels from local branches of national film companies. By the 1930s, some town halls also sponsored local amateur film societies and individual filmmakers. The Bermondsey films were made by three medical men from the Public Health Department, enthusiastic amateurs engaged in filmic *bricolage*. As Medical Officer of Health, radiologist, and chief administrator of the department, they had an intimate knowledge of the bodies and circumstances of the municipality's citizens. Glasgow, as Second City of the British Empire and leader in national and Scottish politics, could afford to pay professional filmmakers and use its cinematographic agenda to encourage Scottish and educational cinema. It had from the outset commissioned local branches of national film companies such as Gaumont but was soon promoting the development of a Scottish film industry with companies such as Campbell Harper

Films Ltd and Elder Dalrymple Films.[14] In the 1930s, it became involved in adult film education and supported the newly formed Scottish Educational Film Association (SEFA). By the 1950s, the corporation finally gave in to numerous offers from amateur film groups and allowed the Glasgow SEFA Production Group to make a number of films on its galleries and museums service with the artist Louise Annand.[15]

Glasgow also sponsored directors associated with the documentary film movement; Donald Taylor made *Give the Kids a Break* in 1937, and a series of health and welfare films were sponsored by Glasgow Corporation for the 1938 Empire Exhibition, not only to illustrate an eminent example of public health but also to demonstrate a model of filmmaking; John Grierson, the founder of the documentary film movement, was their producer. The most substantial municipal documentary was Paul Rotha's 1947 film, *A City Speaks*.[16]

From Street to Empire: Bermondsey Borough Council and Glasgow Corporation Health Films

Of the two main examples of municipal filmmaking and sponsorship discussed in this chapter, Bermondsey focused entirely on public health for fifteen years (1922–37). Although it made almost forty films, after 1937 they consisted mostly of street scenes, municipal events, including one of a March for Russia May Day parade (1937) and a 1939 Air Raid Precautions (ARP) demonstration. Glasgow Corporation's filmic interests were in the main related to their education policy: health films, sponsored mostly in the 1930s, were also in the minority of their overall output of about fifty films made between 1922 and 1980.

For Bermondsey and Glasgow, there were other, political motives for filmmaking besides improving the particularly poor health of their constituents.[17] Each of these cities' councils represented a particular strand of Labour Party politics. In both cases, most likely public health was used to "medicalize"—and as such disguise—their left-leaning political strategies. Glasgow had an established reputation in public health[18] that it wanted to maintain in the context of social unrest during and immediately after the First World War. Meanwhile, Bermondsey, a much smaller, poorer, and newer London local authority created in 1900 used filmmaking to promote its distinctive form of Guild Socialism and approach to the management and treatment of tuberculosis.[19]

The differing circumstances within these municipalities, as well as their chosen means to get films made, produced different styles of films: Bermondsey's were intimate and familiar, addressing a consistently impoverished English working class, while Glasgow's were more distant and general, addressing multiclass, multiethnic and multifaith audiences.[20]

Two examples may be used to illustrate the differences. Bermondsey Borough Council's charming film, *Where There's Life, There's Soap* (1933), is addressed to children. It presents washing as an ordinary daily activity practiced by cats and monkeys as well as humans and it shows the municipal wash baths and laundry, but it doesn't instruct the viewer on *how* to wash. The film is about a way of living, a cleaner everyday life made possible by council facilities. As such it opens a new consciousness about the body and the self and, indirectly, the politics that make it possible. By contrast, Glasgow Corporation's Necessitous Children's Holiday Camp (NCHC) films might not superficially appear to be concerned with the child's body or child health at all. This is despite being motivated by municipal duties under the 1907 Education (Administrative Provisions) Act and the 1921 Education Act to ensure the health of children at school, which included the feeding of malnourished children. The films sponsored between the late 1920s and late 1930s purport to persuade parents to send their children to camp during school holidays. They also served as a collective souvenir for those who had gone to camp the previous summer and also as fund-raisers for the scheme, as it did not have full public funding. But the films also show how plentiful food, rest, and exercise are beneficial for children and how camp gives their parents a breathing space. They inform the viewer how and where to apply to get a place at camp. At camp the children are promised another life—full of sunshine and fun. Nowhere is mentioned the fact that a child had to be "defective" to get a camp place.[21] According to the corporation, every child was entitled to a holiday and presumably for some this meant a municipal holiday. It was the corporation's duty to instill not only the ideal of universal entitlement, but also its practice. Universal entitlement implied services free to the individual consumer, but people still had to be persuaded to use them.

Both of our selected municipalities looked outward for recognition and represented their services as models, though Glasgow, much richer, sought a different reputation, more universal, administrative and technical. Both also shared some fundamental principles buried deep in a Protestant and dissenting culture: education was more important than instruction. An educated person was a responsible person. Knowledge was the key to self-empowerment. Within these two contexts, the meaning, uses, and very contents of health films were quite different, although they shared broadly similar topics guided by legislation.

When Bermondsey Borough Council undertook its antitubercular and general public health publicity campaign in 1924, it presented itself as a pioneer: "Up to the present the work of education and propaganda has been mostly in the hands of voluntary societies, and although a few authorities have made sporadic attempts to spread a knowledge of certain diseases . . . no systematic and sustained attempt at general health propaganda has yet been taken by any Sanitary Authority."[22] This was no exaggeration. Minutes from the Ministry of Health General Policy of the Department on Propaganda for 1920 confirm that, except for propaganda societies already receiving grants, local authorities were to be in charge of health propaganda. It was clear, though, that there was little consistency of interest in propaganda between what the Department called "progressive" and "backward" authorities. As for the ministry, it had five somewhat vague and contradictory functions in health education: decentralization and the guidance of local effort on the one hand, the direction of certain campaigns such as those against influenza on the other; the two other functions being to educate and produce leaflets. Moreover, the new department was not to use the terms *publicity* or *propaganda.*[23]

Two years later ministerial focus was still lacking.[24] So, in 1924 after the first national Labour government came to power and the Independent Labour Party gained a strong victory in the borough elections, the Bermondsey Borough Council found the motivation to launch a comprehensive public health campaign headed by its powerful Public Health Department. It flew under the motto of Prevention is Better Than Cure,[25] to which was added the Beautification Department's own motto, Fresh Air and Fun.[26] The campaign lasted until the Second World War. As part of this, between the wars Bermondsey made some twenty-one health films. There were, for example, two films about exercise (including one of members of the Arsenal football (soccer) team training on their then home grounds in South London); one on public gardens; and another on the structure of the eye, tuberculin-tested milk, cleanliness, the management of tuberculosis, the unsanitary conditions of hop picking in Kent, and most famously its portmanteau film about the borough's services, *Some Activities of Bermondsey Borough Council* (1931).[27] Bermondsey's public health campaign comprised not only filmmaking, which had preceded it with a first film, *School in the Sun* (1922 or 1923) and film lectures on syphilis. It also included the production of lantern slides, leaflets, bookmarks, and electric signs to promote its facilities. These included twelve maternity and child health clinics; a comprehensive health clinic (one of twelve built in Britain in the late 1930s); a maternity hospital; a rest home for mothers in Kent; a tuberculosis dispensary; a purpose-built solarium; a communal bakery and laundry; a tree-planting project; the acquisition and laying out of children's playgrounds; and the building of baths, swimming pools, and public conveniences for children and adults and a new morgue.

Bermondsey's amateur yet serious approach to cinematography contrasted with Glasgow's. The London council made films because they could do what no other medium could do—to show a process. As a medium of scientific demonstration, they could explain how the body worked and the causes of illness in an entertaining way. Self-sufficiency in filmmaking was all-important: vans were converted to screen films; street lamps were fitted with special sockets; and film stock was obtained from Kodak, which also supplied film for radiography. All actors were local and played themselves. Finally, the council's Direct Labour department built an outdoor film set.

As more generally in health education cinema, Bermondsey's municipal films were almost always accompanied by a live lecture. Audience response was part of the lecture. Today's viewers obviously cannot recapture the aural elements of these lectures with silent films—explanation, repetition, argument, interjection, and heckling. In Bermondsey audience numbers for films with lectures eventually tailed off, but the films were screened long after they were needed to convey a health message. If they were in the open air, projected from the back of specially fitted cinema vans, audiences ranged from 250 to 1,000, with children singing council health ditties at the top of their voices.[28] On these occasions, while one council officer gave a filmed lecture, another patrolled the crowd. In 1932 a third of the borough's population saw the films: over thirty thousand people. These performances did much to reimage its environment, including supporting the tree-planting campaign and the building of a garden suburb, both of which survive today.[29] By showing real examples of what was already happening in the borough, they projected a future in the making, visible and plausible.

Glasgow's approach to health-related topics was much more administrative and departmental than Bermondsey's. Glasgow was a large cosmopolitan city with enduring class and religious divides compensated for by a shared belief in the value of education. The costs of sponsoring films were negligible compared to the corporation's overall budget and could be subsumed under educational expenses. By the 1930s, officers and elected members connected to the Education Department had become involved in national debates on film education, sometimes through the Scottish Film Council. They also promoted the establishment of a Scottish film industry by hiring exclusively Scottish film production companies and lobbied for the establishment of what became the Scottish Film Council. They were also involved in setting up the Central Scottish Film Library with funds from the Carnegie Foundation. The library was to supply schools with suitable films to which the corporation may have contributed their own.[30] The aim was to establish a distinctively Scottish, even national, educational film culture. Eventually Sir Charles Cleland, chairman of the Necessitous Children Holiday Camp Fund, became in 1936 the chairman of the British Film Institute and that year its journal, *Sight and Sound*, published an article referring to the corporation's film sponsorship.[31]

By contrast with Bermondsey, Glaswegian audiences and the sites of film shows seem to have been more formal and sedate, although there are few records of audience figures, screenings, or distribution. Most commissions and screenings were for schools' use. Only the films sponsored in 1938 and shown at the Empire Exhibition the same year were recorded in the Council Minutes.[32] Occasionally the Town Hall was used as a venue and, instead of cinema vans, there was an assiduous drive to have film projectors in every school.

Here four films from my selected two municipalities are used to demonstrate their similarities and differences. Two relate the experience of hospitalization: Bermondsey's *Consumption* (1932) and Glasgow's *Stobhill Hospital: The Story of a Modern Hospital* (1938). The other two films demonstrate what was considered to be the best practice in the care of newborn babies.

Consumption and *Stobhill Hospital*

Consumption was the only explicitly antituberculosis film made by Bermondsey, and at over forty-five minutes, it was very long by their standards. Like their other films, it was made by the medical officer of health, the borough radiographer, and the chief administrative officer of the Public Health Department. *Consumption* is about more than the mere diagnosis and management of tuberculosis; it is about a young man's personal quest from tubercular to healthy person, from nineteenth-century man to modern citizen. The opening explains what consumption is (a bacterium), its symptoms (fatigue and coughing blood), and its causes—on the one hand, "self-neglect" and "bad habits" (images of a workingman coughing on his mates and of another man spitting) and, on the other, bad housing, lack of proper food, and "unsuitable work." Thus, tuberculosis is the negative outcome of interaction between unfortunate aspects of the individual's habits, his work, and his living environment. (Unusually, as in the next film introduced here, this motion picture appears to be aimed mostly at men; most health films assumed a female audience.)

The quest begins in the consulting room of a general practitioner (probably, from his appearance, Dr. Alfred Salter, one of the instigators of the propaganda campaign).[33] The viewer (and potential patient) is prepared for uncertainty: from the consulting room he *may* be referred to the Tuberculosis Dispensary. If the case is suitable for treatment, the patient *may* then be sent to a sanatorium where "a small charge will be made relative to the financial circumstances of the family."[34] The next two scenes are of another patient getting off the train in the countryside and finding her way to the King Edward Sanatorium onto its beautiful grounds. At first these appear to be empty, like a noble landscape, but as she approaches the purpose-built structure, figures of men relaxing come into view. The King Edward Hospital featured in *Consumption* was a county hospital to which Bermondsey contributed some of the costs of sending patients. This was not necessarily a deception, as it demonstrated the borough's involvement with mighty and forward-looking authorities such as the London County Council. Similarly, in some Bermondsey films, social housing provided by the London County Council was presented as Bermondsey's achievement.[35]

The therapeutic work regime receives the most footage; it functions both as a method for rehabilitation and as a program for reskilling patients who are mostly laborers. The viewer is told that the patients like work because it means they are improving, that work is graded, and that the aim is to be able to do the heaviest work before returning home. There are many shots of men being retrained as furniture makers and carpenters.[36] We are assured that they are paid trade union rates and work no more than six hours a day. (This is not a workhouse.) Women can also be given suitable work, although it seems to consist entirely of sewing.

The film explains that when patients are considered fit to leave the hospital and start work, they can be accommodated in hostels. The camera lingers over women chatting in a garden, pretty bedrooms, and a dining room decorated with vases of flowers. The penultimate title card informs us that married men are encouraged to "colonize," that is, bring their wives and children to live with them on the estate's large and detached cottages. Our hero has meanwhile returned home, and we see him preparing to go to bed in his outdoor shelter.[37] His wife looks on; she is not joining him.[38] The final title card is an exhortation: "It may therefore be said with confidence that Consumption is preventable.

Consumption is curable." The last shot informs the viewer where to apply for further information from the medical officer of health.

The second film on hospitalization discussed here, *Stobhill Hospital: The Story of a Modern Hospital*, was not explicitly sponsored within the context of a municipal health campaign, although it may have been influenced by the first national health campaign, Use Your Services, in 1938. The film was part of a series of films made around 1938 that expressed the aspirations of the Glasgow Corporation to become part of a larger and more modern cultural movement. Up to this time, in addition to the Necessitous Children's Holiday Camp films (see above), the corporation had sponsored a few films on such topics as its housing program, its parks department, and its educational department's special services. It marks a midpoint between Bermondsey's essentially homemade "local topical" approach and the modern public information film.[39] The idea of making the film and the series may initially have been a response to a somewhat naive application by the Glasgow School of Art to the Clinical Sub-Committee of the Public Health Department in April 1936 to make a film to "illustrate the work of a school clinic and a children's hospital."[40] The corporation, presumably besides having reservations about students filming in hospital wards, was clearly not going to be outdone. The idea was found good enough for the medical officer of health to propose producing eight hundred feet of film the following October on the Public Health Department's Services that could be shown on a portable projector acquired for the purpose.[41] By the following year, the project was transformed into commissioning seven films, including *Stobhill Hospital*, from the Edinburgh-based Campbell Harper Film Co. Ltd.[42] The films were officially premiered in the Magistrates' Room in the autumn of 1938 to members of the Health Committee, although since May they had been screened at the 1938 Empire Exhibition being held in Glasgow.[43] Municipal films had gone imperial, in the sense that they were featuring at the Empire Exhibition and so were part of a broader effort to celebrate and promote imperialism and imperial identity among visitors to the exhibition.[44] It is unknown how this film project was financed, but it certainly represents a change in audience and inevitably of style and approach.[45] Closer to home, copies of these films were already being requested by national charities.[46] The use and delivery of the services the health-related films (*Stobhill Hospital*, *Bathing Baby*, *Child Welfare*, and *Country Homes*) depicted were projected as universal and immutable models of citizenship and administrative good practice. They were not part of a local health campaign but anticipated postwar national centralization and consequent delocalization. The series begun in 1938 made up the last films sponsored by the corporation before the war and altogether were the last health-related films.

Stobhill Hospital: The Story of a Modern Hospital is not about the treatment of an infectious disease but about acute care and so narrates a different hospital experience from the Bermondsey example. But that is not its only difference from *Consumption*. The opening title cards assert that the subject is a corporation hospital with two thousand beds and that a hospital is more than wards. The camera pans the Scottish Baronial exterior of the main building and its beautiful setting.[47] There follows a systematic and somewhat labored description of the complex organization and spaces of the hospital: the store, the dispensary, the telephone room, the records office, and the nursing school. It could be a description of the running of one of the many huge passenger ships built on the Clyde in the period. Perhaps typically for an engineering town, the camera often lingers on machines and technical processes.[48] Some way into the film we are reminded what the hospital is about—*treatment.* Beginning with the admission process, shots of the gradual recovery of a very unwell male patient are threaded within the film to its end. As in *Consumption,* almost as an afterthought, attention is at last given to the needs of women. The viewer is shown the maternity ward and the home for babies and young children. But soon the film returns to the more specialist activities of the hospital: the mobile x-ray unit, the Laboratory, and the Bacteriological Department. Thirty-seven minutes later, as our patient, now almost fully recovered, joins his friends on a walk, the film comes to a close. The final title card announces, "It is the result of such diligent labour that makes it possible for a patient to win back gradually his former good health and resume his place as a happy and useful citizen." Despite their differences (*Consumption* is actually better lit and scripted than the professionally made *Stobhill Hospital*), the similarities of the messages in both films are striking; with the help of modern, freely accessible public services, illness can be an invitation to useful citizenship and a more productive life.

Two maternity and child welfare legislation films may briefly illustrate how the nature of the audience, the social identity of the filmmakers, the standing of municipalities and their relations to institutions outside influenced the style and contents of municipal films. Both municipalities were responding to maternity and child welfare legislation promulgated in 1924.

Bermondsey's *Maternity and Child Health* (1927)[49] and Campbell Harper's *Bathing the Baby* (1938) are instructional films that feature the technique of bathing and dressing a newborn. In terms of professionalism in the handling of a young baby, *Maternity and Child Health* expresses the more relaxed approach.[50] Meanwhile, *Bathing the Baby* relies on a notion of clinical professionalism; the baby is handled by a health professional in a gentle, confident, and respectful way.[51] In *Bathing the Baby,* a uniformed nurse performs the ritual. In both films the babies, when "done," are put back into their cots and briefly cuddled. Baby care films were shown in maternity and child health clinics to mothers-to-be who were to receive further guidance from their health visitor once the baby was born.[52] *Maternity and Child Health* is set in the dark, old-fashioned kitchen of a working-class mother's home.[53] The mother calmly bathes and dresses her baby as her toddler, leaning against her knee, looks on. The baby having been washed and dressed as the film closes, is put to the breast. It is the contrast between the poverty and ordinariness of the setting (in this film water is heated on a coal range) and the modernity of the practice of daily washing a baby (although the contrast is not explicitly drawn; there is no caption board hammering its home) is typical of all of Bermondsey films. The poor did not look modern but could do modern things. *Bathing the Baby* by contrast is brightly lit and set in a state-of-the art nursery, perhaps in a hospital or clinic, but not inconceivably in a modern, middle-class home. A uniformed nurse, using an astonishing array of baby impedimenta neatly set out, methodically attends to a very young child. The mother is absent—as a mother might be in a middle-class home able to afford a nurse.[54] The final title card concludes, "All is made clean and tidy for the next time." One wonders who cleaned up. This film projects a certain aspirational tone. There is a correct way of washing and dressing a baby and it is a middle-class way; to adopt this way is modern and being modern is being—or at least becoming—middle class. In short, the two ways of washing a baby express more than two methods of child care. They make mother and baby pioneers of modern everyday life as expressed in the daily bath and hint at new relationships between social class and modernity.

Conclusion: Health Films in Municipal Context

The municipal health films presented here are just a fraction of the 350 or so other health films produced between the wars. Timothy Boon points to the narrower medical interest of municipal health films whereas here I have introduced their wider agenda: promoting the identity of the municipality and through the services it advertised, of creating a space of consensus resting on equal and universal entitlement.[55] Writers such as David Armstrong have suggested that successive regimes of public health created new spaces of individual identity lying beyond sovereign power.[56] Certainly, it is safe to say, when comparing Bermondsey with Glasgow health films, that models of personal and social identity were being experimented with. As I have hinted, there was not always congruence between appearances and practices, nor between modernity and class—although by the end of the war modernity seems to have inhabited a new idealized lower middle class.[57]

From the outset, a positive connection was made between cinema and the promotion of personal responsibility for health, with municipalities as a major market and venue for health films.[58] Minutes from the Ministry of Health's Department on Propaganda for 1920 mention that the National Council for Combating Venereal Diseases (NCCVD) was "using the cinema." Meanwhile, Bermondsey Council Minutes reveal that a film on venereal disease had been shown at a maternity clinic, and Glasgow Corporation Minutes note the difficulty of finding a suitable venue for *The End of the Road*, an NCCVD film.[59]

Writing in the *Manchester Guardian* in January 1923, Christopher Addison, the former minister of health, made some prescient albeit implicit connections between a self-directed approach to health reforms ("Health reforms can only be made by people themselves becoming reformers"), cinema ("Kinema, although primarily a means of amusement, may also be used as a means of instruction if it is done with tact and good sense"), and the need for a central body for health education.[60] By September of that year, the Society of Medical Officers of Health had sent a memorandum (in answer to a letter from the

Ministry of Health), which proposed the formation of a central authority among whose functions would be "to facilitate the provision of travelling cinemas and exhibitions and the importation of films for the use of local authorities: also to help stocking films."[61] In 1927 such an authority was formed, the Central Council for Health Education (CCHE), supported by voluntary membership from local authorities, although Bermondsey did not belong.[62] The CCHE's Annual Report for 1935–36 boasted that they had arranged for several hundred programs of health film showings in connection with local authority health weeks and that ninety-five thousand adults and children had seen these films. By 1940–41 the council had begun film production on its own account with the aim of improving the general repertoire of health films and to advise the Ministry of Health on its film production. In 1941 the CCHE's film work was transferred to the Ministry of Information.[63]

Whether health films were shown depended on available services and these on the politics of the council in question and the availability of suitable films. Films made or sponsored by a municipality, featuring local scenes and people, could be expected to have a particular local appeal compared to nationally distributed films with such unappealing titles as *The Rat Menace* (1925), made by the Ministry of Agriculture and Fisheries under the 1919 Rat and Mice (Extermination) Act, or *Head Lice*, made in 1943 by the Central Council for Health Education. But when local authorities showed health films, it was within a culture steeped in commercial cinema (more than twenty million people attended cinemas a week) over which they had little aesthetic or political influence despite the fact that they had powerful statutory duties concerning conditions of showing and censorship—which they still do. On the other hand, they could not compete with *Gone with the Wind* appearing on a Saturday night at the local Odeon.

Speaking in 1937 to the Twenty-Third Annual Conference of the National Association for the Prevention of Tuberculosis (NAPT), Paul Scott Rankine, secretary of the CCHE, commented on class attitudes toward the use of public health services: "Among certain classes one finds the impression that the public health services are only for the very poor, that they are not quite respectable, that a free service provided by a municipality must necessarily be less efficient or less effective than paid services, or at any rate that personal consideration for the needs of the individual will be lacking. On the other hand there is a feeling amongst others that some services cannot possibly be free, that some payment will eventually be asked for, however small, which will be embarrassing to be unable to make."[64]

Rankine was speaking prior to the launch in the following year (1938) of the joint national Use Your Health Services campaign by the Ministry of Health and the Board of Education. He announced that a joint production between the CCHE and the Ministry of Education (which now had a Public Relations Department), *Health of the People*, would be shown in the summer at one thousand cinemas to audiences of between ten and fifteen million people. This first national public health campaign heralded the beginnings of a centralized approach that prefigured the creation of the NHS a decade later in 1948. It took almost thirty years and wartime mobilization for people to accept free health care. Municipal health films had played their part in this political education and though they were shown long after the war, they had become unnecessary.

Rankine conceded that generally the owners of big cinema circuits were wary of including health publicity films in their programs as people stayed away because of them. On the other hand, cinema owners were happy to be associated with their local authorities by putting up health posters and distributing leaflets. By then films were accepted as an essential part of any public health meeting, their quality having improved.[65]

Rankine had identified an appropriate place for health films: the municipality. What the municipality did in providing such a place was not only to exercise its duties under late nineteenth-century legislation to improve the mental as well as the physical conditions of the people, but to place health outside the commercial realm. When people watched health films they did so as citizens, not as consumers. Health was a right, not a commodity. It is in this light that we may consider the role of the local state between the wars in promoting universal entitlement to health through cinema.

Notes

Elizabeth Lebas, principal author of this piece, died in 2014. At the time of the "Communicating Good Health" conference, she had been in clear remission between two episodes of the cancer, which finally took her life. I undertook to edit the notes she submitted as a final act of friendship (she had been a dear friend for two decades). I have sought to edit her submission into something like the contribution she would have wanted to make to the volume. This has mainly involved grouping her similar material together and giving it a narrative. It has, unfortunately, been necessary to lose a small number of examples where references were missing.—Tim Boon, December 2014. For an obituary of Elizabeth Lebas, see Anna Goldie, "Elizabeth Lebas Obituary," *The Guardian*, July 1, 2014.

The title of this essay is borrowed from one of the best-known films made by Bermondsey Borough Council. Originally titled *Where There's Life, There's 'Ope*, its final version appeared in 1933. But already by 1929 it was circulating nationwide in voluntary and municipal venues under the aegis of the Central Council for Health Education; see Central Council for Health Education, *Panel of Lecturers, Films, etc.*, October 1929.

1. This essay is based on Elizabeth Lebas, *Forgotten Futures: Municipal Cinema in Britain* (London: Black Dog, 2011) and subsequent research. A number of films made by Bermondsey Borough Council are online. See for example "The Empty Bed (1937) Pt. 1 of 2," YouTube video, posted by Wellcome Library, February 21, 2012, http://www.youtube.com/watch?v=c5NMRRfdKvQ. "The Empty Bed" is also available on the Wellcome Library's website at http://catalogue.wellcome.ac.uk/record=b1803918~S3 (accessed September 6, 2017). The Scottish Screen Archives holds all the films sponsored by Glasgow Corporation, a sizeable number of which

are online at Scotland on Screen, http://www.scotlandonscreen.org.uk (accessed September 6, 2017).

2. On health citizenship, see Harry Oosterhuis and Frank Huisman, "The Politics of Health and Citizenship: Historical and Contemporary Perspectives," in *Health and Citizenship: Political Cultures of Health in Modern Europe*, ed. Frank Huisman and Harry Oosterhuis (London: Pickering & Chatto, 2013), 1–40.

3. Ministry of Health Minute Sheet, August 12, 1920, MH55/78, National Archives, Kew, London.

4. For a timely account of the legislation underpinning municipal provisions just on the eve of the creation of the NHS, see Norman Wilson, *Municipal Health Services* (London: George Allen and Unwin, 1946), 178. Wilson was lecturer in Public Administration at the University of Liverpool.

5. The notion of a municipal cinema as a social cinema really gained ground only after the Second World War. Paul Rotha, *Preface to the 1949 Edition of The Film Till Now* (London: Vision, 1949), 23. Here I am referring to a wider and preexisting context in which local authorities not only made their own films of an informative and reforming nature and showed them to their constituents free of charge, but also regulated the showing of commercial films, including premises, conditions of work, and censorship.

6. Tim Boon's thesis contains a table listing all the 350 films he had identified in 1999. Tim Boon, "Films and the Contestation of Public Health in Interwar Britain" (PhD diss., University of London, 1999). The Ivory Castle League was founded by D&W Gibbs Ltd., toothpaste makers. They produced one film in the mid-1920s entitled *Ivory Castles*, which was mistakenly on Bermondsey Borough Council's list of council-produced films.

7. Bermondsey Borough Council made a phonographic recording for *Some Activities of Bermondsey Borough Council*, 1931, and there is some color footage of public flowerbeds made in the late 1930s.

8. Holidays at Home were entertainments put on by councils during wartime to encourage people to stay at home rather than use train and bus transport, leaving these free for the movements of troops. An example is *Holidays at Home*, Rochdale County Borough, 1942. Some films are in color, the stock believed to have been given to councils by American servicemen.

9. Later, local authorities also made films to be shown outside their boundaries, usually in commercial cinemas and possibly to companies looking to relocate. For example, there is *Turn of the Tide: Liverpool's Emergence as an Industrial Power*, Corporation of Liverpool, 1966. These films, often travelogues, promoted local industry, geographical location, and the district's infrastructural advantages. They may have been subsidized by central government regional policies but this is not clear from surviving archives.

10. See "The Empty Bed (1937) Pt. 1 of 2," YouTube video, posted by Wellcome Library, February 21, 2012, http://www.youtube.com/watch?v=c5NMRRfdKvQ.

11. A detailed account of the local politics of public health before the Second World War has still to be written.

12. Elizabeth Lebas, "The Little Citizen is not at Home: Children in Municipal Cinema," in *The Child in Cinema: Tears, Fears and Fairy Tales*, ed. Karen Lury (London: I. B. Tauris, 2010).

13. Bermondsey produced its own diphtheria immunization film, *Germs* (1931), but it has been lost.

14. Early films were commissioned from local branches of national film companies; for example, a film sponsored in 1922 by Glasgow Corporation titled *Parks Department* was produced by Gaumont. Vanessa Toulmin, Simon Popple, and Patrick Russell, eds., *The Lost World of Mitchell and Kenyon, Edwardian Britain on Film* (London: British Film Institute, 2004). A more recent book by Ian Craven begins to explore relationships between amateur cinema and municipal film sponsorship; see Ian Craven, *Movies on Home Ground: Explorations in Amateur Cinema* (Newcastle upon Tyne: Cambridge Scholars Publishing, 2009).

15. Lebas, *Forgotten Futures*, 140.

16. See Ian Johnson, "A City Speaks: The Story of Manchester's Municipal," *Manchester Sounds* 6 (2005): 109–31. Charlotte Wildman, "A City Speaks: The Projection of Civic Identity in Manchester," *Twentieth Century British History* 23, no. 1 (January 3, 2012): 80–99.

17. In 1924 Bermondsey had the third highest rate of tuberculosis in Britain; the health of Glasgow's citizens remains the poorest in Britain to this day.

18. See, for example, Dr. A. K. Chalmers, *The Health of Glasgow, 1818–1925* (Glasgow: City Corporation, 1930), 462 pages with diagrams. The text is reviewed in *Health and Empire: Journal of the British Social Hygiene Council* 5, no. 1 (1930). See also in Lebas, *Forgotten Futures*, the film commissioned by Glasgow Corporation titled *Health of a City* (1965) to celebrate the centenary of its Public Health Department.

19. Lebas, *Forgotten Futures*. See also Boon, *Film and the Contestation*, 176–204.

20. The great cultural divide in Glasgow was and remains the divide between Protestants and Catholics. From the late seventeenth century onward, it was home to influxes of immigrants from Ireland and the Scottish Highlands, and in the late nineteenth century to incomers from Italy and Eastern Europe.

21. *Glasgow Corporation Minutes*, Committee on Necessitous Children, February 17, 1921, 933. The term did not have a derogatory meaning but was used to mean "lack." That year the Education Department provided 39,496 breakfasts, 116,130 dinners and 32,766 teas a year in addition to 47,721 partly subsidized dinners.

22. Bermondsey Borough Council, Medical Officer of Health Report, 1924, 38. Also cited in Boon, *Film and the Contestation*, 194.

23. Ministry of Health General Policy of the Department on Propaganda, Minute Sheet, August 12, 1920, MH/55/27.

24. "The Weakness of Health Propaganda." Item 10, Public Record Office, MH/55/27 File. Twenty-page report signed by Sir George Knight and dated August 22, 1922.

25. H. Bush and D. Conan, *Better Than Cure: A Handbook on Public Health Propaganda* (London: Douglas, 1927).

26. See Elizabeth Lebas, "The Making of a Socialist Arcadia: Arboriculture and Horticulture in the London Borough of Bermondsey after the Great War," *Journal of Garden History* 27, no. 2 (1999): 219–37.

27. Hop picking in Kent was a mainly London East End working-class practice in which women and children went to Kent in late August or early September to pick hops on farms. There they set up camps and were joined at the weekend by the men. Hop picking was the rural carnavalesque side of Bermonsey's urban misery.

The council made a film in 1930 titled *'Oppin* that warned of the charms and dangers of "hopping."

28. Meeting with members of the Bermondsey Pensioners Action Group, ca. spring 1998. Incidental notes.

29. *Twelve Years of Labour Rule on the Bermondsey Borough Council, 1922–1934* (Labour Institute, 1934). The borough actually built a garden suburb in 1924, but a stop was put to it by the then-Labour government as this caused the displacement of people to neighboring boroughs, leading to complaints.

30. Between 1934 and 1938, the corporation sponsored twenty-five films for schools known as the Carrick Film Series.

31. Thomas Baird, "The Film and Civic Education," *Sight and Sound* 5, no. 17 (Spring 1936): 17–19. Education in civics became a central topic of Glasgow postwar films. The corporation's Education Department sponsored twelve films between 1947 and 1948 under the Civic Series films. Baird was a protégé of John Grierson, who lobbied to have the corporation's films shown at the Empire Exhibition.

32. Four sponsored films, all made in 1938, were shown at the Scottish Pavilion: *Bathing Baby, Stobhill Hospital, Child Welfare,* and *Country Homes.* Lebas, *Forgotten Futures,* chap. 4.

33. Salter had a very large general medical practice in the borough, had been an alderman, was a member of Parliament for Southwark (which included Bermondsey) until the outbreak of war, and was the founder of the Socialist Parliamentary Health Committee. See Fenner Brockway, *Bermondsey Story* (London: George Allen and Unwin, 1949).

34. Film title card.

35. This may also have been the case for other inner London boroughs such as Hackney.

36. This and many other films show practices that can horrify us today, such as tubercular patients smoking. In this furniture-making scene, a patient is spraying paint—without a mask.

37. Here the council is hinting that after discharge it continues in the after care of former tubercular patients. It was not until 1936 that local authorities had a statutory duty to do so. Dr. Salter was an advocate of these shelters; he slept in one in his own back garden.

38. Once home, the hero's self-restraint and self-discipline had to be supported by others, particularly his wife.

39. See Toulmin, Popple and Russell, *Lost World of Mitchell and Kenyon.* The local topical had an element of immediacy; people saw their selves as they were very soon after they were filmed in their own surroundings. They showed the veracity of the life lived by their audiences, while the "pubic information" film had an element of authority that came from without.

40. Glasgow Corporation Minutes, April 8, 1936, Public Health Department Clinical Sub-Committee, Items 3 and 4, 1357.

41. There is no information concerning where this film was to be shown. The Council Chamber and many schools had projectors.

42. A more detailed account of the sponsorship of these films is available in Lebas, *Forgotten Futures.*

43. Two later films, *Vital Statistics* and *Country Homes,* were completed only in 1940.

44. For background on imperial exhibitions, see John Macdonald MacKenzie, *Propaganda and Empire: the Manipulation of British Public Opinion, 1880–1960* (Manchester, UK: Manchester University Press, 1984), 96–120. Paul Greenhalgh, *Ephemeral Vistas: A History of the Expositions Universelles, Great Exhibitions and World's Fairs, 1851–1939* (Manchester, UK: Manchester University Press, 1988). Peter H. Hoffenberg, *An Empire on Display: English, Indian, and Australian Exhibitions from the Crystal Palace to the Great War* (Berkeley: University of California Press, 2001). Alexander C. T. Geppert, *Fleeting Cities: Imperial Expositions in Fin-de-Siècle Europe* (Basingstoke, UK: Palgrave Macmillan, 2010).

45. For a fuller account, see Lebas, *Forgotten Futures*, 136–37. It is not entirely clear just how many films were made.

46. The National Council of Maternity and Child Welfare and the Invalid Children's Aid Association, respectively.

47. It seems that the more modern the council practices, the more traditional the architecture. Bermondsey's Town Hall was in classical style, although both boroughs tended toward Arts and Crafts style for their smaller buildings. In Britain modernism was about practices, not appearances.

48. The film, *Vital Statistics*, sponsored by the corporation that same year, has an almost identical structure, describing the activities of various departments and the values of literacy and numeracy in getting a white-collar job with the council.

49. The film was first made by Dr. King Brown in 1925 and then reedited in 1927. King Brown had been the Medical Officer of Health for Bermondsey and had first proposed making films. He is the filmmaker, with Dr. Guy Bousfield, director of the Camberwell Research Laboratory, of *The Empty Bed* (1938) on immunization against diphtheria.

50. By contrast, footage found in the London Borough of Hackney Archive titled *Day Nursery* (1935), made by Kodak featuring a nurse furiously engaging in the mechanics of undressing, bathing, and dressing a baby, expresses the opposite. No eye contact is exchanged between nurse and bewildered child.

51. This is not unlike a film directed by Miss M. H. Keating in 1935 for the Shoreditch Model Welfare Centre (still extant) titled *Washing and Dressing*.

52. For a comprehensive account of the 150-year-old history of Health Visiting in Britain, see Cheryll Adams, "The History of Health Visiting," *Nursing in Practice*, November 27, 2012, http://www.nursinginpractice.com/article/history-health-visiting.

53. This is a rare film set in a real working-class interior. Interior shots in municipal films were either of middle-class homes or of hospitals, schools, and clinics. Real working-class homes were simply too small and dark to be used for filming.

54. This same great grandmother as the one already mentioned assured me that in "proper households" it was the done thing to hire a nurse during the first two weeks of a mother's convalescence after the birth. Well-off mothers had a nurse from the outset until the child was sent to school around age six.

55. Boon, *Film and the Contestation*, 6, 176.

56. David Armstrong, "Public Health Spaces and the Fabrication of Identity," *Sociology* 27 (1993): 410.

57. See discussion of the Civic Series films sponsored by Glasgow Corporation after the War. Lebas, *Forgotten Futures*, 144–45.

58. See T. Crew, *Health Compendium and Health Publicity* (Leicester, UK: Reader Print Co., 1926), and *Health First, Propaganda (Ways and Means) with Illustrations* (Leicester, UK: Lemuel Bell, 1935). In these two texts, Crew—who was clerk to the Leicester Insurance Health Committee and organizing secretary to the Central Council for Health Education, lists a huge number of health publicity films available for a variety of venues. That local authorities were the preferred venue at which films were shown is made quite explicit by the fact that *Health First* is prefaced by Professor Bostock, chair of the Health Week Committee of the Royal Sanitary Institution. Health Weeks, as "self-help to health," were held during the first week of October and were aimed at the municipal public health departments. Health Weeks lasted until the advent of the Second World War.

59. Ministry of Health General Policy of the Department of Propaganda, Minute Sheet, August 12, 1920, MH/55/27, National Archives, Kew Gardens, London, Item 1. See also Lebas, *Forgotten Futures*, chap. 3. On *The End of the Road*, see also Miriam Posner in this volume.

60. Article by the Right Hon. Christopher Addison, MD, formerly of the Ministry of Health, in the *Manchester Guardian*, January 3, 1923, Public Record Office File MH/55/27 file, item 12.

61. Central Office for Health Education, 1923 MH82/19, National Archives, Kew Gardens, London.

62. For detail, see Boon, *Film and the Contestation*, 109–29. There was also a separate body for Scotland but it is not known whether Glasgow Corporation belonged to it.

63. Central Office for Health Education, MH55/28, Annual Reports for 1935–36, 1940–41, and 1946–47, National Archives.

64. NAPT Transactions of the Twenty-Third Annual Conference July 1–3, Bristol, 1937, 27.

65. Transcription of a speech made by Paul Scott Rankine on the eve of the launch of the national health campaign "Use Your Health Services" at the Twenty-Third Annual Conference of the NAPT, Bristol, July 1, 1937, 24–34.

Part Three

International Reorganization

Chapter Seven

Cinema and Public Health Care in Early Postwar Germany, 1945–49

Ursula von Keitz

Following German capitulation on May 8, 1945, and the country's liberation from National Socialism, the occupation policies of the four victorious Allied powers—the United States, Great Britain, France, and the Soviet Union—paid particular attention to the goal of "reeducating" German society. This aim was to be achieved through an education and propaganda program based on two central ideas: first, the German population must discover the truth about National Socialist crimes; second, they must be persuaded of the advantages of democracy and its institutions. Health education films were a significant category in this undertaking.

This essay explores some of the popular medical short films of the period from 1945 to 1949 ("some" since not every film has survived or is accessible in German archives) as well as one feature film concerning venereal diseases and their therapies, which was shown in all zones and sectors of occupied Germany. I shall inquire what forms of health education films were present and what communication and information strategies these films of the postwar period used. Eventually I shall investigate where this corpus of health education films produced and screened under Allied occupation stands within the wider context of German film culture of the time. The chapter outlines the formal and aesthetic design of the films, their dramaturgy, and their targeting especially the emotions of the audience. The detailed analysis of two examples for the treatment of war veterans and their convalescence also illuminates different approaches of the Russian and Western sectors of Germany to the interaction between medical and administrative institutions, which contribute to the reintegration of war disabled.

Between 1945 and 1949, as the two German states were created, twenty-three medical and health films were produced (some of these got lost while others survived), a corpus defined in part by the peculiar time of political, economic, and social transformations in occupied Germany.[1] One short film focused on gynecology (radiotherapy in uterine cancer), a purely scientific educational film, primarily targeted at professional audiences but for commercial reasons probably shown at fairs. Four films were produced on the subject of domestic hygiene and six films on contagious diseases and epidemics (malaria, typhus, typhoid fever, tuberculosis and syphilis). Two other films were dedicated, one to the issues of nutrition and health and safety and the other to the work of relief organizations like the Red Cross. Three films focused on disabilities (the blind and war invalids) and showed the war-damaged roads to recovery. Finally, one film is concerned the subject of filial anxiety.[2]

All these films are short ones with a playing time ranging from nine to fifteen minutes. They would have been shown, alongside two or three other films (newsreels, other short films, commercials, cultural films, and nonfiction short films), as part of the regular cinema program before the feature film, a format German cinema audiences had been familiar with since the late 1910s. In general these health education pictures can be differentiated from medical or biological training films intended for an expert audience—like those produced from 1946 onward in the American zone by Erich Menzel and the Institute for Scientific Films (Institut für Wissenschaftliche Filme) in Erlangen[3] and in the Soviet zone by Fritz Dick and Erich Schmücker at the DEFA Medicine and Hygiene Production Unit (Medizin- und Hygienefilm-Produktion)[4]—in that the latter were not framed by fictional narratives commonly used in health education films. DEFA was the Deutsche Film-Aktiengesellschaft, the state-owned film studio in the Soviet zone and later the German Democratic Republic.

To begin, the corpus of health films analyzed here raises questions about the image of the medical profession that the films convey, for they were produced at a time when leading physicians and administrators were accused of crimes committed in connection with National Socialist programs of sterilization and euthanasia and so-called scientific experiments on concentration camp inmates. In particular, the Nuremberg Medical Trial in 1947 convicted physicians representing a racist medical system of selecting, abusing, and killing patients.[5] The trial was widely covered by newsreels (Wochenschau) and the judgment marked a historic breaking point in the public perception of the medical profession. The verdict not only revealed the scope of medical atrocities under the NS dictatorship, but it also signaled a need for an ethical reorientation of medicine in Germany. Where NS physicians had focused on the health of the *Volk*, postwar physicians were to focus on the individual patient as stressed by the Nuremberg Code.[6]

Newsreels also suggested that the indictments in Nuremberg represented only the tip of an iceberg.[7] The concern was that some of the most prominent representatives of the medical profession had expressed an outspoken and internalized racism. During the NS period, many registered physicians had taken over the medical offices of ousted or deported Jewish physicians; many had been trained by professors who espoused NS ideology; and many subscribed to eugenic theories. Furthermore, wartime restrictions and medicine shortages for the civilian population had restricted therapy in many occasions. By documenting in film how physicians helped individual patients, moving images participated in the restoration of physicians' professional image, recreating confidence and trust in the profession. This was a fundamental element of any popular health education film in Germany at the time.

If it is important to understand how physicians sought to use film to restore trust in their profession, it is also important to understand the contexts in which these films were commissioned. We have noted the significance of the Nuremberg trial, but another context was also important: the Allied reorganization and reconstruction of Europe. The military governments played a crucial role in commissioning films, alongside local commissioning authorities, so that many of the films produced and distributed in Germany after the war were international films in the sense that they were made or screened by the occupying powers and reflected their various approaches to reconstruction. Evidence shows that Americans, for example, wanted health education films to emphasize the occupying power's role of benevolent responsibility for public health.[8]

Film scholars investigating supporting programs are faced with a highly complex situation: in addition to analyzing films' formal aesthetic structures and characteristics of style and placing them within genre contexts and traditions (which is the primary focus of this essay), they must also consider questions about the conditions and effects of their production, distribution, and reception. The lack of extensive sources for the immediate postwar period makes addressing these issues difficult. While it is likely that opportunities for audiences to see these films were (at least until 1948) limited by zone and sector borders, it is difficult to make reliable statements about territorial coverage with precise statistics on the number of copies, the period in which each film was used, and information on program placement. Also, in the absence of documentation on reception, it is difficult to make reliable statements about audience responses to the films. The major source for such responses are reports by members of film sections attached to the military administrations.[9] However, the scholarship on these sources refers mainly to political reeducation films. Only a comprehensive reception study that would also take into account regional factors could close this research gap.[10]

In the following, it is necessary first to briefly describe the film culture context of the production and reception of postwar health education films. First, I will outline allied programming policies and the resumption of film production within the structures specific to their respective occupation zones and sectors. A second section will provide an overview of the production of health education films in the first four postwar years and will sketch out their themes and subjects. A closer examination and analysis of seven films that address different areas of health information is intended to reveal how their framing of concepts was mobilized for ethical reorientation.

It has already been noted that health films were generally part of a supporting program in cinemas, not the main feature. In this context, it is important to note that one cannot limit an account of how medical and health subjects were disseminated to the supporting films. Audiences did not go to the cinema solely to see these movies, although some feature films touched on medical or health issues, too. Indeed, because supporting programs addressed only a limited range of subjects, it is possible that feature films were sometimes the main source of cinematic health education. For example, the short film *Fear* (*Angst,* 1949),[11] which portrays the treatment of a young boy after an accident, is exceptional in addressing psychological disorders, which were otherwise rarely represented in nonfiction films. Another example of such a film will be addressed in this analysis to examine how prewar traditions of filmmaking filtered into the postwar period: the DEFA feature film on venereal disease, *A Nodding Acquaintance* (*Strassenbekanntschaft,* 1947–48), by Peter Pewas. Screened in all four German occupied zones and sectors of Berlin, the film's analysis will show how gender relations and emotions were modeled at the time and what role medical institutions in particular played in that. *A Nodding Acquaintance* provides good evidence for conclusions about continuity and change in the field of sexual hygiene pictures developed by early postwar medicine in the transition process from dictatorship to democracy.

Finally, this raises the question of whether different health information strategies in film from the East and West can already be observed in this early phase. Uta Schwarz has observed that "while the construction of a democratic healthcare system and the break with the eugenicist focus in National Socialism were part of the fundamental consensus for the founding of the GDR in 1949, in the West, health was now [post-1945] conceived of as individualistic, differentiated both from National Socialism and from the 'collectivism' of the GDR." A final question thus focuses on whether the films discussed in this essay lend support to such a view.[12]

Allied Film Programming Policy in the West and East: Reeducation, Film Shortage, and Divided Resumption of Production

Concepts of reeducation were expressed differently in the various occupation zones and sectors into which the German territory and its capital city, Berlin, were divided. Although all four occupying powers agreed that "they wanted to make democrats of the Germans,"[13] they based their reeducation activities on their particular understandings of democracy. The Soviets permitted the formation of multiple political parties and a comprehensive trade union in the summer of 1945. The United States and the United Kingdom intended to build a political multiparty system and to encourage the recreation of industrial unions. The French showed little interest in a rapid development of political life. Moreover, the Western Allies endeavored to revive the democratic traditions of the Weimar Republic, but without its constitutional deficiencies. Only the Communists rejected the model of Weimar and leaned toward the Soviet model.

If the occupying powers struggled over political orientation, they also struggled to meet the severe social and economic problems after the war. The defeat and division of Germany triggered massive migration of the German population from east to west. Since the escapees and displaced were all without resources, significant problems in their supply and accommodation arose. Furthermore, the division of Germany had major impacts on the German economy and industry. Until the war ended, the eastern territories of Germany had provided the cities of the West with large quantities of agricultural products; industries in central Germany, Berlin, and Saxony had provided intermediary and precision engineering products for heavy industry in the Ruhr, which in turn had produced and provided coal and steel to eastern parts of Germany. All these traditional relationships were interrupted after 1945. In short, industry was seriously damaged and agriculture was not able to provide basic supplies for the German population.

Just as they differed over issues of reeducation, so the four military governments differed over economic policy. The British preferred centralization at the zone level. The Americans wanted a federal structure within their occupation zone. The French aspired to a comprehensive regionalization. And the Russians operated a large-scale economic dismantling on the grounds that "one-third of industrial capacity in eastern Germany was wicked, more than has been destroyed during the war."[14]

What they all agreed on was that the media, and especially motion pictures, should play a key role in reforming the beliefs and attitudes of the population, in easing the transition from dictatorship to democracy, and in helping the people cope with numerous aspects of everyday life in a ruined Germany. In their view, film was especially valuable because it was a particularly effective medium for conveying the knowledge and social codes of conduct and values that should inform legislation, public administration and justice, and public health measures. From the American viewpoint in particular, occupation policy was "media policy to begin with"[15]—the psychological power of National Socialist propaganda had to be broken and the political and moral superiority of democracy demonstrated. "The Germans were expected to assume individual and collective responsibility for the crimes of the Nazi regime . . . and simultaneously to demonstrate their willingness and ability to undergo a democratic transformation."[16]

In particular, the use of film built on the dominant theory that defined the effectiveness of the media in terms of a simple top-down stimulus-response model.[17] In this model, the role of movies in public health education was to provide information on health and hygiene (the stimulus) that audiences would then apply to their own lives (the response) to achieve self-preservation, especially in the war-ravaged cities in which privation and hardship were just as common as poor sanitary conditions. In addition, the commissioning authorities suggested that films allowed audiences to withdraw for a few hours from the depressing living conditions of postwar Germany.

The importance that the administrations of the four occupying powers attached to film as a medium for disseminating and implementing their reeducation goals is underscored by the swift restoration of dubbing units in Berlin and Munich (facilitated by the military film censorship sections) and the rapid reconstruction and reopening of cinemas (at least, those that had survived the war). But policies toward film differed in the West and East German occupation zones. In the West, numerous cinemas in the British and American occupied zone reopened for business as early as July 1945, approximately one month after the occupied zones had been created on June 5, 1945.[18] Their approach to the political "reeducation" and democratization of German society initially gave nonfictional films a significant role.[19] The audience was to (re)learn democracy through documentary films;[20] feature films were to follow later, according to American plans.[21] The military administrations also had responsibility for monitoring film imports from the respective countries of all four occupying powers.[22] Consequently, they determined which programs would be shown on the screens of all of occupied Germany.

Particular challenges existed in the French occupied zone.[23] Although the French had a specific interest in reeducating Germans since France had suffered German occupation, the French occupied area of Germany was economically weak and had little appreciable infrastructure to support the film industry. Former production and now dubbing centers were mainly located in the American and Soviet zones, and until IFU Remagen was founded in 1947, it was not possible to translate imported French films for German audiences. Only from 1947 could the French occupying regime's Section Cinéma, managed by Marcel Colin-Reval, commission dubbing for feature films or produce documentary films for the reeducation program.

The deployment of documentary films was, in the first instance, intended to confront German society with National Socialist crimes, in particular the implementation of organized mass murder in the concentration camps.[24] Cinemas in the British zone screened recordings from the liberated concentration camps in Buchenwald and Bergen-Belsen as early as May 1945: witness the newsreel *British Movietone News Nr. 830: Atrocities—The Evidence.* In June and July of the same year, the American zone ran the British-American newsreel *Welt im Film. KZ Nr. 5,* with images of Nazi crimes and from the liberated camps. On November 29, 1945, the hour-long film *Nazi Concentration Camps* was presented as evidence in the trial against the major war criminals at the International Military Tribunal in Nuremberg. The short film *The Camps of Death* (*Les Camps de la mort*), commissioned by the French Information Ministry and produced by Actualités françaises was shown in cinemas in the French zone in 1945. Hanus Burger's short film *The Death Mills* (*Die Todesmühlen*; 1945) was shown in all the movie theaters of Bavaria in January 1946 and was withdrawn from distribution later that year, evidently because it denied the collective guilt theory.

If the Allied aim in screening these films was to make Germans face up to their responsibility for the Nazi dictatorship, a selection of documentary films from the 1940s were shown in the occupied zones for a different purpose: to give the German public an understanding of everyday life in the United States and Great Britain, the functioning of their democratic institutions, the background to the war, and the Allies' motives. The first programs in the American zone—admittedly not especially successful with their audience—were the documentary and government films that the Office of War Information (OWI) had stipulated in the Operational Plan for Germany of February 5, 1945.[25] Among them were the *The Town*, films from the "Why We Fight" series by Frank Capra, *Autobiography of a Jeep, Power and the Land, A Child Went Forth,* and *A Better Tomorrow.* The Office of Military Government, United States (OMGUS) was closely connected to the Hollywood studios, and their European distribution branches sought favorable sales conditions for their films on the European markets. There were differences of opinion between the exponents of freedom of the press and freedom of speech and anticommunist voices within OMGUS and in the Information Control Division (ICD) about the priorities of the reeducation policy with regard to political goals and the concept of democracy that was to be conveyed.[26] Moreover, the film supply for programs was inadequate: neither the number of original imported films, nor the number of copies of each film, was large enough to supply adequately the growing number of cinema theaters reopening in the American occupied zone: "There were, all in all available only some 30 feature titles in the immediate post-hostilities months, 15 commercial shorts, and about 25 documentaries (all varying from five to six copies each), sufficient to service only something like 150 motion picture theaters, whereas there were actually three times that number found capable of opening for business in Bavaria alone."[27]

In order to alleviate the film shortage and to make programs more attractive to audiences that still demanded mainly German feature films, the Allied film sections organized inspections of confiscated German films produced between 1933 and 1945. The four occupying powers determined censorship criteria through a subcommittee of the Allied Control Council and made decisions about which films should be prohibited or approved.[28] This included compiling a catalogue listing prohibited and approved feature films, kulturfilms, as well as the training and educational films from the National Institute for Film and Image in Science and Education (Reichsanstalt für Film und Bild in Wissenschaft und Unterricht; RWU).[29] Nonfictional or nontheatrical films of German production were monitored for any Nazi content and divided into three categories: the first group consisted of those films that were still permissible; films in the second group had to have obviously Nazi motifs removed; films prohibited in their entirety formed the third group. The first "old" (produced prior to 1945) German films were approved in the American occupied zone by ICD/OMGUS in December 1945[30] and a little earlier in the British and French zones.[31] In 1945 fourteen feature films were screened in the French zone, of which nine were German and five were French productions (with German subtitles). Also in the French zone, there was a requirement that for every screening of a German film, a French film had to be shown and that the opening program had to show the concentration camp film *The Camps of Death* (*Les camps des la mort/Die Todesmühlen*). In 1946, 126 feature films were screened in the French zone, of which 60 were German and 58 were French.

A shift in American occupation policy took place in the course of 1946 from a predominantly punitive focus that emphasized collective guilt to a focus that was intended to highlight the commitment of that occupying power to the task of rebuilding a democratic political system in Germany. This shift was also reflected in American film policy: now fewer subjects relating to politics and more subjects relating to everyday problems were to be shown on screens. Providing solutions to these problems, the Americans hoped, would elicit positive feelings toward OMGUS as a protective and benevolent occupying power. In May 1946, the ICD produced a catalogue of topics for new nonfictional films, which among other things listed "Agriculture; Housing; Tuberculosis; Venereal Disease; A Hungry World and Decartelisation."[32] A film on tuberculosis, which had been initiated in response to the growing concern about the spread of the disease immediately after the war, was never completed because—according to some authors—the biological nature of the disease could not be appropriately realized on film.[33] It was not until 1949 that Kosmos Film, Hamburg, produced the first West German tuberculosis film, *Nur ein winziges Stäbchen* (*Just a Tiny Rod*; 1949),[34] supporting the Central Committee for Prevention of Tuberculosis and its work.

As planning got underway for the new American film policy, the authorities hoped to produce from twenty to thirty nonfiction films in 1947. In order to do this, a "documentary film section comprised of at least three production units" was to be created.[35] In late autumn of 1946, the ICD began production of the first three films, and on November 20, 1946, OMGUS awarded the first three licenses to German documentary filmmakers whose work was to contribute to the emergence of the documentary film as a crucial element of a democratic media culture. In order to counter accusations of propagandist manipulation, the Documentary Film Unit, led by Stuart Schulberg and Joseph Zigman, provided licensed German producers with development aid:[36] "reeducation" was now to be brought about by the Germans themselves.[37] The films were differentiated according to their content as either "functional films" (which also included the area of "public health") or "ideological films."[38] In January 1947, the ICD director, Gordon Textor, authorized another topic catalogue, which also included Public Health.

The problem facing planners in the West zones was that, unlike in Berlin's Soviet sector, there was no focal point for the initiatives surrounding the reconstruction of the film.[39] Many filmmakers were scattered across the entire western occupied zone, and interzonal mobility was extremely difficult. The western occupying powers looked to the production management structures of their native countries to develop film production in Germany, which was to develop in the West within a free competitive market after the breakup of Universum Film AG (UFA). UFA had been the principal film studio from 1917 to 1945, and the authorities in the West wanted to prevent any concentration of power within the German economy. They were less interested in the rapid establishment of a new production industry than in ensuring that future filmmakers displayed democratic convictions. Licensing the first German producers was thus a protracted process.[40] In time, approximately forty production companies and even more distributors emerged, the majority of which were unable to stay in the market due to their inadequate financial footing. Moreover, because of the zonal borders and German territorial losses, the deployment region was much smaller than it had been during the war. However, free film exchange became possible in the western zones from October 1948, after currency reform and the creation of the Trizone—the three western zones that eventually formed the Federal Republic of Germany. The new businesses located themselves in cities that had the necessary ancillary industries—in Hamburg, Munich, and in Berlin's West sectors.[41]

On the East German side, film screening and production was dominated by the Soviet Union. Besides a few full-length Russian documentary films,[42] mainly Soviet feature films were screened in the eastern occupied zone in 1945. This changed in March 1946, when certificated German and Austrian entertainment films from the 1930s and 1940s became available in cinemas through Sovexportfilm, the Soviet film distributor. As regards film production, in August 1945 Filmaktiv, whose task was to initiate the production of a new German film, was formed with the support of the Soviet military administration, SMAD, in Berlin.[43] Filmaktiv maintained close contact with the advisor for movies in the East German Central Administration for National Education (Zentralverwaltung für Volksbildung, ZVV), who was answerable to the administration for cinemas.

Filmaktiv would provide a major focus of film production. On November 17, 1945, in conjunction with their president, Paul Wandel, the Filmaktiv members and numerous directors, authors, camera crew members, actors and technicians resolved to form a new German film company. The financial basis for the reconstruction of the studio facilities was provided by the revenues from dubbing Russian films. How new productions were to be financed remained unclear at first; both restoring the equipment and procuring the raw stock proved problematic because production at the Agfa plant in Wolfen was only slowly picking up.[44] The new (East) German film production industry was to be antifascist and free from Nazi lies and hate speech, as well as "imbued with the spirit of Humanism, international understanding and true democracy."[45]

Filmaktiv began production in early 1946. Director Wolfgang Staudte shot short documentary films about the destroyed Berlin U-Bahn and current events in the Soviet sector—these short films served as stock shots for the archive of the new film company and for a new newsreel, *Der Augenzeuge* (*The Eyewitness*).[46]

A further development occurred on May 17, 1946, when DEFA, the Deutsche Film-Aktiengesellschaft, received its Soviet license from Colonel Tulpanow, director of the Propaganda and Administration Department.[47] Health issues were a subject of filmmaking almost from the start. The short film *Berlin im Aufbau* (*Berlin in Reconstruction*) addressed the generally poor hygiene conditions in the capital city's bombed out buildings, conditions that were exacerbated by a housing shortage and the destitution of refugees. More significant for this study, the protagonist of the first East German postwar feature film, *Die Mörder sind unter uns* (*The Murderers are Among Us*; 1946) by Wolfgang Staudte, is a doctor. This rubble film (Trümmerfilm, a style of film that focused on the impact of war and used the rubble of destroyed cities as a location) from DEFA, which works with stylistic elements of film noir, can be read as a character study of a physician suffering from perpetrator's guilt. Only when the existentially disoriented physician, Mertens, is forced to carry out an emergency operation on a child in the cellar of a bombed out building amid the most primitive of conditions, is a part of his former humanist medical personality restored to him.[48] The physician, placed in a drama of transformation, embodies, as it were, an ethical reorientation, facilitated by his ability to apply his surgical skills with only the barest necessities to hand (which is of course important in war). At the end of the film, he applies for a position in a clinical practice where there is a charismatic leading figure in the form of his former teacher, who is able to give him decisive professional reorientation.

Topics, Subjects and Aesthetics of Health Films in Germany 1945–49

Despite the different approaches to reconstructing a film industry in the Soviet and Western zones, in some ways post-1945 public health films would have seemed familiar to German audiences. Many of the topics they covered were not new, but rather had been the subject of films since at least 1918.[49] For example, films that refer to the rapid spread of venereal disease and the consequences of wartime malnutrition in children exhibit similarities to health films produced between 1918 and 1945, as did pictures addressing domestic hygiene and the prevention of vermin in the home, and especially the treatment and reintegration of the war wounded. Much of the (scientific) knowledge presented in postwar films was little different from that of films made before or during the war, with perhaps the exception of any eugenic content. What gave these films their period characteristic is their aesthetic communication, by which I refer not only to the repeated references to the "here and now" of urban ruins, but more generally the films' sound, commentary, and character dialogue.

In dividing production into different departments early on, DEFA came to dominate the early making of health education films in all zones in divided Germany.[50] From 1945 to 1949, the majority of health education films were shot at the studio's locations in Berlin, Potsdam-Babelsberg, and Dresden, where it operated first as the Section Culture Film (Abteilung Kulturfilm) in 1946–47, then as the Section Short Film (Abteilung Kurzfilm) between 1948 and 1952, and later as the DEFA Studio for Popular Scientific Films (DEFA-Studio für populärwissenschaftliche Filme). Given the shortages in postwar Germany, "genre questions were not discussed." Debates concerned "rather how film ideas could be realised quickly despite raw stock shortages, power supply cuts, transport problems, and inadequate or insufficient technology."[51]

The impetus for producing health education films that dealt with the post-war emergency situation (which featured a dramatic lack of housing, refugee destitution, inadequate nutrition, and poor hygienic conditions) came from the former medical orderly, photographer, and amateur filmmaker Fritz Dick in November 1945. With the author and dramatist, Georg C. Klaren, he had written two short film screenplays on the control of epidemics. The director of *Filmaktiv,* Hans Klering, referred Dick to the director of the Central Administration for Healthcare in the Soviet occupied zone, Professor Maxim Zetkin. Dick was able to persuade Zetkin to finance his films *Fleckfieber droht!* (*Typhus Menace!*; 1946)[52] and *Seuchengefahr* (*Epidemic Threat*; 1946).[53] *Typhus Menace!* was filmed in the partially destroyed studios in Berlin-Johannisthal, and Dr. Kirchberg from the Kaiser Wilhelm Institute Berlin and Dr. Claus Bloehmer from the Central Administration for Healthcare Affairs (Zentralverwaltung für das Gesundheitswesen) acted as scientific advisors for the film. The director was the highly experienced Kulturfilm maker Hans Cürlis;[54] Fritz Dick acted as floor manager, laboratory supervisor, director's assistant, and camera assistant.[55] Filming was complete by the time DEFA's official license came through.[56]

The plot of *Typhus Menace!* unfolds between the present and the immediate past, narrated in three flashbacks, which provide an account of the incubation period of the disease. Photomicrographs from the laboratory and short documentary recordings are set into the fictional scenes. A man, sweating heavily, lies in bed; his wife is extremely worried. Sharp shadows emphasize the dramatic situation in the humble bedroom. The doctor takes the patient's temperature—the thermometer displays thirty-nine degrees Celsius. Two days earlier, the man had come home in a weakened state, but his wife has only now fetched the doctor, who proceeds to inform her that she should have done this after twenty-four hours at the latest. His examination diagnoses typhus. A second flashback shows the man at the table. He is scratching himself. He keeps his underwear on when he goes to bed and puts his nightshirt on over it. The following morning, his wife discovers lice in the shirt. "Little murderers," comments the voiceover during a shot of a test result under the microscope. A final flashback shows how the man became infected from the clothes louse: he had helped a man who was transporting a mattress out of an overcrowded tram. Another shot of lice under the microscope. His wife is advised to buy lice powder. Delousing stations, which also "register evacuees," eliminate carriers of disease professionally, according to the offscreen voice. People undergo a "general cleansing" in a shower. Seams in clothing are ironed, shoes sprinkled with louse powder, the body washed in fine sand. The feverish patient is brought into a hospital. The doctor's good advice turns into an offscreen voice: "Prevent and kill lice, too, or they'll kill you!" Although meant as a tool for denazification, the commentary of the film paradoxically was an echo of NS anti-Semitic rhetoric about "Jewish vermin."[57] However, in *Typhus Menace!* the NS reference to the body of the nation is substituted with a reference to the physical body of the individual attacked by the lice. The problem was that filmmakers could not always predict which way the viewer would interpret the images on the screen.

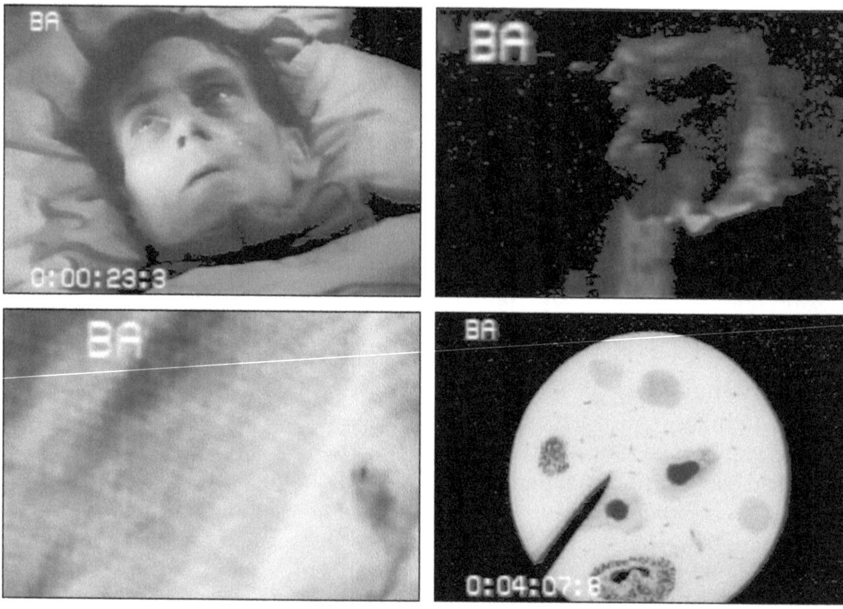

Figure 7.1a–d. Frames from *Fleckfieber droht!* (Typhus Menace!, 1948), dir. Hans Cürlis. Bundesarchiv-Filmarchiv Berlin.

Typhus Menace! describes the interaction between individual and institutional efforts at prevention. It portrays them both as necessary to fight the louse infestation and to prevent typhus by highlighting the interrelationships between inside (the home as a space to be protected) and outside (street/overcrowded trams as the area of contagion), private domain (household), and public domain (delousing station). The work done by the delousing station is explicitly directed toward the "evacuees" coming into the city "from outside." This is visualized in the urban topography through the "relocation" of the louse-infested mattress in the tram.[58] The lice transfer themselves to the man from this "vehicle in a vehicle." The film also locates the preventative care to be taken by the individual in a premedical sphere—in line with the idea that "everyone can do his/her part for hygiene"—and it provides information on how to recognize the infection and when medical expertise is required. Individual and institutional practices are also depicted as analogous: the housewife combats lice in the microsocial realm, the staff at the delousing station in the macrosocial realm. Physician and clinic are there when the illness manifests itself.

The narration in this short film concentrates on an exemplary case study in which the housewife represents the audience in need of instruction, and the film shows her the path of infection and the development of the typhus case through the three short flashbacks. However, *Epidemic Threat* also provides a kind of concise compendium of everyday hygienic measures against infectious diseases such as typhus, typhoid fever, dysentery, and diphtheria. It shows how to protect foodstuffs from contaminants, how to delouse and disinfect textiles, the necessity of boiling water due to risks incurred through war damage to water-pipes, of disinfecting toilets, and so on. "Hitler's criminal war has destroyed ordinary life," says the offscreen voice:[59] "Protect yourself and the community."[60] The film ends with images of rubble women (Trümmerfrauen) and children playing with skipping ropes among the ruins—the "intact life" that the camera finds in the destroyed city is reliant on adherence to the regulations on domestic hygiene conveyed in the film.

Several other short films illustrate the topics, subjects, and aesthetics of DEFA health films at this time. *Vitamine an der Straße* (*Vitamins on the Street*), directed by Hans Cürlis for the DEFA Section Culture Film from a screenplay by Fritz Lafontaine, who also performed the main role, was screened in cinemas from October 18, 1946. The motion picture tells the story of Father Lemke, who gives the hungry city dweller Brösel advice on how he can grow his own vegetables in the city's open abandoned spaces to improve his poor diet. *Hilf mir, Mutti* (*Help Me, Mummy*), which Fritz Schmücker directed for the DEFA Medicine and Hygiene Film Production Berlin,[61] describes the symptoms, causes, and treatment of rickets. After the extremely severe winter of 1946–47, Fritz Dick's film *Diphtherie* (*Diphtheria*), supported by the Saxon Serum Plants (Sächsische Serum-Werke) in Leipzig, appeared in cinemas on April 25, 1947.[62] It highlighted the symptoms, development, and secondary symptoms of this childhood disease and encouraged parents to have their children vaccinated.

In addition to these films, which are representative of the classic supporting program format, DEFA Saxony in Dresden was commissioned by the public health department to produce a series of approximately one-minute-long cinema-health adverts. The two short films *Es ist leider so!* (*Unfortunately, That's the Way It Is!*, 1946) and *Lebensbaum unseres Volkes* (*Our Nation's Tree of Life*, 1947) explained venereal diseases. In 1947, *Der hohe Preis* (*The High Price*) was the first in a series of short- and medium-length road-safety education films, some of which were commissioned by the GDR national police (Volkspolizei) and which depicted more or less graphic examples of road accidents.[63]

DEFA might have dominated film production, but it was not the only producer to release motion pictures on health subjects. Thus, the short film *Ungebetene Gäste der Hausfrau* (*The Housewife's Uninvited Guests*), produced by Gea-Kulturfilm in Hamburg in 1947 and directed by Ulrich K. T. Schulz,[64] a zoologist and biology film pioneer in UFA's culture section, places itself on the boundary between a biology and a hygiene film.[65] It is the only hygiene picture produced in the British sector that has been traced. The title of this "jolly film about biology and combating household pests"[66] reveals its intended female audience. As the "guardian of the hearth," it is the woman's task to keep germ-infested pests away from domestic spaces and from foodstuffs in particular. A cartoon shows insects sitting at a table laden with food. Figured anthropomorphically, they have taken over the house and put themselves in the place of the humans. This image, reminiscent of the work of Ladislaus Starevich, takes up the topos of inverted hierarchies: humans have, as it were, capitulated to inferior creatures.

A pest parade in short scenes follows, their filmic presentation exposing them to the macroscopic and microscopic gaze: rats run around among the ruins of buildings, closeups of rats—intended to arouse the audience's disgust—is followed by the admonition, "Leave the rat infestation to the experts."[67] However, the housewife can "master" insects herself with a variety of pest control methods ranging from soda water to DDT. Bedbugs live behind pictures and wallpaper in the bedroom: they are "stains on a housewife's honour."[68] Their bloodsucking is shown highly magnified, the human body labeled a "crime scene."

The scene in which fleas infect the mothers, all neatly sitting in a row on a bench with their prams, makes use of a similar principle to that in *Typhus Menace!* A man of impoverished appearance and wearing scruffy clothing carries them, much as the mattress carries the lice in the plot of Cürlis's and Dick's film. It is those individuals of no fixed abode who threaten resident individuals and their "homes." As in *Typhus Menace!*, here again Nazi tropes are involved: the racist speech of National Socialism merges seamlessly into the martial rhetoric of the offscreen voice in Schulz's film. The flea is turned into a metaphorical "monstrous mythical creature" and criminalized, yet at the same time, the humorous tone of the commentary makes this linguistic see-saw act the subject of irony: "The dastardly flea uses this razor sharp weapon [its mouth parts] to stab humans."[69] More harmless pests follow this climax: cockroaches are lured with a beer-soaked cloth, which is then plunged into hot water, and moth-infested clothing are laid out in the sun or fumigated thoroughly with paradichlorbenzene. Mother and children are overjoyed to find their clothing undamaged as they unpack. At the end, the woman can contemplate herself with satisfaction.

Occupational safety was an important subject for DEFA from 1947 onward. *Das seltsame Haus* (*The Strange House*, 1947) deals with occupational safety in the home, while *Stürzende Mauern* (*Falling Walls*)[70] and *Warum nicht gleich so* (*Why Not Like That in the First place*) deal with the prevention of accidents in construction and roofing work. Some of the themes in this mini-corpus are illustrated by the two-act short film *Achtung Gefahr!* (*Caution, Danger*, 1948),[71] written and directed by the former UFA director Milo Harbich and commissioned by the Brandenburg government, the Ministry for Health and Social Care, and by the Brandenburg Health and Safety Board (Landesarbeitsschutzamt).

In spite of the warnings of his fellow lodger, a woman, journalist Karsten attempts to repair a faulty electrical socket and fuse, causes a short circuit, and receives a hefty shock. In his profession as a reporter, Karsten participates in a trial in which the accused, a supervisor, who neglected his legal duty of care and left an assistant operator to work alone, is sentenced to a year in prison. At his office, occupational health and safety inspectors help Karsten with his research, telling him that businesses must establish health and safety commissions to look into every accident. A series of case studies, which Harbich stages in the style of a crime film and in part with film montage tricks, reconstruct acts of gross negligence that lead to accidents and show dramatic injuries but also, like instructional films, demonstrate how to handle machines correctly. The message is that occupational safety is as much the responsibility of workers, who often ignore safeguards despite being familiar with them, as it is of corporations, who neglect to put safeguards in place because of the costs. A quick montage of insurance claims highlights the increasing frequency of occupational accidents: "Who's going to pay for all this?—All of us workers!" is the agitprop-style cry,[72] and the film further argues that disability causes economic damage (an important point at a time of economic reconstruction) that could be prevented through occupational safety measures. The journalist ends his research work with the independent medical examiner—none other than the female fellow lodger who warned him before and who now has the corpus delicti lying before her: the faulty electrical socket. At the end of the film, the offscreen voice directs an urgent appeal to "workers, work managers and businessmen" to adhere to occupational safety regulations. The journalist takes on the role of the observer who visits the various supervisory and sanctioning authorities and so stands in for the public (in need of instruction). His questions to those responsible provide the opportunities for the latter to educate the film's audience about the occupational safety measures and responsibilities. The film's cyclical ending provides a double revelation: the realization of his own negligence and the identification of the woman as the medical examiner and as someone whom Harbich can use to confer an erotic tone to the film.

If occupational films were important, so too were movies on the care and support for the war wounded and disabled people. This topic provides an opportunity to compare films produced in the East and the West. My focus will be the DEFA-produced *Zurück ins Leben* (*Return to Life*; 1948) by Werner Bergmann and *Erben der Vergangenheit* (*Heirs of the Past*; 1949) by Ernst Niederreither.[73] These films provide slightly different depictions of the topic in East and West Germany and make clear the differing dispositions of DEFA and the western producers. Both films deal with the orthopedic treatment of and psychological support for war wounded, with physical education through sport, gymnastics, and motor training with prosthetics. However, their titles betray markedly divergent approaches: Bergmann's film emphasizing rehabilitation, Niederreither's film emphasizing the costs of war and the loss of masculinity that faced the war wounded.

In the case of Bergmann's film, the commentary underscores the urgency of care for the wounded; in Berlin alone, with a population of three million, the film tells us, there are 350,000 physically disabled individuals, half of whom are severely disabled through injuries received during the war. With prosthetic aids (e.g., the so-called Sauerbruch Arm), social legislation, and their own willpower, these war wounded can be helped and will be able to find work again. Bergmann[74] also injected the film with an autobiographical note; he, having himself had an arm amputated in the war, at one point steps in front of the camera and shows one of his frustrated actors how to tie a tie with only one hand.[75] This moment of independent care and help among men puts a stamp of authenticity on real situations taking place both in front and behind the camera and focuses insistently on an item of clothing that stands as the quintessential aspect of the civilian appearance. Bergmann's presence in the film—which can be seen as an early example for the participatory mode in documentary filmmaking[76]—indicates the extent to which his own employer was dedicated to a policy of integrating disabled people into the workforce. Moreover, in

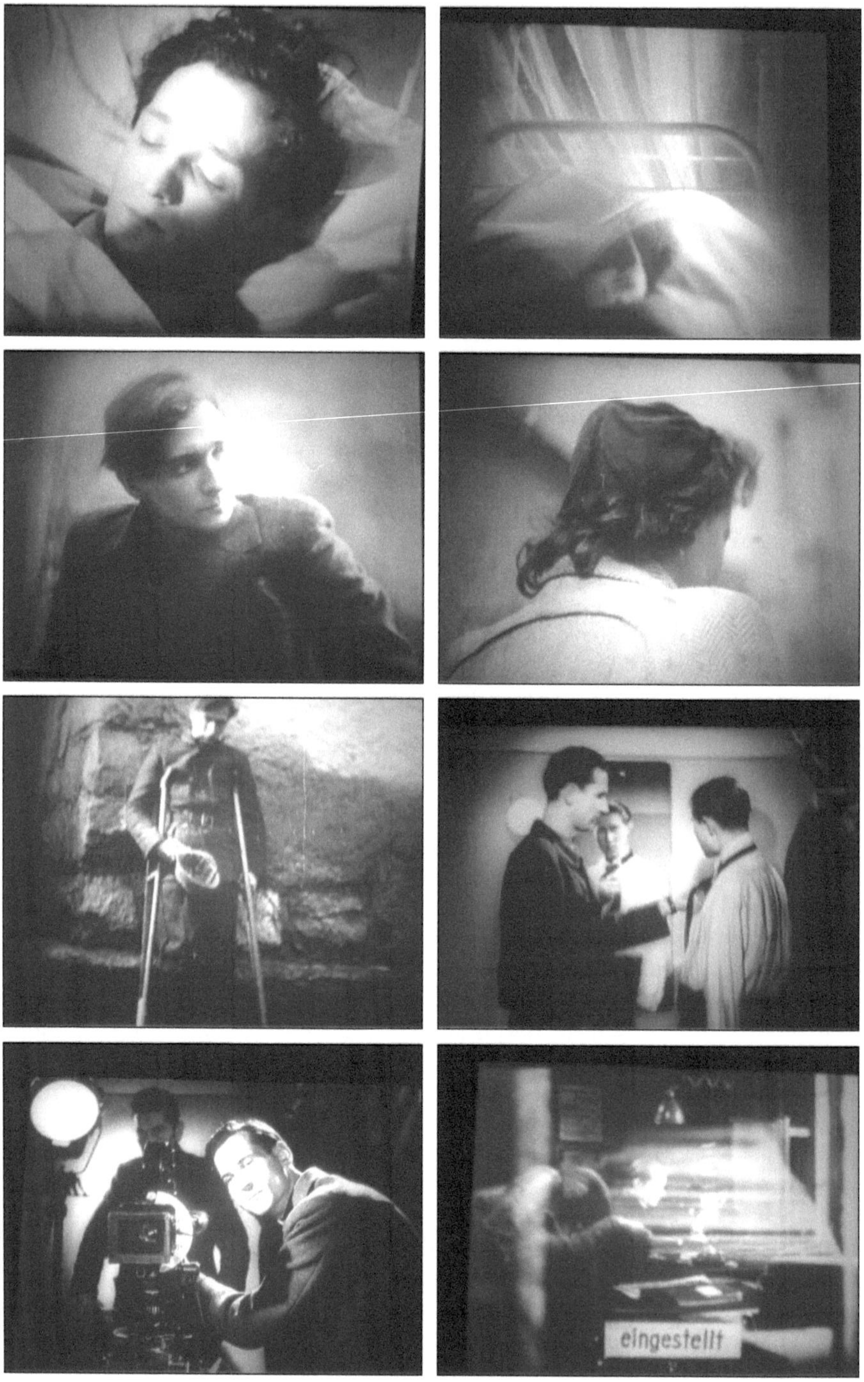

Figure 7.2a–h. Frames from *Zurück ins Leben* (Return to life, 1948), dir. Werner Bergmann. Bundesarchiv-Filmarchiv Berlin.

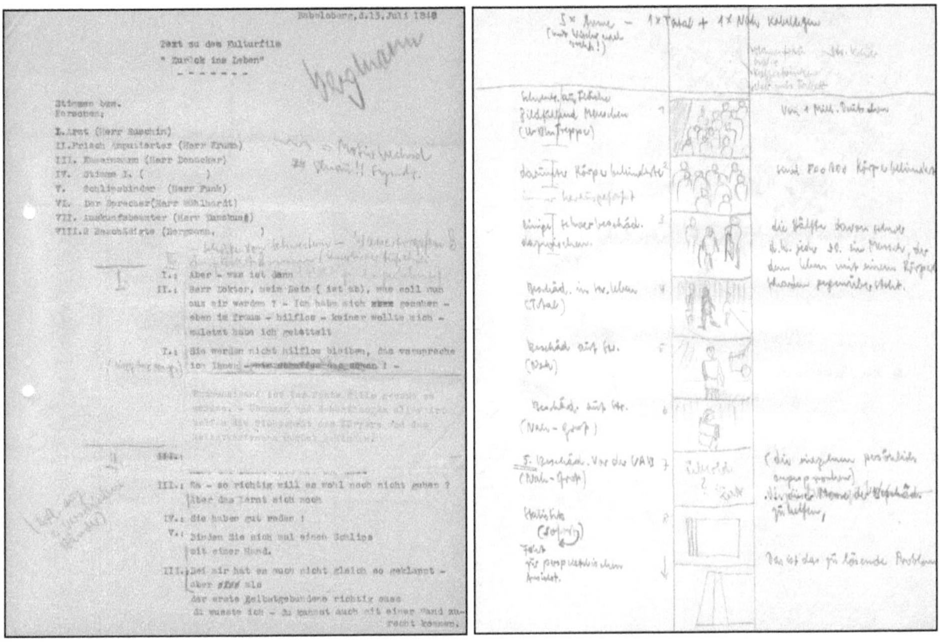
Babelsberg, d.13. Juli 1948

Text zu dem Kulturfilm
" Zurück ins Leben"
- - - - - - -

Stimmen bzw.
Personen:

I. Arzt (Herr [illegible])
II. Frisch Amputierter (Herr [illegible])
III. [illegible] (Herr [illegible])
IV. Stimme I. ( )
V. Schlipsbinder (Herr [illegible])
VI. Der Sprecher (Herr [illegible])
VII. Auskunftsbeamter (Herr [illegible])
VIII. 2 Beschädigte ([illegible],)

I.: Aber - was ist denn
II.: Herr Doktor, mein Bein (ist ab), was soll nun aus mir werden ? - Ich habe mich [illegible] - eben im [illegible] - hilflos - keiner wollte mich - zuletzt habe ich gebettelt
I.: Sie werden nicht hilflos bleiben, das verspreche ich Ihnen [illegible] ! -

[illegible]

III.: Na - so richtig will es wohl noch nicht gehen ? Aber das lernt sich noch
IV.: Sie haben gut reden !
V.: Binden Sie sich mal einen Schlips mit einer Hand.
III.: Bei mir hat es auch nicht gleich so geklappt - aber [illegible] als der erste Selbstgebundene richtig sass da wusste ich - du kannst auch mit einer Hand zurecht kommen.

Figure 7.3a–b. Two pages from the script of *Zurück ins Leben*, written by Werner Bergmann. Courtesy of Werner Bergmann, Filmmuseum Potsdam.

Bergmann's film the detailed description of the craft of prosthesis production and adaptation is interlaced with the reintegration process of prosthesis-equipped working men in new working surroundings, where the adaption of the workplace becomes the visualized "craft" of administration. The department for occupational welfare (Hauptabteilung Berufsfürsorge) takes care of professionally reorienting crippled men after their medical rehabilitation.

By contrast, the film *Heirs of the Past*, produced in Munich, seeks to shock audiences by dramatically emphasizing the loss of masculine physical integrity by following a male leg amputee going through a ruined city, along with a condensed montage of images of (erotic) happiness and unhappiness.[77] It is only after establishing the loss of masculinity that the film begins to focus on rehabilitation, with a depiction of prosthesis manufacture and fitting; men learn to walk again "like children" and pace lines drawn on the ground; a man even breaks down in tears during a walking practice synchronized with the walking aids. There follows a series of images of adept swimmers, cyclists, horseriders, and dancers, which brings the image montage full circle, finishing with images of men returning to work. "Then they come back," intones the offscreen voice, "and resume their positions. They want to be what they were, no more but also no less."

A commonality between the two films is the concept of a "rebirth to new life" made possible through adaptation to and functional training with artificial

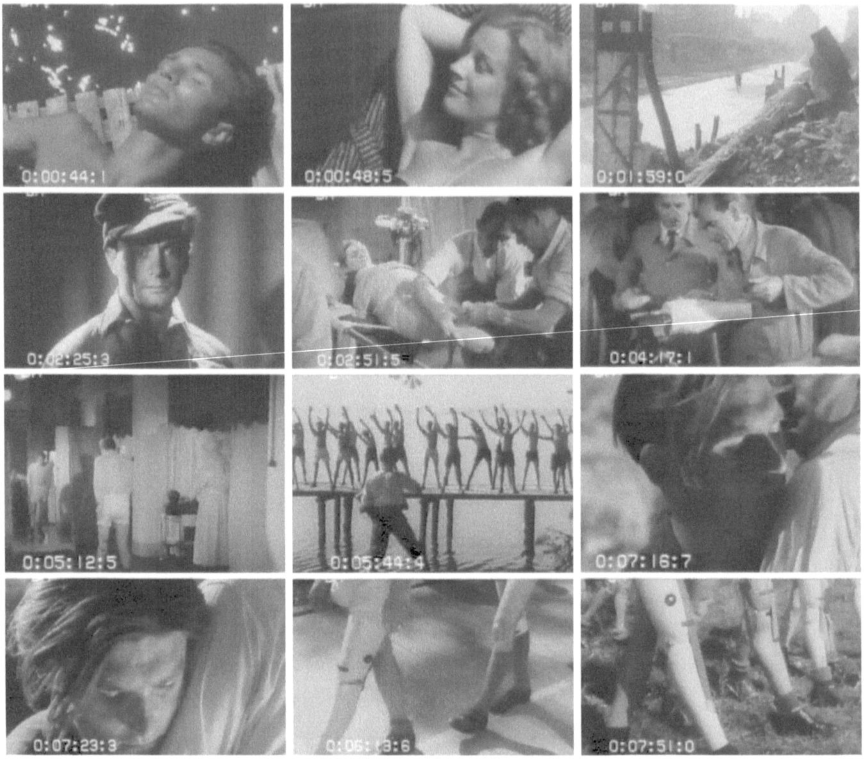

Figure 7.4a–l. Frames from *Erben der Vergangenheit* (Heirs of the past, 1949), dir. Ernst Niederreither. Bundesarchiv-Filmarchiv, Berlin.

limbs. Nevertheless, *Heirs of the Past* configures the war-wounded men as a social group that has the right to regain their identity. The narrative first places the man in a paired configuration, then in stark isolation amid forlorn ruins, and finally taken into employment along with others who share the same fate. However, Bergmann's film individualizes the man through his prosthesis and his acquisition of new motor skills but highlights how the collective takes care of the reintegration of the wounded into society. Concrete statistics provide an argument for the imperative to make the body whole through prosthesis—information that *Heirs of the Past* ignores.

What Body, What Sex, What Freedom?—Venereal Diseases and Reeducation between the Film Genres and Political Spheres of Influence

One of the major public health concerns in postwar Germany was the rapid spread of venereal disease, and films were a crucial part of the campaigns against it. They included the short film *Reaktion: positiv* (*Reaction: Positive*) in 1947, a response by the Documentary Film Unit in the American zone to demands of the health department at OMGUS for a sex education film about syphilis. This new film accompanied the ten-minute-long imported short film *Fight Syphilis* (USA 1942, directed by Owen Murphy), to be shown as well in the American sector—was intended to buttress the projected image of the occupation authorities as "desiring to educate and protect the German population and, to this end, being obliged to police them."[78] The collaboration of the two screenplay writers, Dr. H. Meissner and Karlheinz Schmidt, who also directed the film, followed a tried and tested division of labor between outside expert knowledge and a dramatic narrative form, which had characterized the German sex education film on venereal diseases since the work of Richard Oswald, Curt Thomalla, and Nicholas Kaufmann.

Fight Syphilis illustrates some of the limitations of using American films for a German audience. The motion picture is partly characterized by its commentary, which makes use of martial rhetoric: "People who know how he [the enemy] strikes and how to strike back." There is no consistent plot; instead the film argues that men suffering from venereal diseases weaken the military and economic strength of the United States. It emphasizes the importance of laboratory tests for diagnosing disease and for developing drugs against it. The fictional scenes give structure to the background locations, but at most merely refer to them: a bar and nighttime street as locations of infection, the quacks' advertisements as the false promise of a cure, the healthy family saying grace. The extent to which the film reflects the period of its production, its focus on the US Army and Navy as male groups at particular risk of infection, and its complete omission of the mechanism of action of the pathogens gave it limited appeal to German audiences. Filmmakers would have to present and justify prevention and treatment measures for syphilis very differently in postwar Germany.

Thus, in contrast to the American short film, *Reaction: Positive* integrates its message into a consistently fictional plot: a voice over is used simply to introduce the short flashback that tells the background story to the protagonist's infection. The start and end of the film take place in the doctor's surgery. The professor of medicine holds a row of vials up to the light: "Reaction positive, the patient will be treated in the clinic from tomorrow."[79] In the meantime, the man to whom he is referring is sitting in a bar. As the landlord of the bar serves him a beer, he becomes nervous, runs outside, and is involved in an accident. The man is taken to hospital where he meets the professor, who tells him that he has syphilis. The man believes the disease is incurable.

The flashback tells the story of how he acquired the disease. It shows him returning from the war, having lost his parents and his home. A woman at the next table in a bar befriends him, and he eventually moves in with her. One day he discovers a small ulcer and turns for help to the quack who frequents the cellar bar and offers him a cure, and he spends his remaining money on ointment and tablets. Then he meets an old work colleague outside the cinema and marries her "after two years adrift."[80] However, the disease resurfaces again, and he finally confesses his condition to his wife.

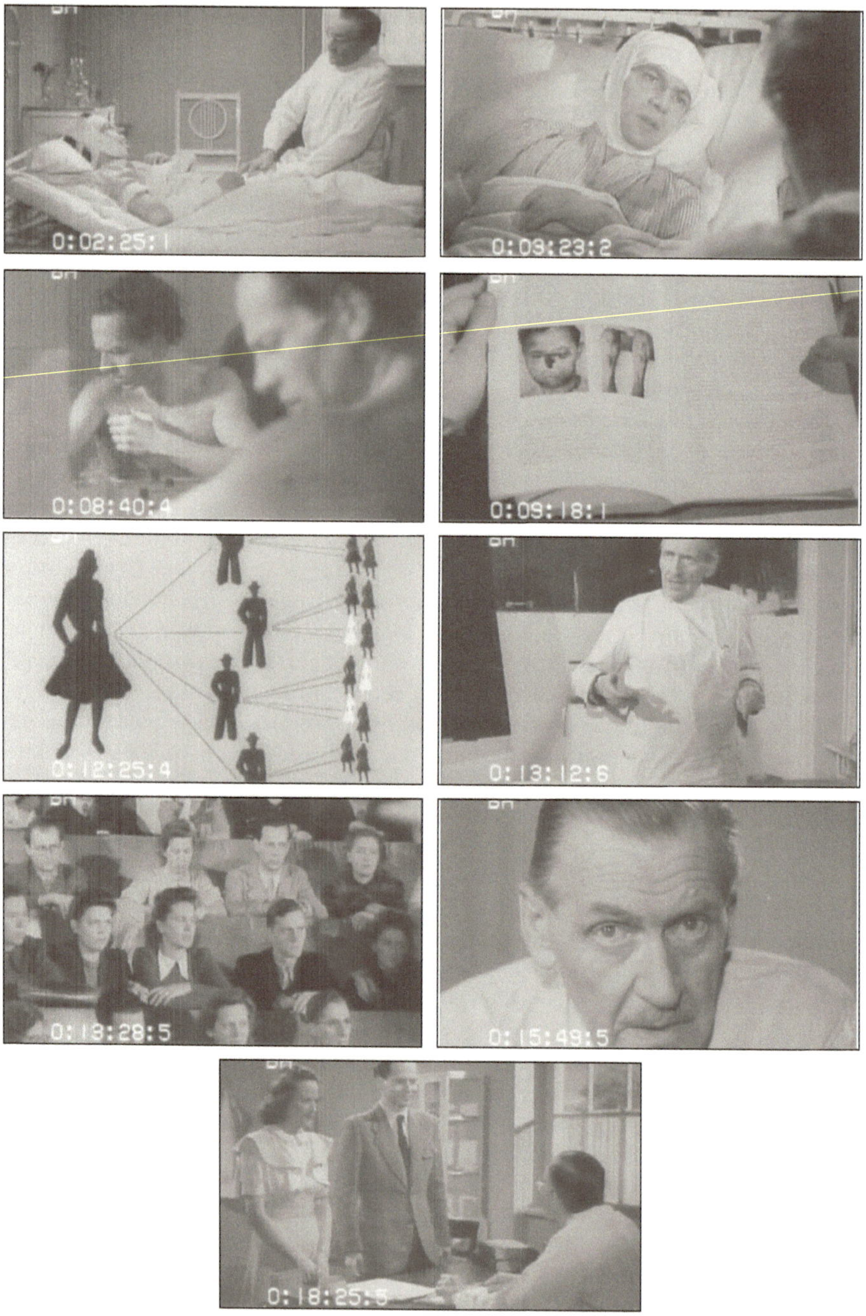

Figure 7.5a–i. Frames from *Reaktion Positiv* (Reaction: positive, 1947), dir. Karlheinz Schmidt. Bundesarchiv Filmarchiv Berlin.

Now we return to the scene with the professor. The professor admonishes him that, as a carrier of syphilis, he could cause immense harm, a point highlighted by an animated sequence that illustrates the pattern of infection: a female silhouette is connected to four smaller male silhouettes and, in their turn, each of these is connected to two smaller female ones. The animation ends and in a live-action sequence in which the professor is shown given a presentation in a lecture hall: "These people spread their fresh infections by having multiple sexual partners. However, the law will deal with people like this."[81] There follows a cartoon sequence that explains the way syphilis pathogens behave in the body, after which the physician, looking directly into the camera, says that the local health authority and the local doctor must be informed of cases of infection and that they will "investigate" such cases. "You can clearly see from your own example where recklessness and false shame will get you."[82] Now the film shows us some of the consequences of untreated syphilis (a boxer who becomes a cripple, a painter who goes blind, and a bridge builder who becomes paralyzed) before we return to the man and his wife, worried about the fate of their child. However, it turns out that all will be well. The professor says that because the woman has already been treated in the early stages, everything will "look much better within a year."[83] The couple visits the professor again: "Reaction: negative!"

The film may be located in civilian life, but it contains clear references to the war in the figure of the directionless man returning home. His isolation and loneliness is confirmed when he permits himself to be picked up by a prostitute. Sex and the desire for comfort and security are closely linked. The woman remains silent, but the signs of wickedness speak all the louder: she smokes while ironing. His rejection of her and finding a new partner more attuned to the expectations of his civilian past represent a transition from a sexually dangerous present to a (monogamous) reproductive family in the future. However, his infection with syphilis imperils this transition, and his body and sexuality need to be cleansed for him to enter into this "new life," something brought about by the doctor and by hospitalization. The period in the hospital thus has a double function. First, it literally brings the man to a halt—his treatment ends his odyssey through the urban space, which climaxes in the accident in the street. Second, the clinic is the site in which he can tell his story and in which a realignment of his consciousness through sexual education can take place. The disease is not labeled, as it is in *Fight Syphilis,* with military metaphorical language as an "enemy," which must be fought with the "weapons" of laboratory medicine. Rather the dissemination of syphilis is criminalized: the aim is to regulate and prosecute sexual behavior through "compulsory registration" of those with the disease and the female carriers through "inquiries." Where the metaphorical discourse in earlier anti-syphilis films criminalizes the pathogen-carrying creature, *Reaction: Positive* shifts into the literal criminalization of the—human—female syphilis carrier. The targets are prostitutes, who are to be kept in check by a "medical police force." This correlates with a pattern of thought that Richard Oswald had challenged in 1919 in his two-part film *Die Prostitution* (*Prostitution*; 1919). However, the motives that cause men to go to prostitutes in the films after

1945 are different from those in Oswald's film: sadness, disorientation, loneliness, rather than a search for amusement and an ignorance toward the dangers of venereal disease as set out in the 1919 film.

Peter Pewas's feature film *Strassenbekanntschaft* (*A Nodding Acquaintance*, 1947–48) shows the effect of the criminalization measures in action. For this 1947 film, DEFA followed the narrative tradition of the sexual education films of the 1920s, using a dramatic structure that links thematically similar "cases" together from different social groups.[84] At the same time, *A Nodding Acquaintance* distances itself from wartime movies by critiquing how, in a crisis situation, medicine legitimizes and carries out its interventions. The fact that the film was shown in all four occupation zones makes it the most significant health education film of the postwar period in Germany. Furthermore, the film is also significant because it took the typical subject matter of supporting program material and turned it into something else.

A Nodding Acquaintance was a feature length film, a format that indicates the gravity of the topic. It focuses on the risk posed to young women and marital relations by venereal diseases. However, the film also projects a critical image of how National Socialism socialized physicians. Their attitudes are in direct opposition to a recently attained freedom for the female body, whose "right of disposal" in a democratic society is guaranteed within the framework of the right to personal physical integrity. This tension becomes a problem for doctor-patient relationships in the postdictatorial situation, given that many physicians would have trained and practiced under National Socialism. In *A Nodding Acquaintance*, a relationship with the body is articulated that links the historic break of the end of the dictatorship with the end of an ideological expropriation of the female body in the name of racial politics and eugenics. This link is expressed in the structure of conflict as well as in character discourse of the film.

Twenty-year-old Erika, who works in a small laundry shop with her friend, falls out with her parents and moves in with Walter, a journalist, whom she knows only slightly. Walter can offer her little except a room, but she wants to dance and have fun. She meets the returning soldier Herbert in the flat of her friend Annemie, who lives well from her business deals with profiteers and brings them girls. Herbert has discovered that his wife did not remain faithful to him and is trying to forget: Erika, tipsy and impressed by Annemie's example, gives in to his advances. Later, in the home of an older aristocrat, Annemie tries to set Erika up with rich men, but she manages to elude them. Then follows a health inspection raid and Erika is diagnosed with a venereal disease; a stay in hospital is prescribed, but she runs away only to return in the end. Meanwhile, Herbert discovers from his wife that he must also be sick because she had tried unsuccessfully to treat herself but has fallen sick again and infected him. During the war, with Herbert absent, she had succumbed sexually to the charms of another man, Henry. Conscious-stricken, Herbert and his wife are brought back together. Erika is cured in the clinic. Walter's devotion to her is great enough for him to forgive her and they are reunited in the end.

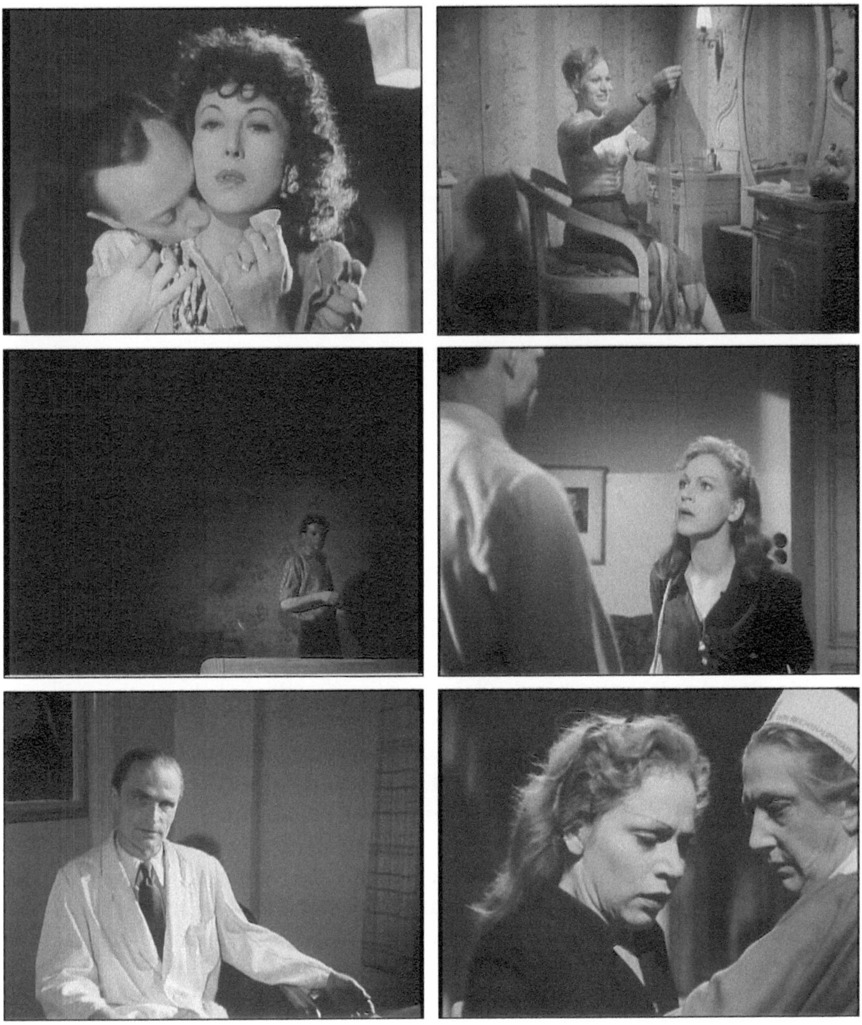

Figure 7.6a–f. Frames from *Strassenbekanntschaft* (*A Nodding Acquaintance*, 1947/48), dir. Peter Pewas (Berlin: Absolut Medien, 2011), DVD.

In a visual aesthetic inspired by the French poetic Realism of Jean Renoir and Marcel Carné that features highly complex camera movements and image layering in the opening sequence, Pewas creates a network of three female characters who cover the spectrum of venereal disease curability and incurability. Pewas takes the openness and coincidental nature of encounters from the street film genre, popular in Germany since the 1920s, in which the street was both a space of violence and a space in which virtues that had ostensibly been discarded by the middle-class found a home among prostitutes and other outsiders. Like the heroes in these earlier films, Erika breaks away from the conventions of the home to seek adventure in the street, only to return to a conventional lifestyle.

In Pewas's film, the space of the street has been appropriated by the women: it is there in order for them to display themselves, and their characters are defined by the way they move in it. Erika, the youngest, experiences the greatest discrepancy between material need, hunger, and her desire for a more pleasurable life. Her self-image is dominated by a tension that exists between her real deprivation and the image of the sexually attractive woman to which she aspires in a space, the street, that permits her to rehearse the behaviors of such a woman and allows her to indulge her sexual curiosity. She imagines this space to be a cost-free paradise, outside of any economic laws, as the femme fatale Annemie comments: "She thinks she'll get everything for free. She doesn't know that everything has its price."[85]

If the street forms one location, Annemie's well-furnished apartment provides another. It is divided by three different illumination values—the evenly and brightly lit living room with its depth of focus forms an initiation space in which profiteers and the girls can satisfy their hunger and thirst, the couples make themselves comfortable on the couch in the low-lit side room, dancing takes place in the dark adjoining room. Annemie's bedroom, on the other hand, is just as brightly lit as her living room when Erika withdraws there with her nylons and, standing so that she is always looking at her reflection in the mirror, slips on the tights appreciatively. Herbert is the voyeur of this narcissistic act. The mortification that Erika experiences through her tough work, her father's blows, and the hesitation of Walter (who represents the moral core of the film) is extinguished in this act of self-reflection. In line with the fundamental rationale of the film where values are internalized, Erika's sexual infection by the unwitting carrier, Herbert, is directly correlated with a false object of feminine desire—the western product of nylon tights, which, as a fetishized commodity compensates for mortification and neglect, turn Erika herself into a fetish. This appropriation of the fetish, embodied in the phallically upstretched leg, releases Erika and Herbert from their positions: subject and object of this curiosity come together in the act of sex and the chain of infected bodies gains a new link.

Erika's body is also contextualized by frustration, neglect, and redress. Just as, during his three-year absence through war and captivity, Herbert's wife had sought sex and comfort with Henry, so Herbert's sexual act with Erika redresses this grievance. His masculine desire does not demand an object that increases erotic attraction, but rather a youthful female body whose sexual possession may be substituted for that of a female body, his wife's, that has become polluted by infidelity. Physiological and psychological characteristics come together in this semantics of infection, which beyond the medical discourse, has always understood venereal disease as a symbol of promiscuity.

The key figure here is Herbert's wife, Marion, whose latent symptoms and the failure to cure them through self-medication are the sign of her infidelity. She can cast a veil over her infidelity by self-medicating, but she cannot blot out its consequences. Marion's body bears within itself the sign, initially illegible because invisible, of having violated sexual norms, which recalls the past of the war and thus also chaotic sexual relations. Her infidelity is revealed gradually, materializing first in the text of Henry's letter to Marion. Herbert, whom the "topsy-turvy" rubble world of Berlin has turned into a housewife, reads it but avoids confronting his unknown rival.

This sign then turns into an internal symptom: the pathogen once again enters into Marion's body as a symbolic sign of self-infection, as a foreign body that has remained preserved in the self. It is also the trace of the primary carrier, Henry, whose own body does not exhibit symptoms of disease, but whose appearance bears an uncanny characteristic resemblance to the physiognomy of a gangster. The fetish object of nylon stockings and the adulterer Henry, which alienate women from those men who are seeking a space and a task in the economic distress of the postwar period, both carry English names, and they cultivate, symbolically or directly, the pathogens that threaten the female body. (Even though the names Marion and Herbert are also Irish and English, they are much more familiarized in the German context and as such do not function as signifiers for foreigners.) Paradoxically, the English and Americans who had helped to liberate Germany from National Socialism are cast as symbolic of the disruption of war, if not invaders themselves of Germany and German women. The war has disrupted Marion and Herbert's relationship. Marion will accuse Herbert, as a distant soldier and conquering member of "the master race," of having had sexual relations with other women, even if these relations have not left any symptoms on his body.

While Erika's and Marion's diseases are cured through medical intervention because they, in line with the dramatic narrative logic of repentance, confess their guilt and submit themselves to a medical regime, syphilitic Annemie is excluded from this dynamic. She is introduced as a vamp figure, whom Erika initially idealizes but then rejects when she perceives the black marks on Annemie's back: these remain offscreen and horrify Erika.[86]

The justification used by the medical educators at the hospital for their raids to investigate and hospitalize young women comes under pressure: Erika and Walter accuse them of false imprisonment, lack of empathy, and bias. While the male doctor argues in favor of such raids exclusively on the basis of statistics on the distribution of the disease, the female doctor tries to understand the sexual behavior of "young people": "You can't expect young people to assume responsibility, they've experienced too much."[87] Pewas's use of lighting provides a clear indication of where the filmmaker's sympathies lay: Erika appears in a clear, soft light, while the doctors are set in the shadows, a visualization of their pessimism. Walter, who as a journalistic observer is also an observer of his own relationship to Erika and remains outside the infection chain, represents the middle-class perspective of "worldly wisdom" and an exemplary model of masculine self-control. He says, "We don't think about tomorrow. Those that come together today, without giving a thought to it"[88]—which is the opposite standpoint to Erika's materialism and "hunger." She is the woman who must be cured twice, from her disease and from her sexual impulses.

These moments of curing do not in fact take place under compulsion; the appeal is to Erika's freedom of choice. Walter admits their cohabitation (legally forbidden, but now openly discussed) and the clinic ultimately proves to be a site of mild severity. It is only the treatment that Erika undergoes in the end that makes her a suitable partner for Walter. In *A Nodding Acquaintance*, medical intervention recalibrates appropriate sexual relations and sometimes even makes them possible. In sum, the film challenges current narratives on different developments in the postwar Germanies: while in both systems different film industries and health systems evolved, the screening of *A Nodding Acquaintance* in all four occupation zones underlines that this did not necessarily result in different ideological approaches to health education films.

Conclusion

This account of post-1945 health films allow us to draw conclusions about the "relationship of control and pertinacity, as well as of experts and nonprofessionals, to social life and body perception."[89] These films should be seen, on the one hand, as a genre that developed a set of constitutive aesthetic and narrative characteristics, which are carried from film to film. They are also, in many ways, films that function on the margins, positioned on the boundary between theatrical and nontheatrical film, circulating within a variety of different contexts.[90] The majority of them—generally single-act short films and commercials, originally produced for the supporting program in cinemas[91]—were commissioned productions whose explicitly formulated aims reveal their functional nature.[92] They aim to influence behavior by giving information about disease prevention and, by portraying diagnosis and treatment for illnesses and disabilities, to demonstrate the work that health care institutions do, thereby promoting trust in them and raising awareness of their efficacy. In formal aesthetic and technical production terms, health films are usually genre hybrids (part feature, part documentary, and part animated films) that link fictional plots with direct instruction. This frequently results in a rupture in the conventional fictional gaze. The basic key phrases most important for the message are, in sound film, often spoken directly into the camera—explicit appeals to alter behavior or to adopt the "correct" behavior just demonstrated visually are directed at the (implied) viewer. While they strive to present evidence and to solicit the attention and understanding of a lay audience, health films, in contrast to medical training films, must also follow the fundamental rules of entertainment. They address viewers' emotions and "work" with them by staging, positioning, and thus also functionalizing knowledge-based elements—factual statements and educational messages—within narratives that usually act as frameworks for these elements.

As this essay has shown, the early divergent development of film production and screening in the East and West occupied sectors of Germany did not result in the development of different systemic ideological positions embedded in the health education films produced in West and East Germany in the immediate postwar period. Curative care and humanism, as well as positive portrayal of paternal authority, characterize the representation of physician figures in both East and West. This is true for physicians in short theatrical films as well as for male aid workers in documentary short films on care and support for war disabled. And it is also true for health education films produced across all military zones of occupied Germany.

Characteristic of both genres (feature and documentary films) is the metaphorical criminalization of harmful influences, which always impinge from outside and whose spectrum stretches from the little louse to the newcomer and the urban homeless. Only the occupational safety film *Caution, Danger!* explicitly emphasizes the consequences of workplace accidents for "all the employed." What this admittedly cursory overview of supporting program health education films also has demonstrated is that in the Soviet occupied zone, the production of health-related films in general played a considerably more important role than in the West. The new community was concerned about the health of its members and the cinema was the site in which the audience learned this.

Notes

1. Johannes Hauser, *Neuaufbau der westdeutschen Filmwirtschaft 1945–1955 und der Einfluß der US-amerikanischen Filmpolitik* (Pfaffenweiler, Germany: Centaurus, 1989).

2. The health education film and its transformation is an important topic in the DFG project "Geschichte des dokumentarischen Films in Deutschland 1945–2005" (The history of the documentary film in Germany 1945–2005), where its socio-political, health policy, and health technology, as well as media technology development processes, is investigated. On these three criteria and the problem of periodization, see Uta Schwarz. "Vom Jahrmarktsspektakel zum Aufklärungsinstrument: Gesundheitsfilme in Deutschland und der historische Filmbestand des Deutschen Hygiene-Museums Dresden," in *Kamera! Licht! Aktion! Filme über Körper und Gesundheit 1915–1990,* ed. Susanne Roessiger and Uta Schwarz (Dresden: Deutsches Hygiene Museum, 2011), 12–49, 27. This contribution is a first step toward setting this out.

3. See the films *Die gynäkologische Kleinraumbestrahlung mit dem Siemens Körperhöhlenrohr* (Gynaecological radiation therapy in small areas with the Siemens body cavity tube; 1947, L.: 593 m), *Achtung, Mücken!* (*Beware, Mosquitoes!*; 1948) on the anopheles mosquito and malaria, which Menzel filmed during his military service in 1940 and which later (after it had initially been confiscated) OMGUS commissioned him to rework as a popular scientific film. This film was a pure prestige product that Stuart Schulberg valued highly for the quality of its microcinematographic images. See Brigitte J. Hahn, *Umerziehung durch Dokumentarfilm? Ein Instrument amerikanischer Kulturpolitik im Nachkriegsdeutschland, 1945–1953* (Münster, Germany: Lit-Verlag, 1997), 280. *Eiweiß—eine Lebensfrage* (*Protein—A Vital Issue*, 1949, L.: 392 m) shows the effect of protein in the body and makes predictions for the food economy in light of a growing population.

4. See the films *Feind und Freund: Ein Film vom Schimmelpilz* (*Foe and Friend: A Film on Mildew*, 1948, D.: Erwin Schmücker, L.: 429 m) and *Leuchten wir einmal hinein! Ein*

Aufklärungsfilm über die Lungentuberkulose (Let's shine a light on this! An educational film on pulmonary tuberculosis; 1948, D.: Erwin Schmücker, L.: 257 m). The first part of the film *Malaria* (1948, D./S./C.: Fritz Dick, L.: 533 m) on the development of the pathogen in the anopheles mosquito and its transmittal to humans was based on a Bayer Group film; the second part demonstrated prophylactic measures against malaria. This was followed in 1949 by the training films *Beckenaplasie* (Pelvic aplasia; D./S./C.: Fritz Dick, L.: 150 m) and *Congenitalis Vitium Cordis* (D./S./C.: Fritz Dick, L.: 250 m). On DEFA, see Ralf Schenk, ed., *Das zweite Leben der Filmstadt Babelsberg: Zur Geschichte der DEFA, 1946–1992* (Berlin: Hentschel, 1994).

5. Till Bastian, *Furchtbare Ärzte: Medizinische Verbrechen im Dritten Reich* (Munich: C. H. Beck, 1995), 15–33.

6. Ibid., 8–9.

7. The term *inner racism* refers to a range of measures from the outlawing of curative care for physically and mentally disabled people to their murder under the euthanasia program of the National Socialists, while the term *racism* means the degradation, outlawing, and murder of persons on the basis of their ethnicity. On these terms, see Gisela Bock, *Zwangssterilisation im Nationalsozialismus* (Opladen, Germany: Westdeutscher Verlag, 1986).

8. On this, see the third section of this article.

9. See Hauser, *Neuaufbau der westdeutschen Filmwirtschaft*. Hahn, *Umerziehung durch Dokumentarfilm?*

10. See Schwarz, "Vom Jahrmarktsspektakel," 27.

11. P.: Attila Film GmbH, D.: Herbert B. Fredersdorf, L. 514 m.

12. "Während der Aufbau eines demokratischen Gesundheitswesens und der Bruch mit der rassenhygienischen Ausrichtung im Nationalsozialismus zum antifaschistischen Grundkonsens der DDR-Gründung 1949 gehörten, war im Westen Gesundheit nun individualistisch, in doppelter Abgrenzung zum Nationalsozialismus und zur 'kollektivistischen' DDR konzipiert," Schwarz, "Vom Jahrmarktsspektakel," 27.

13. "Man aus den Deutschen Demokraten machen wollte," quote from Gabriele Clemens, "Umerziehung durch Film. Britische und amerikanische Filmpolitik in Deutschland 1945–1949," in *Mediale Mobilmachung II: Hollywood, Exil und Nachkrieg*, ed. Harro Segeberg (Munich: Fink, 2006), 245.

14. Cay Rademacher, "Die Männer aus Moskau," *Geo Epoche* 64 (2014): 29.

15. Sabine Hake, "Erziehung zur Demokratie: Trümmerfilme made in Hollywood," in *Im Banne der Katastrophe: Innovation und Tradition im europäischen Film 1940–1950*, ed. Johannes Roschlau (Munich: Edition Text & Kritik, 2010), 94.

16. "Von den Deutschen wurde erwartet, individuelle und kollektive Verantwortung für die Verbrechen des Nazi-Regimes zu übernehmen . . . und zugleich ihre Bereitschaft und Fähigkeit zur demokratischen Wandlung unter Beweis zu stellen." Hake, "Erziehung zur Demokratie," 95.

17. Ramón Reichert, *Im Kino der Humanwissenschaften: Studien zur Medialisierung wissenschaftlichen Wissens* (Bielefeld, Germany: Transcript, 2007).

18. On the asynchronous restoration and reopening of cinemas in the two zones, see Clemens, "Umerziehung," 252.

19. Hauser, *Neuaufbau*. Sabine Schubert, "Die Filmpolitik der amerikanischen Militärregierung 1945–1949: Vorbereitung, Organisation und Durchführung

eines amerikanischen Programms mit Fallbeispielen aus Bayern" (master's thesis, University of Munich, 1988). Hahn, *Umerziehung durch Dokumentarfilm?*

20. Heiner Roß, ed., *Lernen Sie diskutieren! Re-education durch Film* (Berlin: Cinegraph Babelsberg, 2005).

21. Feature film screenings continued to be prohibited until the end of July 1945 in the American occupied zone.

22. On the feature film imports from the United States, Great Britain, and France during the years 1945–48, see the lists in Peter Pleyer, *Deutscher Nachkriegsfilm 1946–1948* (Münster, Germany: Fahle, 1965), 444–58. On the Soviet import films, see Bundesarchiv-Filmarchiv/DEFA-Stiftung, ed., *Ausländische Spiel- und abendfüllende Dokumentarfilme in den Kinos der SBZ/DDR 1945–1966* (Berlin: Bundesarchiv, 2001), 12–55.

23. Peter Gleber, "Kino als Überlebensmittel: Anfänge und Bedeutung dieses Mediums in der französischen Zone unter besonderer Berücksichtigung der Großstadt Ludwigshafen am Rhein 1945–1949," *Zeitschrift für die Geschichte des Oberrheins* 145 (1997): 403–29.

24. Hauser, *Neuaufbau*, 189, 191.

25. See the complete list and rubrication in Hauser, *Neuaufbau*, 186–87. In addition to 35mm prints, 16mm prints were also made of these films for screenings outside the cinema. In terms of the subject matter or title, there was no differentiation between a "theatrical" and "nontheatrical" program; the sole classification criteria were the format and form of distribution. The British initially only used *The Crown of the Year, Clydebuilt* and *New Zealand* in 1945. On further developments in the British zone, see Clemens, "Umerziehung," 257–58.

26. Hake, "Erziehung zur Demokratie," 94.

27. Albert Norman, *Our German Policy: Propaganda and Culture* (New York: Vantage Press 1951), 60, as cited in Hauser, *Neuaufbau*, 151.

28. For the criteria, see Clemens, "Umerziehung," 255–56.

29. See John F. Kelson, K. R. M. Short, and Zonal Film Archives, eds., *Catalogue of Forbidden German Feature and Short Film Productions* (Trowbridge, Wiltshire, UK: Flicks Books, 1996).

30. In his filmography, Bauer appends these prohibition notes to the end of each film title's entry, and he also provides information on the so-called Überläufer (defector) films, i.e., those productions that remained incomplete at the end of the war or that had not been screened before the war's end on May 8, 1945. See Alfred Bauer, *Deutscher Spielfilm-Almanach, 1929–1959* (Munich: Filmbuchverlag, 1960).

31. On the film screening statistics until 1949, see Gleber, "Kino als Überlebensmittel," 419.

32. Hahn, *Umerziehung durch Dokumentarfilm?*, 170n198.

33. Ibid., 170.

34. D.: Walter Fredersdorf, L.: 125 m, see Deutsches Institut für Filmkunde, ed., *Katalog der westdeutschen Kultur- und Dokumentarfilme, 1945–1951* (Wiesbaden, Germany: Deutsches Institut für Filmkunde 1952), 115.

35. Hahn, *Umerziehung durch Dokumentarfilm?*, 174.

36. The Documentary Film Unit modeled itself on the production groups initiated by John Grierson in England in the 1930s, which frequently undertook work

commissioned by public institutions. The model established by Grierson in Canada in the 1940s was designed to provide publicly funded productions.

37. At the same time, production was separated into three tiers: films with a clearly recognizable American message were demarcated as OMGUS productions, which were to include German film crew members ("overt productions"); licensed German producers were to carry out commission work for OMGUS under monitoring by Erich Pommer's film agency ("sponsored/contracted productions"); finally, independent German production proposals would be permitted after approval through OMGUS ("independent productions"). Films on aspects of American democracy and the American way of life, however, would continue to be imported from the United States. The reorganization of feature film production started in the American occupied zone in conjunction with this. *Und über uns der Himmel* (And above us the sky) was produced in the summer of 1947 under the supervision of OMGUS as the first German feature film in this zone.

38. See Hahn, *Umerziehung durch Dokumentarfilm?*, 277.

39. The facilities at Filmstudio Munich-Geiselgasteig, which had remained intact, served as garages, but approval by the American military authorities was not conceivable at first.

40. License applicants had to complete questionnaires and submit to psychological tests. See Pleyer, *Deutscher Nachkriegsfilm*, 37.

41. On the beginnings of the new German feature film production, see Pleyer, *Deutscher Nachkriegsfilm*, 28–48.

42. Films that ran in 1945 were *Berlin* by Juli Raisman about the liberation of Berlin, *Stalingrad*, a film produced in 1942–43 by Leonid Warlamov, and the popular scientific nature film *Das Gesetz der großen Liebe* (The law of great love), produced in 1944 by Boris Dolin. It is hoped that future research will demonstrate how the import situation was experienced in the short film sector and, if possible, which short films of Soviet provenance relevant to health education were shown in this phase.

43. It comprised five members who had emigrated to Moscow during the Nazi period and had returned immediately after the end of the war.

44. *Filmaktiv* occupied a former UFA administration building while doing preliminary work. Film technicians began the clear-up operations in the former Althoff studio and in Johannisthal. The UFA Studios Neu-Babelsberg remained occupied by the Soviet military administration. Dubbing took place in a former costume stock room.

45. "durchdrungen von dem Geiste des Humanismus, der Völkerverständigung und der wahren Demokratie," as cited in Pleyer, *Deutscher Nachkriegsfilm*, 32.

46. Begun in February, *Der Augenzeuge* initially ran as a monthly show, then with new issues on a fortnightly cycle and finally as a weekly newsreel. At the same time, filming was taking place on the first documentary and training films. The short films *Berlin im Aufbau, Der Gewerkschaftskongress* (The trade unions congress), *Einheit* (Unity) and *Der 1. Mai 1946* (the first of May 1946) appeared in the cinema early on under the production label Deutsche Film-AG (DEFA).

47. For greater detail on the terms of its licensing, see Christiane Mückenberger, "Zeit der Hoffnungen, 1946–1949," in *Das zweite Leben der Filmstadt Babelsberg: Zur Geschichte der DEFA, 1946–1992*, ed. Ralf Schenk (Berlin: Hentschel, 1994), 9–49, esp. 10–16. In the autumn of 1947, the liberal officers of the Leningrad group of SMAD were replaced and DEFA was turned into a Soviet corporation. The majority

of shares went into the hands of the USSR Ministry for Film. See Pleyer, *Deutscher Nachkriegsfilm*, 36–37, and Thomas Heimann, *DEFA, Künstler und SED-Kulturpolitik* (Berlin: Vistas 1994), 58ff.

48. Ursula von Keitz, "Between Dramatization and Epicization: The Portrayal of Nazi Crimes in Exemplary German Films from the Late 1940s to the 1970s," *New German Critique* 102 (Fall 2007): 45–60.

49. See, for example, the film *Krüppelnot und Krüppelhilfe* (Hardship and help for cripples; 1919, P.: UFA, D.: Nicholas Kaufmann) and the films *Erben der Vergangenheit* (Heirs of the past; P.: Filmstudio Leckebusch, D.: Ernst Niederreither) and *Zurück ins Leben* (Return to Life; P.: DEFA, S./C./D.: Werner Bergmann) from 1948, which are discussed more fully here.

50. The division of labor in the studios for the production of feature films, newsreels, and documentary films, as well as for popular scientific films, reflected the tripartite program structure introduced in cinemas.

51. Gerhard Knopfe, "Kalendarium einer deutschen Spezies. Der populärwissenschaftliche Film der DEFA," in *Schwarzweiss und Farbe: DEFA Dokumentarfilme 1946–1992*, ed. Günter Jordan and Ralf Schenk (Potsdam, Germany: Filmmuseum Potsdam, 1996), 295–342.

52. There are several versions of *Fleckfieber* in the Bundesarchiv-Filmarchiv Berlin, either with the verb *droht!* (menace) or without it. The actors in the short scenes are Ewald Wenck, Margarete Kupfer, Isolde Laugs, and Elisabeth Rower. L.: 276 m (10 min.), first released December 13, 1946, nearly a year after filming began. The inspected print was 250 m (9 min.) long.

53. L.: 364 m (13 min.), first released September 26, 1946; a short version was also distributed with the title *Achtung Seuchengefahr*! (Beware epidemic threat!).

54. Hans Cürlis was considered to be politically untainted and had at first offered to create large display placards for the Soviet military authorities, which would document the beginnings of the reconstruction of Berlin. In July 1945, Paul Wegener, president of the Division of Filmmakers, appointed him director of the Non-feature Film Department. His task was to restart the production and distribution of nonfiction films. On November 6, 1945, he received permission from the American military authorities to continue the Kulturfilm-Institute in Berlin-Steglitz, which he had founded in 1919. See Ulrich Döge, *Kulturfilm als Aufgabe: Hans Cürlis (1889–1982)* (Berlin: CineGraph Babelsberg, 2006), 52–53. After DEFA was founded, Cürlis—who had turned down the directorship of its Culture Film Department—was contracted to work for it.

55. Fritz Dick started the production series "Medicine/Hygiene/Health Propaganda" at DEFA and worked as author and director cameraman on nearly three hundred medical university and training films from 1947 to 1981. Dick employed the surgeon Ferdinand Sauerbruch and the gynecologist Kraatz, among others, as expert consultants for these films.

56. The production costs amounted to 45,200 Reichsmark. See Knopfe, "Kalendarium," 297.

57. See Paul Weindling, *Epidemics and Genocide in Eastern Europe, 1890–1945* (New York: Oxford University Press, 2000).

58. Cf. the transport and meaning of the mattress in Billy Wilder's *A Foreign Affair* (USA 1947).

59. "Der verbrecherische Hitlerkrieg hat das Leben zerstört."

60. "Sich selber schützen und der Allgemeinheit nützen."

61. L.: 397 m.

62. L.: 424 m. In 1948 the Munich film studio Leckebusch, in collaboration with the University Children's Hospital, also produced a film titled *Diphtherie* (L.: 121 m, 11 Min., D.: Walter Leckebusch). A sick boy is examined in the epidemiology ward of a children's hospital, the symptoms of diphtheria are shown, and the boy is treated with serum. Another boy is saved by a tracheotomy. The final part shows how serum is manufactured in the Behring works in Marburg. The film was later used as an educational film.

63. For example, films such as *Mir passiert nichts* (Nothing'll happen to me; D. Max Kerstan, L.: 135 m), *Vorsicht! Augen auf!* (Careful! Keep your eyes peeled!), and *Wer hat Schuld?* (Who's fault is it?), all produced in the same year.

64. Schulz worked for UFA until the end of the war, and then earned a living as a gardener. After the UFA company was dissolved, he was also a scientific assistant for the Russian Technical Office for Cinematography. See the bio-filmography of Ulrich K. T. Schulz at http://www.difarchiv.deutsches-filminstitut.de/ dt2tp0146.htm (accessed May 31, 2012).

65. L.: 447 m. The BA-FA copy viewed for this contribution gives the "Laboratorium für hygienische Zoologie Berlin-Dahlem" (Laboratory for Hygienic Zoology Berlin-Dahlen) and the "Biologische Zentralanstalt für Land- und Forstwirtschaft" (Central Biological Institute for Farming and Forestry) as scientific advisors.

66. "heitere Film über die Biologie und Bekämpfung häuslicher Schädlinge"; the quoted paratext is in Deutsches Institut für Filmkunde (ed.) 1952, 65. Gea-Kulturfilm produced several pest control films up to 1949, including ones on bark and potato beetles as well as scale insects.

67. "Die Rattenplage überlasse man dem Fachmann."

68. "Flecken auf der Hausfrauenehre."

69. "Mit dieser messerscharfen Waffe bohrt der Floh meuchlings den Menschen an."

70. A film with the same title on the dangers faced by those who collect wood among the ruins was also produced by Herold Film and directed by Eugen von Burghardt in 1947 (L.: 220 m).

71. L.: 780 m, in cinemas from 8.11.1948, camera: Walter Roßkopf, music: Hans Otto Borgmann, with Harry Hindemith, Knut Hartwig, and Ilse Maria Milde. A short version was also distributed, L.: 513 m.

72. "Wer zahlt das alles?—Wir alle, die arbeiten!"

73. 1949, P.: Filmstudio Walter Leckebusch, L.: 392 m.

74. As a cameraman with DEFA he was a key influence on the company's visual style, for example, in Konrad Wolf's *Der geteilte Himmel* (*Divided Heaven*; 1963) and Frank Vogel's *Julia lebt* (*Julia's Alive*; 1964).

75. See Knopfe, "Kalendarium," 302–3.

76. As it is theorized by Bill Nichols, *Introduction to Documentary* (Bloomington: Indiana University Pres, 2010).

77. The tendency of the Trümmerfilm to treat body and city as reciprocal and psychologically significant metaphors is already apparent in *Die Mörder sind unter uns*. In *Erben der Vergangenheit*, this rhetorical mode becomes immediately apparent.

78. "Die deutsche Bevölkerung aufklären und schützen zu wollen und dazu auch kontrollieren zu müssen," in Hahn, *Umerziehung durch Dokumentarfilm?*, 281. A film like this had been planned even before the *Unit*'s foundation, but correlating the correct presentation of the medical subject and conveying it in a generally comprehensible manner proved problematic. By September of that year there were fifteen draft scripts. The film was ready at the end of 1947 and was released on July 1, 1948, in Großostheim. *Zeit im Film* (Time in film; Berlin/Munich-Geiselgasteig) was the commissioning authority, L.: 546 m (20 min.), camera: Karl Hasselmann, music: Hans-Otto Borgmann. See the entry for the film on filmportal.de, accessed on May 25, 2012, http://www.filmportal.de/film/reaktion-positiv_ed55fed86acc475b96e-3da85922a1ddb. The 35mm print kept in the BA-FA that was viewed for this research bears the opening credit text "Das Landesgesundheitsamt zeigt" (The Public Health Authority presents).

79. "Reaktion positiv, der Patient wird ab morgen in der Klinik behandelt."

80. "Nach zwei haltlosen Jahren."

81. "Durch wechselnden Geschlechtsverkehr verschleppen die Menschen ihre frischen Infektionen. Aber mit dieser Sorte Mensch wird das Gesetz fertig werden."

82. "An Ihrem eigenen Beispiel sehen Sie ja, wohin Leichtsinn und falsche Scham führen." *Falsche Scham* (False shame) is the title of the feature length film by Curt Thomalla and Nicholas Kaufmann on venereal diseases and their treatments, which the UFA Culture Department released in cinemas in 1926. It gave the paternal doctor a similar role to that in the film *Reaktion: Positiv,* which may well have prompted memories of films in older audience members. Anita Gertiser, "Falsche Scham: Strategien der Überzeugung in Aufklärungsfilmen zur Bekämpfung der Geschlechtskrankheiten 1915–1935" Göttingen Vandenhoeck & Ruprecht, 2015.

83. "In einem Jahrsieht schon alles besser aus."

84. *Strassenbekanntschaft* was based on a screenplay by Artur Pohl, produced on commission by the Central Administration Board for Public Health and, like *Fleckfieber droht!,* Dr. Claus Bloemer acted as an advisor for the film. A cross-section dramatic structure, which shows a complex of figures in parallel conflict situations and relates them to each other through sexual relationships, is at the basis, e.g., of the feature films *Die freudlose Gasse* (The joyless alley; D 1925, G. W. Pabst) and *Kreuzzug des Weibes* (The woman's crusade; D 1926, M. Berger). On Pabst's film, see Ursula von Keitz, "Körper—Fleisch—Ding: Zur weiblichen Figur in G. W. Pabsts Die freudlose Gasse," in *Wien, die Inflation und das Elend,* ed. Armin Loacker (Vienna: Filmarchiv Austria, 2008), 77–107.

85. "Sie meint, sie kriegt alles umsonst. Sie weiß nicht, dass die Dinge ihren Preis haben."

86. Even the first shot of Annemie in which she looks at her reflection while her lover, standing behind her, kisses her neck—which she brushes off with the comment "Das Kleid macht mich alt" (This dress makes me look old)—echoes symbolic representations of vampirism and depictions of woman and death.

87. "Mit Verantwortung können Sie der Jugend heute nicht kommen, die hat zuviel hinter sich."

88. "Wir denken nicht an morgen. Was findet sich heute zusammen, ohne nachzudenken."

89. See Schwarz, "Vom Jahrmarktsspektakel," 14.

90. In the later stages of the Weimar Republic and during the Nazi period, nonfiction films were shot and copied on 35mm film, but with the expansion of the educational and training film business in the 1930s, and increasingly with the development and improved quality of 16mm safety material as well as mobile projectors, they were also screened in locations other than cinemas.

91. The catalogues of West German culture and documentary films and of the DEFA, which I examined for this essay, do not provide any information about the 16mm editions. They only give details of the 35mm editions. See Deutsches Institut für Filmkunde, *Katalog der westdeutschen*; Manfred Lichtenstein, ed., *Defa 1946–1964: Studio für Wochenschau- und Dokumentarfilme – Filmographie* (Berlin: Hentschel, 1969). As well as *Defa 1946–1964: Studio für populärwissenschaftliche Filme (und Vorläufer)-Filmographie* (Berlin: Henschel, 1997). A study of their historical reception in the period between 1945 and 1949 remains a desideratum, an important element of which would be to determine which films produced on health, medicine, and hygiene in the years of Allied occupation were original productions, imported, or approved for rerelease and which reached their audience via the large number of mobile cinemas deployed in cities and in the countryside. See Clemens, "Umerziehung," 252.

92. They thus take up health policy aims already formulated under the Weimar Republic.

Chapter Eight

International Animation Aesthetics at the WHO

To Your Health *(1956) and the Global Film Corpus*

Kirsten Ostherr

At the inaugural meeting of all representatives of the World Health Organization—the World Health Assembly—in July 1948, the delegation of the United States of America submitted a resolution sponsored by the Association of American Medical Colleges (AAMC) on "the Importance of Stimulating the Production, Use and Exchange of Films and Other Audio-Visual Media in Medicine, Health and Their Related Sciences."[1] Endorsing the WHO Constitution's stated objective of "promot[ing] improved standards of teaching and training in the health, medical and related professions," the AAMC argued that films are "powerful tools" for instruction, and therefore the WHO director-general and Executive Board should actively promote the use of films in health education.[2] In the decades to come, the WHO took up the challenge, producing a wide range of films that covered major disease eradication campaigns, captured important meetings and historic events, and disseminated the ideals of good health. Although plenty of the WHO's activities took place far from the silver screen, the organization also produced a substantial corpus of films whose content and style provide a window onto the prevalent methods for communicating ideas about global health in the postwar period. Moreover, because the organization contracted with various international filmmakers to make their movies, the WHO corpus also reveals slivers of other cinema corpora that these studios created. As a sponsor of films that were explicitly intended to circulate worldwide, the WHO might be seen as a curator of global styles in persuasive media, though the absence of a cohesive, centralized film program at the WHO makes this impression somewhat misleading. Instead, one might think of the WHO film corpus as a random sampling of instrumental techniques from two major genres of sponsored cinema in the postwar era: documentary and animation.

From this vantage point, the boundaries of the WHO film corpus shift, depending on emphasis: while all of the films commissioned by the WHO are linked by content ("world health"), their form and style may suggest that other aspects, such as genre and aesthetics, are more salient indicators of the work that these films actually do. In other words, the WHO film corpus might serve as the archive of concerns that drove this idealistic organization in its early years: health campaigns centering on malaria, tuberculosis, sexually transmitted diseases, maternal and child health, environmental sanitation, and nutrition.[3] But an exploration of the work of the WHO that focuses solely on the content of its publicity without attending to the methods of presenting that information would miss the more engaging features of these films as they were viewed by audiences. For the many thousands of WHO film viewers worldwide, this collection of motion pictures was not recognizable as a unified corpus; instead, it was part of a broader international media circuit defined by different and overlapping corpora. Unlike many industrial film producers that explicitly branded their training films as marketing tools by highlighting corporate identity within the film itself, most of the WHO films only mentioned the sponsoring organization in a brief opening or closing credit. In this light, the success of the most popular WHO films would depend on their effective use of genre and aesthetics as vehicles for audience engagement rather than on the appeal or importance of viewing "a WHO film" per se. Animated health films sponsored by the WHO would be viewed in relation to other animations exhibited in a given film market, regardless of whether they were shown theatrically for commercial gain or nontheatrically for educational purposes. Indeed, the animated film *To Your Health* (1956) was one of the most celebrated, widely distributed, and long-lived of the WHO films, in part, I will argue, because of its place in an international aesthetic movement.

While the productivity of the WHO films may result more from their generic corpus than their production corpus, the total archive of films commissioned by the World Health Organization nonetheless serves as a unique form of evidence for understanding twentieth-century biocultures as media formations. Moreover, as an archive that includes the health film equivalent of the blockbuster as well as many less notable entries, the WHO film corpus provides a rich and complex instance for considering the methodological question of the corpus and the exemplary case. Through a discussion of the unique attributes of animated health films as distinct from their documentary counterparts, this chapter will consider how postwar styles of health communication come to serve different interests in the global public sphere. An in-depth examination of *To Your Health* (Halas and Batchelor/WHO, 1956) will frame analysis of the production and reception of the total WHO corpus while raising broader questions about the utility of animation as a technology of representation, persuasion, and biomedical documentation.

This study is fundamentally concerned with the productive tensions of the corpus as a methodological frame. It asks, "What can we learn by considering the WHO films as a corpus containing an exemplary "blockbuster"? What can we learn about audio-visual health campaigns by examining one film in depth, or many films in aggregate? On what basis should representative films be selected? Particularly in the case of sponsored films, it may be impossible to conduct large-scale comparative studies of the sort that might shed the most light on recurring production practices, reception, or population-scale effects (these films were made as "health interventions," after all). In the absence of this sort of "quantitative" study, on what basis might we construct a comprehensive account of the role of sponsored films in shaping health practices in the mid-twentieth century?

The impetus for this study came from research on historical health and medical films produced by the WHO, the American College of Surgeons, the US Public Health Service, and others. Part of this work involved viewing of hundreds of health and medical films from the early twentieth century onward, and the ubiquitous use of animation in the postwar period seemed to indicate that these films were responding to a new set of representational concerns. Moreover, the complex status of the animated sequences within the instructional or educational films in which they appeared suggested a paradigm shift in frameworks for visualizing health and disease that demanded further examination. While highly creative uses of animation occurred in health films starting at least in the 1920s (and possibly earlier), the function and aesthetics of the form took on radically different characteristics in the postwar period, as demonstrated by the animated films of the World Health Organization. Because detailed records exist documenting the production, exhibition, and reception of these films, they can serve as a powerful case study of a pivotal period in global health history. These films can simultaneously serve to illuminate an important period in cinema history, crossing the genealogies of animation, documentary, sponsored film, and health/medical film. One goal of this study, then, is to assess how the international field of animation as a whole changed during and after World War II, in order to explain how changes in the techniques and economics of representation impacted health and medical media. To understand the changing status of animation in this subfield of sponsored film, this chapter will consider what cultural, industrial, and technological developments may have enabled these changes to occur, exploring their consequences in relation to larger debates about the role of visual media in health campaigns.

Epistemologies of Medical Animation

Initially serving as a means to visualize organisms or processes that could not otherwise be captured with a camera or seen with the naked eye, early medical animation often appeared as an interlude between live-action segments of a film. Many of the early examples of medical animation demonstrated ingenious solutions to problems of representation (for instance, how to visually depict the living body's interior decades before the development of effective laparoscopic cameras), and some of these solutions were so cleverly actualized as to seem indistinguishable from documentary footage.[4] Employing a range of stop-motion and hand-drawn animation techniques, the artistic (and nonmechanical) quality of these images was often highlighted in publicity for the films. But in terms of their evidentiary status, the animated sequences were nonetheless treated as continuous with the more overtly scientific (noninterventionist, mechanically produced) parts of the film; that is, they were treated as enhancements of the film's technical and educational merits rather than as departures from these objectives.

Although animation continues to serve the function of creatively expanding the documentary field of vision in midcentury health and medical films, this period is also marked by the proliferation of a different type and function of animation—the 100 percent cel animation film that exploits the medium's capacity for abstraction and reduction of visual detail, in contrast to the use of animation to fill in otherwise invisible details. Not only did these fully animated postwar films exhibit an alternate aesthetic (described as "modernist" by some, more on this below), they were often produced for different audiences as well, usually targeting mixed specialist and nonspecialist audiences, including the general public. In contrast, the earlier films that deployed animation as a scientific mode of imaging tended to target medical specialists exclusively. This stylistic distinction signals a deeper division between health and medical films, akin to what Scott Curtis has described as the distinction between educational films and research films.[5] Implicit in this distinction, Curtis argues, are the films' "presumptive modes of viewing": in the research film, "scientific observation connotes an attentive, measuring gaze" and "the *production* of knowledge," while educational film viewing presumes a more passive "spectatorship" and "therefore implies the *consumption* of knowledge."[6] At the level of explicit WHO rhetoric, the presumed film viewers might start off as passive spectators of educational films, but through the films they would learn to implement the featured health interventions, thus attaining the status of experts in a locally situated sense. However, the flow of knowledge about health problems and their solutions remained unidirectional in this era, as film commissions originated at the WHO headquarters in Geneva, Switzerland, not in the provinces served by regional offices. Thus, even the spectators of successful educational films would continue to embody the "untrained eye" of the lay viewer. As we will see, this status had important implications for cinematic techniques in animated health films in this era.

For the purposes of the present discussion, the postwar period marks a decisive shift in animation practices and aesthetics for two major reasons: the World Health Organization was founded in 1948, and most of the European animation studios with whom the WHO contracted to produce films were similarly born in the postwar moment. However, the transition actually begins during World War II, when the field of animation entered into the realm of sponsored industrial films, often through government service, just as many producers of other types of nontheatrical films also did during the war. For example, United Productions of America (UPA), the animation studio that scholar Michael Barrier has called the "Disney" of 1950s animation design (its aesthetic influence on other animation studios mirrored Disney's stylistic dominance in the 1930s–40s), was originally founded in 1943 to produce an industrial film teaching welding to shipyard workers. Reflecting this strategic orientation, the studio initially operated under the name Industrial Film and Poster Service and was commissioned to produce a series of films for the US Army and Navy from 1945 to 1947.[7] The studio also produced animated films for other government agencies, such as the State Department and the Office of War Information, before it moved into commercial work when such contracts dwindled during the postwar recession (especially for studios with obvious leftist political orientation, such as UPA).[8] But the end of government commissions did not mean the end of industrial work for this studio; on the contrary, UPA produced films in the early 1950s for the American Petroleum Institute, the American Cancer Society, CBS Radio, Aetna Casualty and Surety Company, and AT&T.[9] Similarly, the studios that produced the films under consideration in this essay also worked extensively in sponsored film.

As the UPA example demonstrates, most of the successful postwar American animation studios produced both commercial entertainment and industrial films, often gaining attention through work in advertising that led to commissions for educational films. Although sponsored films have historically been treated as an aesthetically impoverished domain of production, comparing unfavorably to the riches of independent art film production, from the perspective of the animators the sponsored projects often allowed for greater creativity and stylistic innovation. As Bill Hurtz, director of industrial films at UPA recounted, "Not only did the corporate sponsors offer generous production budgets, but the films were also creatively challenging because the sponsors knew and cared little about animation, which afforded the artists freedom to experiment with different styles."[10] Hurtz goes on to describe the additional levels of creativity required when working with sponsors whose values the studio abhorred. In one case (the American Petroleum Institute), the animators decided to put the objectionable messages of their sponsor into musical form in an effort to undermine the potency of the rhetoric. An important lesson from the UPA example, then, is that the politics of sponsored filmmaking cannot be read transparently off the surface of the film, as the values and objectives of the sponsoring organization may be radically transformed when translated into the medium of film.

Instead, Thomas Elsaesser's "rule of the three A's" (from the German *Auftraggeber*, *Anlass*, and *Anwendung* or *Adressat*) offers an alternate strategy for analyzing the sponsored animation under discussion here. Elsaesser discusses the need for attention to three central issues in analyses of nonfiction films: who commissioned the film, the occasion for which the film was made, and the use to which it was put or the audience to which it was addressed.[11] The case studies presented here were all commissioned by the World Health Organization. While the occasions for these films and their uses and audiences varied, they were all made for continuous use in educating diverse audiences (including nonspecialists) about health-related issues (that is, they were made for widespread distribution and exhibition, unlike other sponsored films that were made for very specific occasions).

One question the current study immediately raises for Elsaesser's framework is that of aesthetics. While Elsaesser's method explicitly aims to avoid the pitfall of assuming that the meaning of an industrial film can be learned from examination of the film's style and content alone, he may go too far in avoiding attention to the mode of representation as potentially reflective of a larger production context. This issue is particularly vexing in studies of sponsored films, which are often only available for study as orphan films whose production, exhibition, and reception histories may be irretrievably lost. However, in dialogue with Elsaesser's argument, Vinzenz Hediger and Patrick Vonderau offer a strategy for addressing these stylistic concerns:

> The industrial film is a format that, by its very nature, demands serial analysis . . . comparative analysis of a large corpus of film materials. Among other things, such an analysis can yield insight into possible stylistic and rhetorical patterns and parameters that are used recursively, i.e., that reappear regularly with only minor variations. . . . If the recursive patterns of style that a serial analysis focuses on turn out to be conventionalized in the sense that they occur regularly and reliably in different industries, places, and time periods, they can then be analyzed with regard to what you might call their organizational functionality.[12]

This approach may enable the present study to determine whether different uses of animation in health and medical films (as exemplified by *To Your Health* and the rest of the WHO corpus) constitute recursive stylistic and rhetorical patterns which could, in turn, yield insight into broader patterns of conceptualizing and defining health and disease through visual representation. As Elsaesser concisely notes, "The industrial film [is] one of the very special resources for our knowledge about the forces that have shaped the 20th century," and it is a core premise of this study that educational-biomedical-industrial films likewise are a unique resource for understanding the privileged role of visual media in shaping the functionality of contemporary biopower through discourses of health.

Citing the work of JoAnne Yates, Hediger and Vonderau further argue that "the modern corporation depends on the emergence of new media such as the telegraph, the telephone, the typewriter, and the tabulation machine, as well as through the coordination of these media in a *Medienverbund*, i.e., the coordination of several media in a media setup."[13] Understood as particular types of modern corporations, the same could be said of the hospital, medical clinic, or public health department—the organizational entities meant to be served by the animated films under discussion here. Indeed, Joel Howell has made this case in "Technologies Transforming Health Care: X Rays, Computers, and the Internet,"[14] where he argues that the typewriter, the telephone, and the automobile should be understood alongside the x-ray, electrocardiogram, and insulin as technologies that were integral to the modernization of medicine in the late nineteenth and early twentieth centuries. As Hediger and Vonderau note, "Industrial films are perhaps best understood as *interfaces* between discourses and forms of social and industrial organization."[15] Thus, we might consider animation alongside other types of medical imaging devices as a technology that transformed biomedical communication—and therefore transformed biomedical organization—in the middle of the twentieth century.

Postwar Sponsored Film and Global Health Initiatives: *To Your Health* (1956)

While international health efforts long predate World War II, the postwar era saw a dramatic expansion of this work, most visibly in the creation of the World Health Organization in 1948. As I have discussed elsewhere, the global scale of the WHO's pursuit of public health after World War II created an enormous demand for personnel trained in specialized health surveillance techniques, which in turn presented the need for what was called a "universal" language of international communication.[16] The shortage of experts available to respond to the suddenly urgent demands of world health prompted investment in efficient and mass-reproducible technologies of instruction; the transnational dissemination of training in the techniques and ideology of world health could only be accomplished through the use of audiovisual aids.[17] Consequently, the medium of film attained a uniquely privileged status in promoting world health during and after World War II.[18] (Indeed, the US Centers for Disease Control launched its own film production studio after the war, and when new headquarters were constructed for the CDC in 1960, an entire building was dedicated to the audiovisual unit, containing two large sound stages, several darkrooms, and a state-of-the-art sound department.)[19]

The WHO's first commissioned film was *The Eternal Fight*, a mixed animation and documentary style film produced for the United Nations Film Board in 1948.[20] Since World Health Day was first celebrated in 1950, the WHO has often commissioned a short film (when finances permit) for the upcoming year's theme; for example, *Smallpox, Merciless Traveler* was produced for the 1965 theme, "Smallpox, constant alert."[21] The WHO commissioned twenty to thirty films in the two decades after it was formed, engaging various US, Eastern, and Western European documentary filmmakers and animation studios for these productions. While no comprehensive catalog of WHO films exists, other early titles include *Somewhere in India* (1952) and *World Without End* (1954), the award-winning documentary produced by Paul Rotha and Basil Wright for UNESCO. Like other allied United Nations agencies, UNESCO produced films that dealt in part with the work of the WHO, and these films might be considered as part of the broader WHO corpus, although they were usually distributed by UN organizations other than the WHO.[22]

By the time the WHO celebrated its twentieth anniversary in 1968, at least fifteen of the organization's films were actively circulating (as advertised in WHO publications), and several were in production.[23] Although the organization had commissioned or produced additional films by this date, titles were regularly withdrawn from circulation for the same reasons that health and medical films in general often had short lifespans: new research discoveries deemed them obsolete or harmful, a better film on the same subject became available, public interest had waned, or new media technologies superseded the old, and only the most requested titles were transferred to the new medium. The films contained in the 1968 film catalogue therefore represent either new releases or those titles that had stood the test of time.

Six of these fifteen films were animated, as was one of the three films in production. The films were:

Table 8.1. Films listed in *World Health: The Magazine of the World Health Organization* (January–February 1968).

Year	Title	Director	Producer	Location	Topic	Animated
1955	*We Have the Cure*	Unknown	Realist Films	London	Campaigns against treponemal diseases worldwide, but especially in the tropics	No
1956	*To Your Health*	Philip Stapp	Halas and Batchelor Limited	London	Alcoholism	Yes
1958	*La Lutte Contre La Lèpre*	Unknown	Actua Films	Geneva	About the fights against leprosy in central Africa	No
1958	*Open Your Eyes*	Gunther von Fritsch	Actua Films	Geneva	Eye disease in Morocco	No
1958	*People Like Maria*	Harry Watt	World Wide Pictures Ltd.	London	Celebrates the tenth anniversary of the WHO, describes "how better health is brought to many peoples"	No
1958	*Waters of Affliction*	Unknown	Alfred Wagg Pictures, and Audio Productions	Washington, D.C., and New York	Pilot project for control of bilharziasis in the Philippines	No
1961	*Water*	Philip Stapp	Center for Mass Communication of the Columbia University Press	New York	The world water crisis	Yes
1963	*The Monster and You*	Boris Kolar	Zagreb-Film	Zagreb, Yugoslavia	Tuberculosis	Yes

1964	*Doctors in the Making*	Jo Muras	Documentary Programs Inc.	Hamburg, Germany	Education and training of Congolese medical students in France and public health personnel in Ethiopia	No
1965	*Man Alive*	Janine Hamel-Minne	United Nations	unknown	Overview of the work of the WHO	No
1965	*Operation Beheira*	Tadeusz Jaworski	Documentary Film Studio	Warsaw, Poland	WHO project to control bilharziasis in the province of Beheira in the United Arab Republic	No
1965	*Smallpox, Merciless Traveller*	Vaclav Bedrich	Czechoslovak Film Studios	Prague, Czechoslovakia	The history of smallpox worldwide	Yes
1965	*Speciosa*	Tadeusz Jaworski	Documentary Film Studio	Warsaw, Poland	Training of nurses in the newly independent African nation of Burundi	No
1965	*Visit in the Desert*	Tadeusz Jaworski	Documentary Film Studio	Warsaw, Poland	WHO project to control communicable eye diseases in Sudan	No
1967	*False Friends*	Alison de Vere	Interfilm Limited	London	"Dependence-producing drugs," specifically, opium addiction	Yes
1967	*Little Man—Big City*	Gyula Macskassy and György Varnai	Pannonia Studios	Budapest, Hungary	Urban health problems	Yes

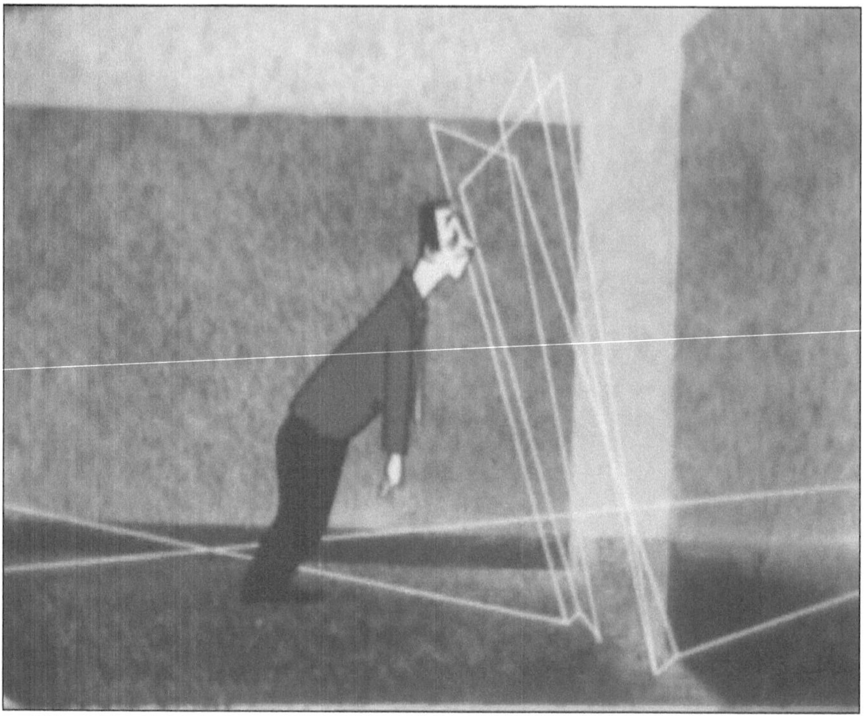

Figure 8.1. The inebriated "any man" protagonist of the film stumbles home from a party through a swaying doorframe. *To Your Health* (Halas and Batchelor/WHO, 1956).

The animated films on this list were produced in Zagreb, New York, London, Prague, and Budapest. As noted above, many of these studios were engaged in a range of sponsored film projects and commercial advertising. Television markets played a central role in the explosion of animation studios in the United States during the 1950s, when, according to some estimates, one out of every four advertisements on television was animated.[24] However, this arrangement was not typical of the international animation scene. As Giannalberto Bendazzi argues in *Cartoons: One Hundred Years of Cinema Animation* (1994), the status of animation in the postwar era was sharply divided by the Iron Curtain. While the rapid growth of advertising on television provided economic and creative opportunities for animators in capitalist countries, in the socialist states of Eastern Europe, "all efforts were directed toward the development of national cinemas. . . . Working as the sole producer, promoter and distributor, the State sponsored only certain kinds of animation, resisting market forces and using cinema for educational purposes."[25] (Adolf Nichtenhauser notes in his unpublished manuscript, "A History of Motion Pictures in Medicine," that many national cinemas, especially in Europe, got their start through state-sponsored educational

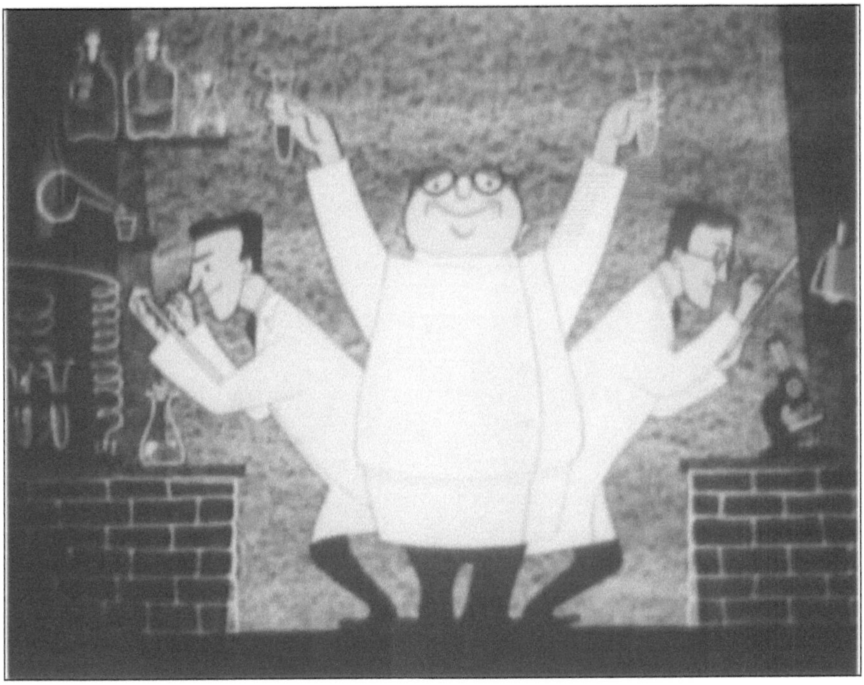

Figure 8.2. A team of scientists attempts to explain alcohol. *To Your Health* (Halas and Batchelor/WHO, 1956).

filmmaking, and he argues that health and medical films made up a significant portion of these films.[26] In this light, the histories of state-sponsored animation and state-sponsored medical film may be institutionally interwoven in important ways.)

Hungarian émigré John Halas founded the British animation studio Halas and Batchelor with his partner Joy Batchelor in 1940. The studio produced many wartime propaganda films for the British government and earned international acclaim for its postwar adaptation of George Orwell's *Animal Farm*, released in 1954 as Britain's first animated feature film.[27] Two years later, the studio released *To Your Health*, a nine-minute animated film about alcoholism, for the World Health Organization. The film production was supervised by a scientist, Professor E. M. Jellinek, whose studies of alcohol defined the research-based approach to the disease in the 1950s. Jellinek was a WHO consultant for the "Expert Committee on Mental Health, Alcoholism Subcommittee."[28] The film presents alcoholism as a social problem and a medical problem, describing through humorous didacticism how alcohol consumption affects the body and how it can impact a person's health, livelihood, and relationships.

While *To Your Health* follows one character as he converses with scientists throughout the film, the content is not structured as a narrative, but rather

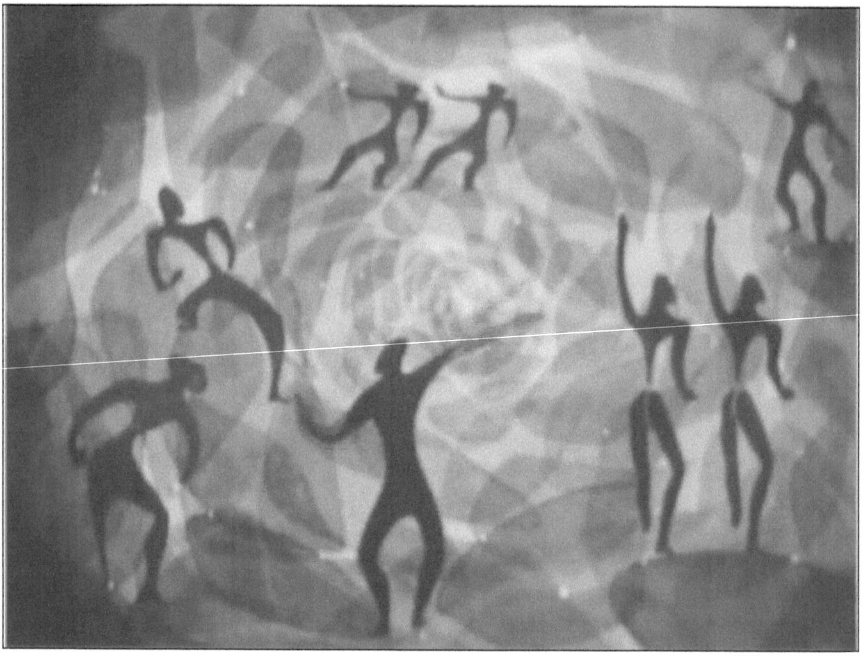

Figure 8.3. Abstract renderings of the interior of the human brain. *To Your Health* (Halas and Batchelor/WHO, 1956).

as a series of informative facts. Viewers meet the film's "any man" protagonist, named "John, Johann, Juan or Jacques," in a party scene where he alternately charms and argues with the other guests, eventually breaking a bottle of wine before he floats out of the scene (fig. 8.1). As a voiceover asks, "What is alcohol, anyway?," a series of figureheads appear in the background to present ideological responses ranging from puritanical condemnation to commodification, leading the frustrated "John" to ask for some "unprejudiced opinions, some facts." At this point a team of laboratory scientists enters the scene, offering up the requested hard data by explaining how alcohol is made, how it enters the bloodstream when consumed, how it causes drunkenness, diminishes mental and physical faculties, and eventually leads to loss of consciousness (fig. 8.2). Each of the film's "factual" explanations is visualized through highly stylized renderings of chemistry and anatomy (figs. 8.3–8.4).

Admitting that very few people die from taking too much alcohol, the scientist cautions against other dangers, such as drinking and driving. This leads "John" to ask, "Why do people drink?" After explaining that most people drink because it is the socially accepted thing to do, the narrator presents a harrowing case of the exception: the tortured alcoholic who begins with a "deep internal conflict" and ends by losing his family and his job before landing in prison or the hospital, "depending on whether his community understands that he is not

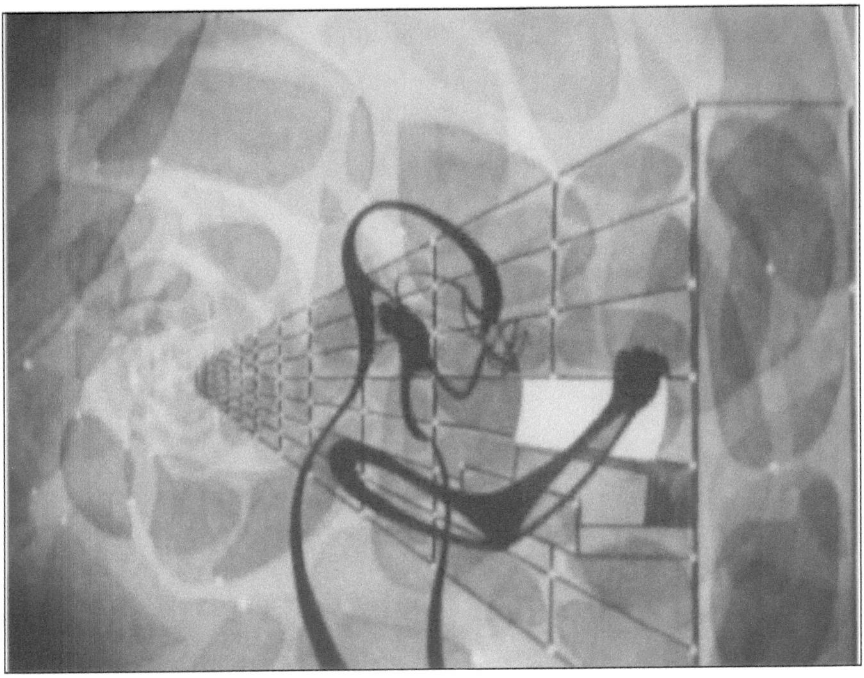

Figure 8.4. The brain's executive function and memory bank. *To Your Health* (Halas and Batchelor/WHO, 1956).

a criminal, but a sick man" (figs. 8.5–8.6). Finally, the long social history of drinking frames the open-ended conclusion of the film, which asks, "The problem stands: will alcohol control us, or can we control alcohol?"

To Your Health was directed by Philip Stapp, an American animator who had worked with Halas and Batchelor on *Animal Farm*. Stapp produced many sponsored educational films, including a series on South American countries for the US government, and film archivist Geoff Alexander has described the unique qualities of his style: "As opposed to the static animation style inherent in many contemporary educational films, Stapp's figures instead float, split apart, dissolve, spin, and vaporize in a constant state of metamorphosis."[29] Stapp's work in the 1950s stood out for its abstract, highly stylized renderings of human figures that "often exist on Tanguy-like watercolor-washed plains containing surrealistic elements, changing states through shifting line, color, and shape."[30] In contrast to earlier health films that folded realistic animation into a scientific, documentary format, I contend that the marked lack of realism in *To Your Health* played an important role in the global success of the film, as we can see from the following discussion of the film's distribution, exhibition, and reception.

While most of the films in the 1968 WHO catalogue list only one or two distributors, *To Your Health* had distributors in Denmark, Finland, France, Japan,

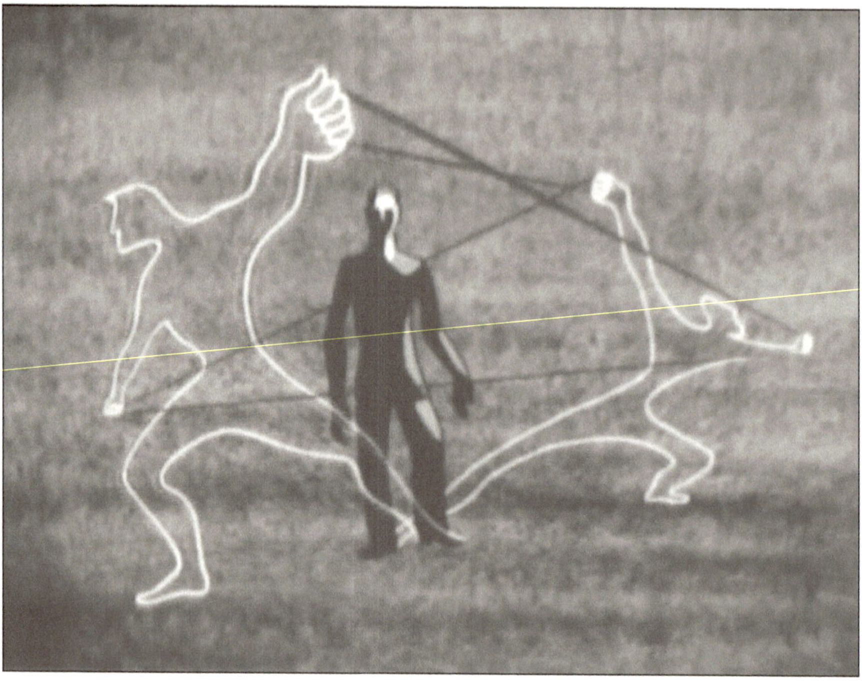

Figure 8.5. Stylized rendering of the alcoholic's internal conflict. *To Your Health* (Halas and Batchelor/WHO, 1956).

New Zealand, Portugal, South Africa, Sweden, Switzerland, the United Kingdom and Ireland, the Americas, and the USSR. Versions of the film were available in the dominant languages of these countries, as well as Greenlandic and Faroese. Any request to produce a new language version of the film was granted, provided the solicitor would pay the costs of translation. Usually, the translation was undertaken independent of the WHO and Halas and Batchelor.

Around the world, *To Your Health* was shown to national and regional health organizations, health professionals, the general public, societies for mental health, alcoholism clinics, AA groups, secondary school children, temperance societies, police officers, church groups, and others. In New Zealand alone, copies of the film were requested as soon as it was released for showing at the Otago Medical School in New Zealand, the New Zealand equivalent of Alcoholics Anonymous, and at the meeting of the Australian and New Zealand Association for the Advancement of Science.[31] The film had considerable commercial success in this country, and by 1961, the 20th Century Fox Film Corporation had secured exclusive rights to distribute the 35mm version of the film throughout New Zealand.[32] Significantly, the film drew audiences interested in the problem of alcoholism as well as film society audiences who were attracted by the film's animation auteurs.[33]

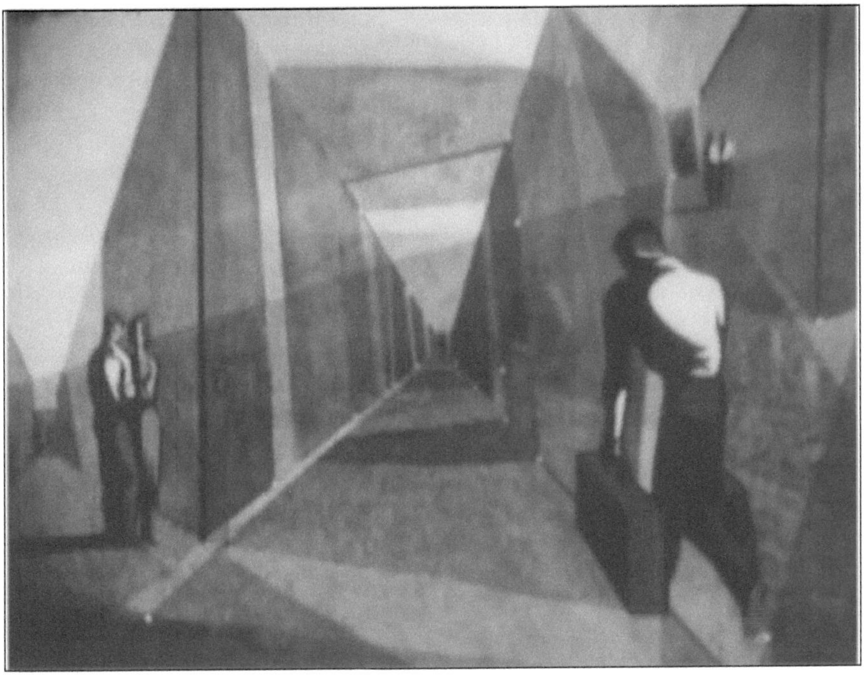

Figure 8.6. Surrealistic depiction of the protagonist's social isolation and decline. *To Your Health* (Halas and Batchelor/WHO, 1956).

Similar accounts of the high demand for this popular film can be found in other countries worldwide, from Japan to South Africa, reaching many thousands of viewers in each setting. *To Your Health* was also shown to thousands of college students in India through a series of screenings in 1962.[34] The Bahrain Petroleum Company ordered a copy in 1970.[35] In 1976 a copy was requested for use in the School of Nursing and Obstetrics in Mexico,[36] and another copy was requested that same year by the head mistress of the East Sussex County Grammar School for Girls in the UK.[37] In 1977 over two thousand viewers saw the film in Ireland.[38] The Italian Red Cross purchased fifteen copies of the film in 1980.[39]

To Your Health seemed to function equally well among crowds of urban sophisticates and in far-flung missionary outposts, suggesting that reports of its success were not merely selecting for positive results among strategically targeted audiences. After a Danish version of the film was made in 1959, the Statens Filmcentral (national film board) proudly informed the WHO that the film would have its premiere in fall of 1960, and that "it will have its first performance at the most fashionable cinema of Copenhagen early in September together with a Danish feature film [*Panik I Paradis*] which means that we may safely assume already now that the film will be seen by a maximum of filmgoers."[40] By

1961 the Swedish Board of Temperance Education had already purchased and distributed 121 copies of the film in that country alone,[41] and an additional forty copies had been purchased by 1963.[42] Various Swedish temperance organizations requested copies to be sent to Kenya and the Republic of Congo, and they requested a version to be made in Swahili.[43] A Portuguese missionary in Angola requested a copy of the film in 1958, explaining that "this is for use among the indigenous peoples of whom alcohol is enemy No. 1."[44] The widespread use of *To Your Health* for such "civilizing" missions demonstrates the film's textual ambiguity; as discussed below, far from condemning all use of alcohol, the film actually makes fun of ideologue reformers.

In 1957 the producer-in-chief for the Commonwealth of Australia, Dept. of Interior, Film Division suggested, "The film should be shown on television, for nine out of ten sets in New South Wales are in hotel bars!!"[45] Indeed, *To Your Health* aired on television in the Netherlands in 1960, in Norway in 1962, in Spain in 1973, and probably in other countries as well.[46] By the mid-1980s, *To Your Health* had been translated into twenty-six languages, and over three thousand prints were still in use.[47] In this era, the WHO received numerous requests for permission to make videotape copies of deteriorating 16mm celluloid prints of the film.[48] WHO agreed to this practice for noncommercial purposes.[49] The film was distributed on videotape as late as 1999, but by 2003 it was no longer in regular or backlist circulation (the section of the WHO Video Catalogue on "substance abuse" exclusively contained anti-tobacco films; none were on alcohol).

Pleasure and Pedagogy

What might account for the tremendous international popularity of *To Your Health*? The film's lack of overt branding or sponsorship may have played a role in enabling audiences to enjoy *To Your Health* as entertainment rather than as a sponsored health message. While this film predates the earliest experiments in the field of "entertainment education," Stapp, Halas, and Batchelor, and perhaps the WHO as well, seemed to have an intuitive grasp of the power of pleasure over pedantry when it came to educational films. Indeed, the WHO remarked on the film's subtlety as promotional material in its celebration of the film's success:

> A film enterprise unique of its kind was the animated cartoon on alcoholism, produced in colour in 1956. This film, entitled *To Your Health*, makes no mention of WHO, but aims exclusively at presenting the problem of alcoholism in a way that will engage the interest of the general public and enlarge popular understanding of the alcoholic's behavior. It has been well received by the people most closely concerned with this problem in many countries, and over three hundred prints in English and French were sold within twelve months of its release. German and Swedish versions have been produced by private

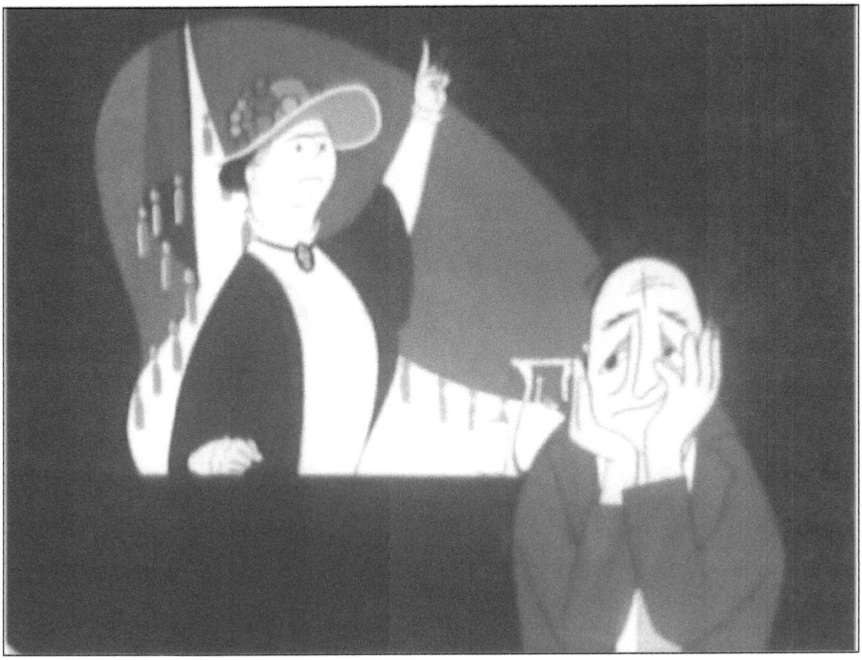

Figure 8.7. The temperance reformer denounces alcohol. *To Your Health* (Halas and Batchelor/WHO, 1956).

> organizations, at their own expense. It seems likely that the demand for this film will continue for many years."[50]

Moreover, the novel fact that the film was the first fully animated, color film commissioned by the WHO also accounted for some of its appeal. Twelve years after its release, the WHO counted the film a success that paved the way for further experiments with animated health films. As noted in a celebration of the WHO's achievements at its twentieth anniversary, "Experience with animated cartoons has been favourable. A short colour cartoon is often more successful than an ambitious feature film and presents no major language problem. *To Your Health*, a cartoon film on alcohol and alcoholism made in 1956, is still in wide use; 160 copies were sold in 1966 alone."[51]

As an animated film, *To Your Health* was able to traverse boundaries of language more fluidly than a documentary film, but the specific qualities of the film's animation style also played an important role in underscoring two other vital aspects of its mode of address: its sense of humor and its lack of narrative closure. Employing animation's innate capacity to transcend the laws of physics that more strictly govern spatial and temporal relationships in live action cinematography, *To Your Health* is able to present the negative effects of alcohol consumption in a lighthearted manner that would allow audiences to enjoy the

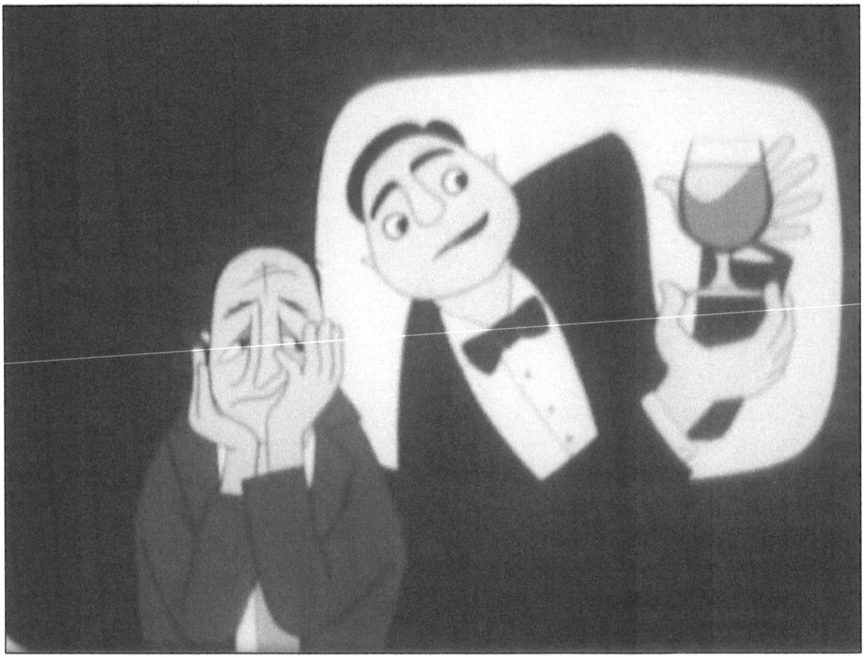

Figure 8.8. Television advertisements lure viewers. *To Your Health* (Halas and Batchelor/WHO, 1956).

cartoon even as it presents a serious message. For instance, the film shows the protagonist "John" in a fight scene and a car crash without delving into the more somber consequences of those events. While documentary realism might have a more profound impact on its viewers, it might also force them to confront the subject matter of the film in all of its unpleasantness—a form of spectatorial engagement that health communications experts and media producers alike have found to be the least likely to result in effective "interventions."[52] John Halas and Roger Manvell have described this effect in relation to *Without Fear*, an animated film about totalitarianism:

> These facts of life would normally be repellent or boring or unintelligible or at the least uncomfortable for the average citizen to absorb during his leisure—far too much like work or formal education for him to bother to look up from the sports page and take note. But these films were also entertainment and so made their point painlessly—either deriving a dramatic impact from the subject or winning the sympathy and good humour of the public because of what was in effect the aesthetic impact of the film, the graphic charm or force of its presentation.[53]

The "good humour" of *To Your Health* extends to its treatment of the traditional lay "experts" on alcoholism, thus positioning *To Your Health* as an amused observer of the punctilious temperance reformer (fig. 8.7) who proclaims, "Alcohol is the root of all evil! Down with king alcohol!" Next, the smiling television spokesman (fig. 8.8) asks, "Have you tasted the delicious flavor of Bacchus sparkling nectar?" The puritanical teetotaler opines, "It's drinking causes most of the world's misery!," and the angry workingman asserts, "It's the miserable state of the world that causes so much drinking!" All of these statements leave "John" clutching his head and begging for "unprejudiced opinions," which the scientists happily provide, even as their unbiased research practices are made comical through their dance-like movements in the laboratory, accompanied by quirky musical punctuation.

While *To Your Health* offers a lighthearted approach to a serious subject, the impact of its humor is enhanced by the open-endedness of its narrative.[54] As noted above, the film proceeds according to a didactic format rather than a classical narrative structure and consequently abandons the standard arc that moves from conflict to resolution through the logical cause-effect chain that characterizes traditional storytelling.[55] Instead, the core conflict—"will alcohol control us, or can we control alcohol?"—is only presented at the film's conclusion, leaving the audience with an open question to ponder rather than a strict prescription for proper behavior. Of course, the correct answer is clearly that "we control alcohol" rather than the reverse, but the specific implementation of that directive is left entirely to the viewer's interpretation. Indeed, the film acknowledges that for many people, alcohol consumption is a harmless social pleasure, and by offering this viewing position coupled with an open ending to the film, *To Your Health* simultaneously warns against the dangers of alcoholism and invites the audience to enjoy a drink. Using a conventional toast—"To your health!"—as its title, the film manages to preserve the pleasure and camaraderie of drinking while also signaling that too much pleasure can be harmful to one's health.

Working in tandem with the film's humorous tone and its open narrative structure, the graphical style of *To Your Health* also features techniques that may have played an important role in the film's broad success. Specifically, the film's abstraction, lack of photographic referentiality, metamorphosing human figures, and surreal backgrounds placed its aesthetics within the international, cosmopolitan design movement of the mid-twentieth century that rejected the dominant Disney animation aesthetic of the 1930s–40s as "firmly entrenched in nineteenth-century pictorial realism with the aim of creating an 'illusion of life.'"[56] In contrast, the mid-century modernist aesthetic that many animation studios (including Halas and Batchelor) adopted in the 1950s broke from the Disney style:

> Designers discarded the earlier reliance on circle and oval graphic formulas and created cartoon characters with a variety of sophisticated "modern" elements, including hard-edged Cubist shapes and organic biomorphic forms reminiscent of Miró, Calder, and Noguchi. . . . Fifties animation featured a more stylized, often abstract, approach to movement. . . . Backgrounds were drawn with little attempt at re-creating a three-dimensional setting, and academic perspective was considered old hat. . . . Background layouts were no

longer painted with realistic textures and photographically accurate shadows and lighting effects."[57]

Despite Disney's self-promotion as a "universal" style of entertainment, the abstraction of 1950s animation may have functioned as a powerful code for viewers, offering through alternate conceptions of realism a more open textuality that could embrace a broader range of international viewing positions. While "John" is clearly a white male figure who speaks English with an American accent in the original version of the film, the visualization of *To Your Health* did not limit the character to his "native" milieu. Instead, the protagonist was seen as amenable to reinterpretation through the simple translation of the soundtrack. In other words, "John's" American or western European characteristics were malleable enough to be easily converted into different national or regional characteristics, as evidenced by the many different language soundtracks and the film's wide success among the audiences for the translated versions.[58] As John Halas and Roger Manvell explained in *The Technique of Film Animation* (1959), "Where live action particularizes, animation generalizes, and in the process makes what it seeks to explain universal."[59]

Conclusion

How does *To Your Health* fit in with the rest of the WHO corpus? What can we learn about the corpus from focused attention to one exemplary film? As noted in the introduction to this essay, the WHO film corpus did not emerge as a result of a master plan or with a clearly defined set of objectives. Instead, films were made to serve a variety of specific needs for high priority health campaigns. Sometimes the films addressed topics of broad concern that traveled well, such as *To Your Health*, and at other times, films were made on local issues that only existed in specific parts of the world, such as *Waters of Affliction* (1958), which addressed "a pilot project for control of bilharziasis in the Philippines."[60] Furthermore, some of the films were documentaries, others were animated, and as I have argued above, the specific mode of address in *To Your Health* played an important role in the success of the film, suggesting that audiences would respond quite differently to a documentary on the same topic. While the WHO and other educational film producers clearly embraced animation as a powerful educational tool in this era, even among the animated films none was as successful as *To Your Health*. The crucial point, however, is that the success of this exemplary film was a model for the impact a health film *could* have, an ideal that undoubtedly shaped decisions large and small concerning future WHO film productions. From this perspective, the study of any film corpus can be greatly enhanced by close examination of an exemplary film that demonstrates the ideals to which the total corpus aspired.

As an exemplary film, *To Your Health* also offers the possibility of standing for a particular approach to health visualization that functioned as an "interfac[e] between discourses and forms of social and industrial organization" in the postwar era.[61] I have discussed elsewhere the tendency in some postwar health and medical films to pursue "authenticity" through indexical representational techniques that seem to close the gap between scientific and fictional modes of representing disease, especially in films that require the use of animation to visually represent invisible contaminants. *To Your Health* demonstrates a different use of animation, perhaps more in keeping with the goals of postwar commercial advertisement to please the largest number of eyeballs, rather than present a technically accurate depiction of disease. Amidi notes that in the 1950s, "Animation played a crucial role in Madison Avenue's efforts to break away from the antiquated 'hard sell' advertising technique and instead woo viewers with light-hearted wit and whimsy."[62] I would suggest that *To Your Health* may signal a broader tendency in postwar global health campaigns that mark a divergence of public health from biomedicine and animation from documentary. To explore this possibility, exemplary films should be identified from the larger corpus of postwar health and medical films, to be compared with one another and the broader corpora. The known, existing sponsored health films of the mid-twentieth century should be systematically reviewed to identify how many of them utilized animation, and to what ends. While such a project would undoubtedly face the challenges of incompleteness, lack of comprehensive catalogues, and missing documentation that plague all studies of sponsored film, it would enable scholars to begin a thorough analysis of the organizational functionality of animation in relation to other practices of medical visualization.

Notes

1. First World Health Assembly, July 15, 1948, 12.1.7.1.11 Technical Education, "Resolution of [the] Association of American Medical Colleges on the Importance of Stimulating the Production, Use and Exchange of Films and Other Audio-Visual Media in Medicine, Health and Their Related Sciences," *Official Records of WHO*, vol. 10, 12.
2. Ibid.
3. Kelley Lee, *Historical Dictionary of the World Health Organization* (London: Scarecrow, 1998), 11.
4. Kirsten Ostherr, "Operative Bodies: Live Action and Animation in Medical Films of the 1920s," *Journal of Visual Culture* 12, no. 2 (2012): 352–77.
5. Scott Curtis, "Images of Efficiency: The Films of Frank B. Gilbreth," in *Films That Work: Industrial Film and the Productivity of Media*, ed. Vinzenz Hediger and Patrick Vonderau (Amsterdam: Amsterdam University Press, 2009), 90–91.
6. Curtis, "Images of Efficiency," 91.
7. Amid Amidi, *Cartoon Modern: Style and Design in Fifties Animation* (San Francisco, CA: Chronicle Books, 2006), 112–13.
8. Ibid., 117.
9. Ibid., 126.
10. Ibid., 126.

11. Thomas Elsaesser, "Archives and Archaeologies: The Place of Non-fiction Film in Contemporary Media," in Hediger and Vonderau, *Films That Work*, 23.

12. Vinzenz Hediger and Patrick Vonderau, "Record, Rhetoric, Rationalization: Industrial Organization and Film," in Hediger and Vonderau, *Films That Work*, 37.

13. Ibid., 38.

14. Joel Howell, "Technologies Transforming Health Care: X Rays, Computers, and the Internet," in *Cultural Sutures: Medicine and Media*, ed. Lester Friedman (Durham, NC: Duke University Press, 2004), 333–50.

15. Hediger and Vonderau, "Introduction," in Hediger and Vonderau, *Films That Work*, 11.

16. Kirsten Ostherr, *Cinematic Prophylaxis: Globalization and Contagion in the Discourse of World Health* (Durham, NC: Duke University Press, 2005).

17. Ralph Chester Williams, *The United States Public Health Service, 1798–1950* (Richmond, VA: Whittet and Shepperson, 1951), 401.

18. A crucial—and rare—source of information about the wide distribution and exhibition of public health films is the work of Adolf Nichtenhauser, an early promoter of motion pictures as medical and public health training tools. See Adolf Nichtenhauser, "A History of Motion Pictures in Medicine" (unpublished manuscript, ca. 1950), Adolf Nichtenhauser History of Motion Pictures in Medicine Collection, MS C 380, Archives and Modern Manuscripts Program, History of Medicine Division, National Library of Medicine, Bethesda, MD.

19. As the postwar assistant surgeon general proudly proclaimed in his history of the USPHS, "The most complete and up-to-date equipment available for production of superior films, filmstrips, and slide series has been installed in the audio-visual production services of the center and well-trained technicians in this field have been employed. A film library is maintained which lends training films and filmstrips to health agencies and schools throughout the world." Williams, *United States Public Health Service*, 402. See also Elizabeth Etheridge, *Sentinel for Health: A History of the Centers for Disease Control* (Berkeley: University of California Press, 1992), 111.

20. For an extended discussion of this film, see Kirsten Ostherr, "Contagion and the Boundaries of the Visible: The Cinema of World Health," *Camera Obscura* issue 50, vol. 17, no. 2 (2002): 1–38.

21. World Health Organization, *The First Ten Years of the World Health Organization* (Geneva: Palais des Nations, 1958), 293.

22. Ibid., 449. See also *The UNESCO Courier* 7, nos. 4–5 (1954): 40–45.

23. *World Health: The Magazine of the World Health Organization* (January–February 1968).

24. Amidi, *Cartoon Modern*, 12.

25. Giannalberto Bendazzi, *Cartoons: One Hundred Years of Cinema Animation*, trans. Anna Taraboletti-Segre (Bloomington: Indiana University Press, 1994), 151.

26. Nichtenhauser, "A History of Motion Pictures in Medicine."

27. In recent years, historians have discovered that the US Central Intelligence Agency (CIA) played a central, though behind-the-scenes, role in this production. See Daniel J. Leab, *Orwell Subverted: The CIA and the Filming of Animal Farm* (University Park: Pennsylvania State University Press, 2007).

28. World Health Organization, Technical Report Series No. 42, Expert Committee on Mental Health, Report on the First Session of the Alcoholism Subcommittee, Geneva, December 11–16, 1950.

29. See Stapp filmography at Academic Film Archive at http://www.afana.org/stappfilms.htm (accessed April 25, 2016).

30. Ibid.

31. Archives of the World Health Organization, October 24, 1956, letter from W. B. Harris, Supervisor of Teaching Aids, New Zealand Education Department, National Film Library to WHO. Folder: *To Your Health*; Distribution: New Zealand; Visual Media Unit.

32. Ibid., Sept 26, 1961, letter from 20th Century Fox Film Corporation [N.Z.] Ltd. to Mary Losey, WHO. Folder: *To Your Health*; Distribution: New Zealand; Visual Media Unit.

33. Ibid., December 18, 1957, letter from Ian McEwan, National Society on Alcoholism, NZ to Mary Losey, WHO: Folder: *To Your Health*; Distribution: New Zealand; Visual Media Unit.

34. Ibid., October 29, 1962, letter from Mr. K. Peterson, National Temperance Society of India, Bhubaneswar, Orissa. Folder: Film: WHO: *To Your Health*; Distribution: India.

35. Ibid., August 12, 1970, Telex: From Caltex, London. Folder: *To Your Health;* Distribution: United Kingdom.

36. Ibid., May 4, 1976, letter from El Director de la Escuela de Enfermería y Obstetricia, Orizaba, Veracruz, Mexico, requesting copy of film. Folder: *To Your Health*; Distribution: Spain; Visual Media Unit.

37. Ibid., July 31, 1976, letter from Miss I. J. Brown, Head Mistress, East Sussex County Grammar School for Girls. Folder: *To Your Health*; Distribution: United Kingdom.

38. Ibid. Wexford Community Services Council, Wexford, Ireland, December 22, 1977. Folder: Film: WHO: *To Your Health*; Distribution: Ireland.

39. Ibid., February 28, 1980, letter from Croce Rossa Italiana to WHO. October 8, 1980, letter from Croce Rossa Italiana. Folder: *To Your Health*—Italy.

40. Ibid., August 22, 1960, letter from Statens Filmcentral to Losey.

41. Ibid., May 2, 1961, letter from Nils Sundberg, Swedish Board of Temperance Education, to Losey, WHO. Folder: *To Your Health*; Distribution: Sweden; Visual Media Unit.

42. Ibid., February 14, 1962, letter from Nils Sundberg, Swedish Board of Temperance Education, to Losey. March 26, 1963, letter from Nils Sundberg, Swedish Board of Temperance Education, to Losey. Folder: *To Your Health*; Distribution: Sweden; Visual Media Unit.

43. Ibid., August 15, 1963, letter from Grand Lodge of Sweden, IOGT (Godtemplarorden, Sveriges Storloge AV IOGT) requesting purchase and shipping of English version of film to Nairobi, Kenya. March 20, 1972, letter from Sveriges Blåbandsförbund, Medlem av Internationella Blå Korsfederationene, Örebro requesting purchase of French version of film, to be shipped to Komono, Rep. Pop. du Congo. October 3, 1967, letter from IOGT requesting price for English copy of film and asking availability of Swahili version. Folder: *To Your Health*; Distribution: Sweden; Visual Media Unit.

44. Ibid., letter of October 3, 1958, from James D. Ormiston, Missão do Dondi, Bela Vista, Angola to WHO. Folder: *To Your Health*; Distribution: Portugal.

45. Ibid., January 30, 1957, letter from Stanley Hawes, producer-in-chief, Commonwealth of Australia, Dept. of Interior, Film Division. Folder: *To Your Health*; Australia.

46. Ibid., May 3, 1960, Memo of agreement between WHO and Nederlandse Televisie Stichting, Bussum concerning the television exhibition of the motion picture *To Your Health*. Folder: Film: Alcoholism; Distribution: Holland. September 17, 1962, letter from Norsk Rikskringkasting, Oslo to WHO. Folder: To Your Health; Distribution: Norway; Visual Media Unit. October 19, 1973, letter from Hoffmann to Christina Navarro, Spanish Television, "Semanal Informativo," Madrid. Folder: *To Your Health*; Distribution: Spain; Visual Media Unit.

47. Vivien Halas and Paul Wells, *Halas and Batchelor Cartoons: An Animated History* (London: Southbank Publishing, 2006), 37.

48. Ibid., September 3, 1982, letter from Western Australia Alcohol and Drug Authority. Folder: *To Your Health*; Australia.

49. Ibid., September 22, 1982, from Hoffmann. Folder: *To Your Health*; Australia.

50. World Health Organization, *The First Ten Years*, 450.

51. World Health Organization, *The Second Ten Years of the World Health Organization, 1958–1967* (Geneva: Palais des Nations, 1968), 294.

52. On the modes of spectatorial engagement with realist documentary film, see Bill Nichols, *Representing Reality* (Bloomington: University of Indiana Press, 1992). On the effects of pleasure in health interventions, see Sheila T. Murphy, Lauren B. Frank, Meghan B. Moran, and Paula Patnoe-Woodley, "Involved, Transported or Emotional? Exploring the Determinants of Change in Knowledge, Attitudes and Behavior in Entertainment Education," *Journal of Communication* 61, no. 3 (2011): 407–31.

53. John Halas and Roger Manvell, *The Technique of Film Animation* (London: Focal Press, 1959), 133.

54. Debates about the historicity and meaning of the "open text" comprise an extensive body of scholarship ranging from the work of Roland Barthes, Jacques Derrida, and Umberto Eco in the 1960s to the present. For a concise overview, see Catherine Belsey, *Poststructuralism: A Very Short Introduction* (New York: Oxford University Press, 2002).

55. For an overview of classical Hollywood narrative structure, see David Bordwell and Kristin Thompson, *Film Art: An Introduction*, 10th ed. (New York: McGraw-Hill, 2012).

56. Amidi, *Cartoon Modern*, 12.

57. Ibid., 10–11.

58. For a useful counterpoint, see Ramón Reichert's discussion of abstraction in the animated management film, a subgenre of the animated sponsored film. Ramón Reichert, "Behaviorism, Animation, and Effective Cinema: The McGraw-Hill *Industrial Management* Film Series and the Visual Culture of Management," in Hediger and Vonderau, *Films That Work*, 284, 287–88.

59. Halas and Manvell, *Technique of Film Animation*, 134.

60. *World Health* (January–February 1968).

61. Hediger and Vonderau, "Introduction," 11.

62. Amidi, *Cartoon Modern*, 12.

Part Four

Constructing Audiences

Chapter Nine

Measuring Knowledge and Emotions

Audience Research in Educational Films at the Beginning of the Twentieth Century

Anja Laukötter

Introduction

The End of the Road, a 1918 film on venereal diseases directed by Army Lieutenant Edward H. Griffith of the War Department's Committee on Training Camp Activities, addresses the dangers of infection with sexually transmitted diseases. Like the venereal disease films *Fit to Fight* and *Fit to Win* (1918–19), it was produced by a close cooperation between the American Social Hygiene Association (ASHA) and the United States government to educate both military and civilian audiences.[1] Together, these films were the beginnings of a wider film production corpus on venereal diseases by the US Public Health Service (PHS) that would continue throughout the next decades. Like most of the films in the corpus, *Fit to Win* and *The End of the Road* were produced with the involvement of physicians. But what is remarkable about them is that, unlike the others in this corpus, psychologists were also involved in the production. As Katherine Bemet Davis remarked (here in respect to *The End of the Road*, but this is also true for *Fit to Win*): "The scenario has been most carefully worked out in consultation with physicians on the side of fidelity to medical fact, and with teachers as to the psychological effect."[2]

The involvement of physicians in the making of health education films has been well documented, but the involvement of psychologists might come as something of a surprise. This chapter aims to explain why both groups were involved in the making of these films, how they shaped the films' production and distribution, and what this tells us about the concerns of various stakeholders at a time when the place of film in public health education was up for grabs.

In the first place, I argue that although some health educators were eager to include films like *Fit to Win* and *The End of the Road* into campaigns against sexual transmitted diseases, they tended to regard motion pictures as an unruly technology. Movies could endorse the educational messages that they were commissioned to promote, but equally they could undermine such messages, and it was not always possible to predict how an audience might respond. Other historians have highlighted such concerns among public health educators.[3] However, what made the health educators who used the films *Fit to Win* and *The End of the Road* different was that unlike most other filmmakers, they turned to experimental psychologists for answers.

In the second place, I argue that experts in the burgeoning field of experimental psychology became interested in film as an object of their research for their own reasons. In particular, I argue that psychologists like the well-known behaviorists John B. Watson and Karl S. Lashley came to see film as a way of establishing the authority of their newly emergent field by exploring how the medium worked on both informational and emotional levels. Out of a broader self-created corpus of venereal disease films, the two researchers selected *Fit to Win* and *The End of the Road* because these films provided them with valuable opportunities to explore these issues. Thus, these motion pictures became the focus of the first substantial psychological film research projects in which the films were screened to a socially stratified audience with the aim of measuring emotional reactions and knowledge transfers. This chapter will analyze in detail how Watson and Lashley set up and conducted their research project to assess the effectiveness of the films from their perspective as psychologists (by using specific questions and methods of investigation, selecting films to create a corpus, creating audiences, and presenting results).

The chapter argues that psychologists used the film in two ways. They not only aimed to help the health educators answer questions about the effectiveness of film but also aimed to use the cinema as "experimental setting" in which they could answer questions of more general interest to psychology. This collaboration between health educators and psychologists in "objectifying" the effectiveness of these films provided a new way of constructing an audience and its perception (the calculated emotional reaction) that still has followers today. Indeed, the story of Watson and Lashley had implications beyond the field of health education. Audience research of the sort undertaken by these psychologists also became common in the commercial entertainment film business.

A final point needs to be made concerning the corpus. Although this work focuses on two films, these can only be understood as part of broader corpus of VD films identified by Watson and Lashley as potential subjects of study. As part of their research, the two psychologists first compiled a list of venereal disease movies that might be used in the study and then selected two that seemed to fit best with their research objectives. Indeed, constructing a corpus was crucial to

Watson's and Lashley's research methodology, and their research results were, I suggest, structured by their evaluation of the films within the corpus and how they fit their research objectives. Neither *Fit to Fight/Fit to Win* nor *The End of the Road* were ideal for research purposes, according to Watson and Lashley. They were, however, the best of the bunch, and Watson and Lashley did not allow their limitations to stand in the way of an evaluation of audience responses to information and emotion in public health films.

VD campaigns and Educational Film

It is well-known that venereal diseases became a major health and social problem in the United States in the late nineteenth and early twentieth centuries, and that vast public education programs were developed to teach people about these diseases and interventions against them.[4] In their view, public ignorance of the disease—how it was transmitted, what could be done to prevent it, and how it could be treated—undermined efforts to combat the venereal diseases and aided their spread, as did a general reticence among the public about the subject.

The entry in 1917 of the United States into the First World War reinforced such concerns. Venereal disease had long flourished during war, and military planners were concerned about its effect on military efficiency, effectiveness, and morale, with thousands of young men away from home and open to sexual encounters. A result was a renewed attention to health education to forestall the expected epidemic, which began in earnest after July 9, 1918, when the US Congress passed the Chamberlain-Khan Act. It ordered the allocation of $2 million to fight venereal diseases, and a division of the PHS that focused on the prevention of the spread of venereal diseases was created.[5] Under the direction of C. C. Pierce, clinics were built and educational programs were set up.[6] The explicit intention of these health education campaigns was to control venereal diseases not only among soldiers and sailors but also within the civilian population: to take care of "the men behind the men behind the guns."[7] As a commentator in 1919 noted, referring to anti-venereal disease programs: "Recognizing the tremendous social and economic losses resulting from venereal diseases even in time of peace, the program has been intensified and accelerated by the extraordinary conditions arising out of the war."[8]

The health campaigns that were part of this program turned to visual techniques to reach and inform different audiences (employees, soldiers, housewives, adolescents (both male and female), and rural and urban dwellers).[9] Thus, in the following years posters and illustrated pamphlets were widely circulated by the PHS in cooperation with local institutions and the American Social Hygiene Association.[10] Printed materials were adapted to target a variety of different groups: illustrated versions were produced specifically for the "coloured population" (assumed to be illiterate), and educational materials were printed in Yiddish, Spanish, and Italian as well as English.[11] In 1919 the PHS also funded up to eight thousand lectures at different institutions including schools, social and medical organizations, and women's clubs.[12] In addition, building on a growing enthusiasm for film as a quintessential modern tool of mass education, a dozen sex hygiene motion pictures were made available.[13]

These educational films were shown at a variety of venues (schools, universities, exhibition halls, theaters, war camps, and so on) and to different audiences, sometimes selected according to gender and belonging to specific social groups.[14] In order to adjust to their audiences, they were often shown in slightly different versions in which titles and names were changed and scenes were cut or inserted.[15] The venereal disease films *Fit to Win* and *The End of the Road* belong to this corpus, even before Watson and Lashley began their research.

The educational efforts of the special division in the PHS were influenced by H. E. Kleinschmidt, the American Social Hygiene Association's director of exhibits. In his influential essay *Educational Prophylaxis of Venereal Diseases* (1919), Kleinschmidt discussed the respective merits of appeals to fact and to emotion in public health campaigns. Although published after the wartime expansion of anti-venereal disease campaigns, this essay captured some of the issues that had dogged the campaign since its beginning. Thus, on the one hand, Kleinschmidt claimed that "perhaps the strongest factor in influencing the actions of men is knowledge—pure, unadorned knowledge of the facts concerning sex and venereal disease. On the foundation of correct knowledge the superstructure of right action is built."[16] On the other hand, he also argued that as "the appeal to reason" does not work for everyone, "the element of fear" needed to be exploited: "Fear of disease forms the backbone of practically every preventive medicine educational campaign."[17] In other words, emotions were the key to promoting knowledge for Kleinschmidt: "Knowledge is the electric wire which becomes a transmitter of power only when it has become activated by the living spark of determination."[18] And for Kleinschmidt, determination was often promoted by emotion. In Kleinschmidt's view, films were of particular interest to health education because of their ability to use drama (and hence emotions) to stimulate action.[19]

Kleinschmidt's comments on the emotional impact of film was an intervention in a much broader debate in the 1910s about the role of emotion in enhancing the educational value of film. For example, the psychologist and film theorist Hugo Münsterberg had argued in *The Photoplay: A Psychological Study* (1916) that one of the main ways in which films promoted their educational message was by evoking emotional responses in their audiences.[20] As the introduction to this edited volume sets out, Münsterberg had written *The Photoplay* in response to the moral condemnation of moviegoing, notably suggestions that it weakened the work ethic. For Münsterberg, movies were a particularly effective tool in reaching audiences because of their ability to circumvent voluntary effort. Motion pictures, he claimed, had a direct connection with involuntary mental functions, in part because cinematic techniques nearly mirrored some aspects of inner mental processes. Münsterberg was primarily interested in entertainment films, but his interest in the role of film in mirroring and stimulating emotional or mental processes would be widely taken up by advocates of the use of the medium as a tool of both social reform and education.[21] In Münsterberg's hands, movies thus became an emotional "psycho-technique," a concept that he had developed in his applied psychology monograph *Grundzüge der Psychotechnik.*[22]

Kleinschmidt's and Münsterberg's arguments about film as a tool of education were widely circulated and discussed in the 1910s, and they gained many followers. Others, however, expressed skepticism about the idea that drama (and the emotions it generated) could educate, that perhaps drama veered too far in the direction of entertainment. Of particular relevance to my argument, critics raised concerns that film in general and even more dramatized "sex films" would entertain but not educate, and worse yet might damage people's health.[23] These films with their potential to distract and mislead people seemed an uncontrollable danger to anti-venereal disease campaigns and the public they were said to serve.

Whether educational films should remain strictly informative, or whether they should also have an entertainment or emotional function, was therefore a continuing matter of debate.[24] And it was in this context that Watson's and Lashley's study was commissioned. None of the claims and counterclaims about the role of film entertainment and emotion in public health education were based on psychological research on audience responses. Watson and Lashley's study was to change all that. Kleinschmidt and Münsterberg might have opened the question of the emotional impact of film, but Watson turned it into an extensive research project.

Moreover, the idea of measuring efficiency was widely spread at that time. Promoted by Hugo Münsterberg's "psychotechnics," studies on the efficiency of work and labor were extensively explored in several experiments in the beginning of the twentieth century.[25] Besides Münsterberg, Frank and Lilian Gilbreth were "well-known efficiency experts," as Scott Curtis describes them. This couple became known between 1910 and 1920 because they had advanced Frederick Taylor's ideas of scientific management.[26]

Audience Research: Psychologists Measuring Knowledge (Transfer) and Emotional Reactions

Watson is widely regarded as one of the founders of behaviorism, the dominant school in American psychology during the 1920s. In his 1913 article "Psychology as the Behaviorist Views it," Watson presented what he called "purely objective" methods for the "control of behavior" and emphasized the necessity of a stimulus-response analysis.[27] In his view, predicting and controlling behavior were the main aims of psychology.[28] Drawing on a wide range of intellectual influences in a newly expanding field of research on emotions, including the work of Wilhelm Wundt and William James, Watson developed his concept of emotions. Drawing on William James's physiological model of emotion, he defined emotions in the following way, quoting James explicitly: "the bodily changes follow directly the perception of the exciting fact and . . . our feeling of the same changes as they occur *is* the emotion."[29] He went on to outline the connection of emotions with physiological processes in a later article.[30] Watson's approach to emotions is well-known to historians. But what is important for my essay is that his study of audience reactions to film made little use of either this definition of emotion or the theoretical assumptions about their relation to the body. Instead, it tended to refer to emotions in much the same way as Kleinschmidt as motivations for learning.

Watson's study of audience reactions was one of the first substantial studies in experimental psychology on the informational and emotional effects of health education films used in public hygiene campaigns on their audience.[31] It started when Watson applied for funding to the US Interdepartmental Social Hygiene Board on May 20, 1919, to undertake "a research which has for its object the determination of safe and scientific conclusions upon the informational and educative values of certain picture films."[32] The application, including the requested grant of $6,600, was accepted.[33] It had the backing of the committee, which included psychologists Adolf Meyer (Johns Hopkins Hospital), Shepherd Ivory Franz (Government Hospital for the Insane), and R. S. Woodworth (Psychology Department of Columbia University) and by the ASHA (including H. E. Kleinschmidt). For reasons that will be discussed later, Watson and Lashley chose *Fit to Win* and *The End of the Road* out of a huge corpus of health education films as particularly valuable for a study that would research the informational impact of the medium, as well as the emotional reactions and longer-term effects they had on viewers' everyday lives.[34] In comparison to other experimental settings at that time, the test audience was to be exceptionally large, with 4,800 members.

Watson and Lashley's goal was to test the idea that the transfer of knowledge was strongly linked to emotions. As they wrote in their published results in 1922, they viewed popular education on sex hygiene issues as striving to achieve two goals:[35] to increase knowledge on sexually transmitted diseases and to "arouse an emotional attitude in the public which will stimulate real application of the information assimilated, since it is doubtful if any amount of information without accompanying emotional factors will lead to significant changes in behavior."[36] Although the "need of information and emotional training for the public is universally recognized," it was still unclear, they claimed, which information should be the subject of a film, and which emotions should be stimulated in order to achieve permanent modifications of behavior. Consequently, they divided their research into three parts to measure respectively informational value, emotional effects, and modifications of behavior,[37] using methodological tools such as audience observation, interviews, and questionnaires. With the help of seventy-three voluntary field workers (physicians, social workers, and others) for the main study, and "various agencies" ("racially" divided) for a second, smaller testing group, the so-called town experiment, they studied the persistent effects of the films using follow-up interviews.

The proposed project was not without its critics: during the review of the proposal in 1920, PHS official C. C. Pierce, for example, voiced some criticisms about the planned approach of the research. But the overwhelming feeling on the Interdepartmental Social Hygiene Board was in favor of the proposal. Thus, T. A. Storey, the executive secretary of the board, emphasized the originality of Watson's research project. In his view it was "one of the best presentations of a research problem that had reached us."[38] He elaborated: "It has been our practice to make our appropriations on the basis of the promise of results that seems to be carried in a research program proposal, and even more importantly we have based our appropriations on scientific training and scientific reputation of the man from whom the application comes." It was with this backing that Watson and Lashley began their research.[39]

How *Fit to Win* and *The End of the Road* Were Selected

One of the first questions that Watson and Lashley had to address was which films they should study. They began by undertaking a preliminary survey to determine what medical knowledge health experts wanted to be included in public education film. As Watson and Lashley put it, they wanted to "obtain from medical men and women who have had most to do with problems in sex education and the actual treatment of venereal infections judgments and opinions as to what it is wise and safe to present to the public."[40] Thus, they sent questionnaires to members of three medical associations featuring forty-five questions on general sex education matters (parts one and two) and on health campaigns against venereal diseases (part three).[41] Parts one and two included such questions as: "Should information given to men and women differ?" and: "How frequent, in your experience, are cases of serious emotional shock at first coitus in women?"[42] Part three included such questions as: "Should the prevalence of venereal disease be emphasized?" and: "Will the belief in the only partial effectiveness of medical prophylaxis discourage its use?"[43] Watson and Lashley later published some of the results, including examples of actual answers (along with the names of the respondents) and sometimes short summaries of all answers were given.

The idea behind such questions was to identify a coherent body of knowledge that would be an aid for those who produced and evaluated new campaign material. Even more important, it could be used for checking whether the "facts" in existing educational material were "in harmony with medical opinion." Watson and Lashley argued that the study would focus on the "types of facts presented" so as to allow an examination of the "proper emphasis and the evaluation of the methods employed in various presentations."[44] Assuming an analytical distinction between knowledge and emotions, Watson and Lashley indicated that emotions function as highlighters of certain "facts" and, at the same time, as transmitters of "facts" to the audience.

Almost from the start, Watson and Lashley encountered difficulties. In particular, their survey revealed that there were several questions related to sex education and venereal disease campaigns on which *no* consensus of medical opinion existed. For example, medical respondents offered very different opinions as to whether "morbid fears" might result from the film, whether "self-applications of prophylaxis" should be included, and which facts introduced in films would be suitable for which age groups.[45] Despite such problems, however, Watson and Lashley concluded that *Fit to Win*, and *The End of the Road*, would work for their purposes, since these films sought to educate audiences in a variety of topics that were largely uncontroversial to medical experts, including the dangers of the disease, how it spread, its bacterial origin, and the health benefits of continence.[46] *Fit to Win*'s major problem was that it did not fully explain the possibilities and facts related to cure and prophylaxis.[47] In that sense, the films chosen were not regarded as "perfect." They were simply the best available—a pragmatic approach that also protected their results.

Fit to Win is a film that chronicles the sexual desires of five friends and their involvement with prostitutes and addresses the themes of morals and crime. While one among the group of five, Billy Hale, resists temptation, his four friends are exposed to the disease. Out of these four, only one, Kid McCarthy, uses medical prophylaxis and stays healthy, while the others get infected. Ultimately, Billy Hale and Kid McCarthy are both recruited for service abroad while the others are dismissed as unfit to serve and sent to the hospital. The version aimed at the military, *Fit to Fight* (1918), ended with these scenes and emphasized the importance of prophylactic measures. By contrast, in the adaptation for civilian audiences, *Fit to Win*, these scenes were shortened.[48] An epilogue was also added to the civilian version where Billy is seen returning from France as a captain, advising his company to be wary of prostitutes, carrying the medal for bravery of Kid McCarthy (who died in war) to his partner before marrying his own sweetheart.

While *Fit to Fight/Fit to Win* tells the story of male friends, the focus in *The End of the Road* is on the destiny of two young women who have different lifestyles. First, we encounter Mary Lee, who has left for New York to train as an army nurse after undergoing a liberal education. Her life is guided by strict values including sexual continence, which is rewarded, at the end of the war, with the great love of Dr. Bell, who epitomizes the ideal physician. Second, we encounter Mary's childhood friend, Vera Wagner, who is advised by her mother to marry a rich New York man in order to climb up the social ladder. Working in a department store, her life is governed by low morals and her desires bring her in contact with the "gigolo" Howard Lord, which leads "in the end to disease, desertion and disgrace" as the writer of the screenplay Katherine Bement Davis pointed out.[49] According to Davis, Vera is one of the girls who "through ignorance, through emotion, take steps which will lead to bitter regret."[50] With the help of her friend Mary, she agrees to get medical treatment and is cured. The main focus of the films is on Mary, who is presented not only as properly morally educated (she is sexually abstinent before marriage, although challenged about this by her friend Vera) but also as a determined and ambitious young woman.[51]

Although Watson and Lashey's preliminary survey concluded that both films might be appropriate for the planned research, the question was not resolved until the full study was about to begin. Thus, the full study reviewed a list of sex hygiene films that were "prepared" and "published" by the American Social Hygiene Associations:

Table 9.1. The corpus of films compiled by Watson and Lashley from which *Fit to Win* and *The End of the Road* were selected

And the Children Pay	*Some Wild Oats*
Birth—The Duties of Motherhood	*Open Your Eyes*
Cleared for Action	*The Scarlet Trail*
Damaged Goods	*The Solitary Sin*
The End of the Road	*The Spreading Evil*
Fit to Win'	*Venereal Diseases—Their Origin and Results*
How Life Begins	*Men's Lecture Film*
Know Thy Husband	

Source: Karl S. Lashley and John B. Watson, *A Psychological Study of Motion Pictures in Relation to Venereal Disease Campaigns* (Washington, DC: United States Interdepartmental Social Hygiene Board, 1922).

Most of the films in this corpus (put together by the researchers) addressed the subject of venereal diseases, though some, such as *Birth—The Duties of Motherhood* or *How Life Begins* were mainly focused on reproduction. It appears that most of these films (not all of those named above have been found yet) combined a feature story with medical-scientific discourse. The corpus includes commercial films such as *Damaged Goods* and *Spreading Evil*, and films such as *Fit to Win* and *The End of the Road* that were campaign films sponsored by the ASHA and the USPHS. Unlike the others, *Fit to Win* and *The End of the Road* were specifically produced to educate soldiers and domestic audiences in the context of the war effort.[52] The reasons why *Fit to Win* and *The End of the Road* were picked among this comprehensive corpus of venereal disease films are explicitly stated in the description of the project.[53] The films sought to impart "information and a definite emotional attitude," provide data in a very direct way and without an accompanying lecture, and used "dramatic methods for emphasizing some educational features." Moreover, the films addressed the "danger of disease and value of prophylaxis without stressing the moral aspects of the sexual problem." The survey singled out some of the "bad effects" of these films: the language was considered "crude," and they included scenes thought to be almost pornographic. Finally, the authors of the study argued that "in the clearness of its presentation of the causes and effects of venereal infection the film is inferior to others which have been produced, but these in turn lack the dramatic interest of 'Fit to Win' and are less typical of the majority of films produced."[54] In other words, while *Fit to Win* had some limitations in the sorts of knowledge it sought to impart to audiences, it allowed the researchers to explore the impact of drama and emotion on the educational value of film. Moreover, the film's structure appeared representative of that era's educational films, with a long introduction providing basic medical information followed by a short story of five men who encounter syphilitic prostitutes.

Ultimately, Watson and Lashley tried to choose movies that reflected the widest possible of range of arguments in the then-ongoing debate on the use of film in health education. Their extensive deliberations on these films and their selection for the study can also be understood as efforts to underline the scientific value of their work.

The Research Setting: Information and Emotions under Supervision

Watson and Lashley did not just select two films out of their venereal disease film corpus; they also created specific audiences for the screenings. For the purposes of the main study, the audience was divided along social and professional lines. There was a Medical Group (around forty physicians and nurses), an Executive and Clerical Group, a Literary Club Group, a mixed audience (250 men and women from a village in Pennsylvania), a Car Men Group (which comprised railway employees from New York City), a Merchant Sailor Group, and a Soldier Group.[55] By contrast, in the so-called town experiment, the audience was divided along lines of gender and race. Research for the town experiment was conducted in two small and "ultraconservative" (as they called them) towns on the Eastern Shore of Maryland to provoke "antagonism" to the films and their messages. In this town experiment, they showed *Fit to Win* to men and *The End of the Road* to women, segregated according to sex and race: "In the two towns 730 white men, 920 white women, 208 Negro men and 450 Negro women were reached."[56] For the researchers, the film's potential emotional effects included fear of infection, sexual desire, aversion toward men and toward sexual education, and fears involving aesthetic or religious traditions.[57] To measure these emotional effects, they adopted four methods that mixed observations of behavior in combination with the question-and-answer technique:

1. Questionnaires used before and after the screening.
2. Observations of the immediate behavior of the audience during the screening.
3. Interviews directly after the screening.
4. Study of the long-term effects together with physicians and social workers.[58]

Interestingly, psycho-physiological data on the bodily expression of inner conditions (such as heartbeat, blood pressure) often collected after the turn of the century were applied in later audience research projects (such as the Payne Fund Studies) but not in this study.[59] The measurements of such inner conditions required specific technical equipment that would have been difficult and expensive to use on such a large group as planned in the Watson project.

Watson and Lashley were worried about certain methodological problems. For example, they discussed the proposed technique of observation, concerned that the interpretation of the behavior and emotional reaction of the audience might be shaped by research team's preconceptions. Such concerns were not new: they had been debated in the course of discussions since the end of the nineteenth century over how emotions could be objects of empirical measurements.[60] In this case, Watson and Lashley asked the research team to document, but not interpret, the behavior (individual reactions of interest, boredom, embarrassment, collective reactions), comments made on the film, and facial expressions (such as crying, shock) of the audience.[61] Their work can be understood as employing emotions as a "commodity of exchange" (as Brenton J. Malin described it),[62] something triggered by the film and passed on to the audience, where they could be "read" by the researcher with his scientific tools.

In the first step of the main and town experiment, the research team used questionnaires and interviews in order to measure what members of both groups of each audience knew about the causes and effects of venereal diseases. By comparing the replies of individuals to several questions pertaining to the dangers of the disease, means of infection, and prophylaxis before and after the screening, they hoped to quantify the facts learned as a result of watching the films, thereby measuring the films' informational effects.[63] In spite of some internal disagreements, the research team regarded their sample as large enough to provide reliable information on the "average middle-class American."[64] The results of the preliminary and subsequent questionnaires indicated that the respondents had accumulated general information regarding communicability, seriousness, and so on rather than detailed knowledge.[65] A strongly positive impact was observed among audience members who had been completely ignorant and uninformed prior to watching the film. They seemed to have acquired information on the disease by watching the film, which Watson and Lashley argued had occurred when that information was "accompanied by the arousal of some emotional attitude." Several different emotional attitudes were examined:

1. Fear of infection.
2. Pride in physical fitness.
3. Patriotism and desire to keep fit to fight.
4. Interest in a possible sweetheart and the desire to keep clean for her sake.
5. Sympathy for innocently infected persons and the desire to protect them, apparently an appeal to the parental instinct.[66]

For the researchers, these emotions were intentionally "calculated" in the films in order to prevent the spread of venereal diseases. Yet they also commented that these imposed emotions could lead to "social maladjustments." For example, there were concerns that the "fear of infection" could be transformed into a "phobia" or into "disgust of the infected"; "continence in sex relations" might lead to "abstinence from marriage"; mentioning "sex topics" might increase interest in sexual intercourse, and so on.[67]

Watson and Lashley argued that strong if varied emotional effects were produced in the main study. The medical group, they reported, was bored, regarding the films as exaggerated and overly dramatic. The mixed audience had mixed reactions, from laughter (described in quotation marks as "horse laughter") to "frank embarrassment and discomfort," which led to a "disastrous" presentation. The car men "reacted rather strongly to the suggestive parts of the picture." The seamen showed an unforeseen appreciation of the film, while the soldiers were instructed to stay silent, orders they succeeded in obeying except for laughter at the bawdy house scene in *Fit to Win*. Regarding the "town experiment," a stronger emotional appeal was recognized in the "negroe audience." They were "more interested and enthusiastic than the whites in their immediate response to the picture" and more of them later sought medical advice.[68] Although the "town group" was regarded as ultraconservative, no religious or moral objections were voiced regarding the treatment of sex topics.[69]

To examine the emotional reactions in more detail, sixteen questions were addressed to each gendered group. Audiences were asked to check a list of possible emotional responses to the film, and far more negative emotions than positive ones were suggested as response, perhaps because these were the responses that most concerned the psychologists, or possibly the ones that they expected the most. One of these questions is most remarkable as it had a "great deal of affective value for the men" and generated "empathic" answers: "Would you want your sister or sweetheart to see such a picture?"[70] Another question, for women, suggests that the researchers either felt that women had a wider range of emotional responses than men (who are never given the range of possible emotional responses provided in this question) or that they needed help in determining which emotional response to choose: "Check the words that describe the way the picture made you feel": "Frightened, Interested, Indifferent, Sick, Fatigued, Unhappy, Excited, Disgusted, Angry, Indignant, Shocked, Amused, Skeptical, Bored, Resentful, Surprised, Tired, Blue, doubtful of the facts, Angry at being shown the picture."[71] Interestingly, sexuality-related emotional reactions (such as fear), which often came up in the discussion, were not mentioned explicitly in the audience responses.

The authors acknowledged that they could only measure the "relative effectiveness" of emotions but knew that there was no clear-cut experimental solution to that problem.[72] In the long term, Watson and Lashley argued, the results showed clearly that no "case of morbid anxiety, excessive curiosity, or any antagonism toward the performance" emerged.[73] In other words, the film did not cause "pathological" reactions—as some critics had argued. Moreover, no evidence was found to suggest that the films aroused sexual stimulation or antagonism, and no excessive emotional reaction was recognized.[74] At the same time, the emotional effects in both research experiments were regarded as merely temporary, showing few signs of causing persistent modification of behavior.[75] The researchers concluded that there was no evidence that (highly) dramatized scenes increased the informative value of the film: "Scenes like the bawdy house in 'Fit to Win' and the attempted rape in 'The End of the Road' have little educative value and unless they are handled with extreme skill and shown under careful regulation there is danger that they will have some erethitic [meaning arousing] effect . . . the dramatic parts are evanescent and without important effects upon behavior."[76] The researchers suggested that educational films should therefore provide greater detail and more accurate information.[77] Ultimately, the question of whether educational films should simply provide information or whether this information should be coated with emotional appeal was answered in the following way: "As used in the existing film the emotional appeals are not effective in modifying sexual behaviour, but they are effective in imparting realization of the need for educational and social reform."[78]

Fit to Win and *The End of the Road*—Educational Failures?

The researchers' conclusions suggested that providing medical information should be the main aim of these films and that appealing to emotion was not conducive to changing behaviors. These findings contradicted the common opinion of some health educators, who expected educational films to do more than just promote an "appreciation of the need for education" and to actually cause a change in the viewer's behavior. Watson and Lashley might have regarded *Fit to Win* and *The End of the Road* as educational failures, but their opinion did little to dent the popular appeal of these films.

All the films discussed here (*Fit to Fight, Fit to Win,* and *The End of the Road*) were widely shown to the public both before and after this research was conducted. Until 1924 all of them could be purchased from the Signal Corps, US Army, Washington, DC.[79] *Fit to Win* was also shown to soldiers and civilians alike, and recommended by the surgeon general in April 1919 for "the widest possible circulation in New York and elsewhere."[80]

According to the (questionable) numbers by Thomas C. Edwards, *The End of the Road* was shown to eight million people.[81] Jean B. Pinney claimed that it was even screened to a paying audience of twenty thousand people within ten days in Toronto in 1932.[82] After some objections by Public Safety Commissioner S. T. Fredricks, the film, originally produced for an all-female audience,[83] got its first private screening for men—namely, for two thousand Boston officers and enlisted men in February 1919.[84] Yet a few months later, in May 1919, the National Association of the Moving Picture Industry declared the film "morally unfit," and in August 1919 the ASHA asked the film distributor to dissolve their contract for commercial screenings.[85] In Pittsburgh, both *Fit to Fight* and *The End of the Road* were banned in 1921.[86] Other health education programs continued to use *The End of the Road,* and box office sales hint at a positive public response.[87] Box office numbers had long been used as an indicator of whether a film worked. As the figures suggested that the films were a success with the public, these numbers could be used for an argument that the films worked—though what "worked" meant when defined by box office receipts is less clear. It worked for theater owners who saw box office receipts fill their coffers; in similar ways it may have worked for the distributors and makers as well. But what it meant to the public is less clear—was it titillation and entertainment, or learning, education, and motivation for a change of health behavior, or even a mixture of both sides? As Miriam Posner notes in another essay in this collection—the commercialization of an educational films about VD was highly problematic in the postwar period. Paying for a movie about sex was akin to paying for sex.

Another indication of the complex response to the movie is that of H. E. Kleinschmidt, who interviewed some viewers after screenings in Boston in February 1919.[88] Based on their comments, Kleinschmidt concluded that the film was suitable to be screened for a "mixed audience." Watson and Lashley might have suggested that the long-term effects of the film were negligible, but for Kleinschmidt what was important was that the film managed to hold the civilian viewers' interest (though he conceded that it was too long for soldiers).[89] Others also disagreed with Watson and Lashley. The *New York Times*, for instance, called *The End of the Road* "the most valuable motion picture of its kind yet produced."[90] The reviewer had a strong opinion on the film's impact: "One feels clean after seeing it." At odds with Watson's findings, the cathartic effect he reported echoed the health educators' view of these films.

Conclusion

This essay has shown that scientifically based audience research had different meanings to different groups. Health educators hoped that it would establish the value of a controversial medium for their campaigns, while experimental psychologists mainly hoped to establish a new discipline in applying their expertise to a newly arising field of public concern. Although *Fit to Win* and *The End of the Road* were chosen from an educational film corpus after careful consideration, the results of the study indicated that the films were not as effective as hoped. In setting up their research agenda, the psychologists developed their own construction of how emotions should be studied scientifically, how educational effectiveness should be assessed, and what an audience is. This chapter has argued that others assessed the effectiveness quite differently. Still, Watson's and Lashley's approach left a mark. The question of how educational films should work (on both an informational and emotional level) first addressed with reference to these films, was followed up by later health educators and psychologists throughout the twentieth century. The perception of film as a medium with a "powerful emotional appeal"[91] has lingered on a discourse level and remains inherent in the idea that films can change public behavior. It is therefore not surprising that similar studies were conducted in other countries and that Watson's audience research project was received enthusiastically beyond the United States, despite its generally cautious assessment of the impact of emotion on learning.[92]

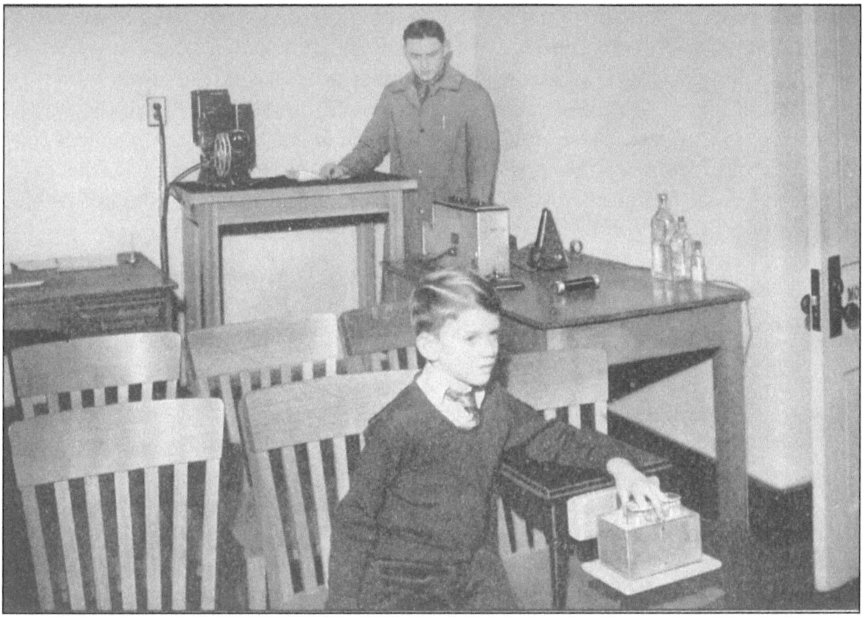

Figure 9.1. The use of the "psychogalvanograph" in Wendell S. Dysinger and Christian A. Ruckmick, *The Emotional Responses of Children to the Motion Picture Situation* (New York: Macmillan, 1933), plate 2.

The idea of measuring emotional effect scientifically was developed further in the late 1920s as the question of the effect of mass media (newspaper, radio, film) became a major focus of scientific and commercial interest, as did studies of the effect of different media in the classroom.[93] Regarding motion pictures, it is worth mentioning the 1928 "New York Experiment," in which the Columbia University psychologist William Moulton Marston tried to measure "romantic love" in "blondes" and "brunettes" watching romantic movies. Marston, a disciple of Hugo Münsterberg, measured women's reactions with a sphygmomanometer (to measure blood pressure) and a pneumograph (to measure breathing).[94] (Marston had invented the lie detector shortly before these experiments in New York but did not apply this measuring technique in this setting.)[95] The Payne Fund Studies, a set of thirteen psychological studies mainly conducted on children, published in 1933, went even further.[96] Disregarding the question of documentary versus fiction under the premise that "facts can be as emotional in their effect as fiction,"[97] they investigated the overall psychological effect of film. In addition to interviews, questionnaires, and behavior observation, techniques such as the "hypnograph"[98] and the "psychogalvanograph"[99] were employed to measure emotional effects. As these experiments were used in marketing strategies, they can be regarded as a form of "scientific marketing" to create "a realm of calculability"[100] in an economic sense. In this line of thought we can also read

Watson's research on the films *Fit to Win* and *The End of the Road* as an effort to calculate emotions for educative (economic) reasons. In that sense, health educators and psychologists shared an interest in the evaluation of the effects of educational films. Thus, both groups "discovered" the audience in a new way as it became an important reference figure in their fields. Ultimately, the fact that *Fit to Win* and *The End of the Road* found an audience despite their failure on a scientific level is neither a contradiction nor a surprise; it merely shows that the effectiveness of film can be appraised on different levels.

Notes

1. Robert Eberwein, *Sex Ed: Film, Video, and the Framework of Desire* (New Brunswick, NJ: Rutgers University Press, 1999), 21–22.

2. Katherine Bement Davis was a sociologist and director of the War Departments Committee on Protective Work for Girls. Katherine Bement Davis, "Social Hygiene and the War, Part II: Woman's Part in Social Hygiene," *Journal of Social Hygiene* 4, no. 4 (October 1918): 525–60, 558.

3. David Cantor, "Choosing to Live: Cancer Education, Movies, and the Conversion Narrative in America, 1921–1960," *Literature and Medicine* 28, no. 2 (2009): 278–332. Scott Curtis, "Dissecting the Medical Training Film," *Beyond the Screen: Institutions, Networks and Publics of Early Cinema*, ed. Marta Braun, Charlie Keil, Rob King, Paul Moore, and Louis Pelletier (Bloomington: Indiana University Press, 2012), 161–67.

4. Alexandra M. Lord, *Condom Nation: The U.S. Government's Sex Education Campaign from World War I to the Internet* (Baltimore: John Hopkins University Press, 2010); Eberwein, *Sex Ed*; and Allan M. Brandt, *No Magic Bullet: A Social History of Venereal Disease in the United States since 1880* (New York: Oxford University Press, 1985).

5. Gertrud, Seymour, "A Year's Progress in Venereal Disease Control," *Journal of Social Hygiene* 5, no. 1 (1919): 54–56.

6. Alexandra M. Lord, "'Naturally Clean and Wholesome': Women, Sex Education, and the United States Public Health Service, 1918–1928," *Social History of Medicine* 17, no. 3 (2004): 423–41.

7. Seymour, "A Year's Progress," 61.

8. Seymour, "A Year's Progress," 61; and "Battle Opens Here," newspaper clip, August 31, 1918, RG 112 290/44/24/00 General Correspondence Files, 1917–27, box 421, National Archives, Washington, DC.

9. RG 112 390/16/30/5 Entry 31, World War II Admin Records, box 1274, National Archives, Washington, DC.

10. RG 112 390/16/30/5 Entry 31, World War II Admin Records, boxes 1274–81, box 1277, National Archives, Washington, DC.

11. William F. Snow, General Director, American Social Hygiene Association to Thomas A. Storey, US Interdepartmental Social Hygiene Board, June 30, 1920, RG 90 130/63/2/5-6 Interdepartmental Social Hygiene Board, General Records, box 3, National Archives, Washington, DC.

12. Lord, "Naturally Clean," 428.

13. Eberwein, *Sex Ed*, lists of film, p. 236. On the enthusiasm for films see Martin S. Pernick, "Thomas Edison's Tuberculosis Films: Mass Media and Health Propaganda," *Hastings Center Report* 8, no. 3 (June 1978): 21–27; Martin S. Pernick, *The Black Stork: Eugenics and the Death of "Defective" Babies in American Medicine and Motion Pictures since 1915* (New York: Oxford University Press, 1996); Martin S. Pernick, "More than Illustrations: Early Twentieth-Century Health Films as Contributors to the Histories of Medicine and of Motion Pictures," in *Medicine's Moving Pictures: Medicine, Health, and Bodies in American Film and Television*, ed. Leslie J. Reagan, Nancy Tomes, and Paula A. Treichler (Rochester, NY: University of Rochester Press, 2007), 19–35; Miriam Posner, "Communicating Disease: Tuberculosis, Narrative, and Social Order in Thomas Edison's Red Cross Seal Films" in *Learning with the Lights Off: Educational Film in the United States*, ed. Devin Orgeron, Marsha Orgeron and Dan Streible (New York: Oxford University Press, 2012), 90–106; Stacie A. Colwell, "The End of the Road: Gender, the Dissemination of Knowledge, and the American Campaign against Venereal Disease during World War I," *Camera Obscura* 29 (May 1992): 91–129; Susan E. Lederer and Naomi Rogers, "Media" in *Medicine in the Twentieth Century*, ed. Roger Cooter and John Pickstone (Amsterdam: Harwood Academic Publishers, 2000), 487–502; Lisa Cartwright, *Screening the Body: Tracing Medicine's Visual Culture* (Minneapolis: University of Minnesota Press, 1995); and Adolf Nichtenhauser, "A History of Motion Pictures in Medicine" (unpublished manuscript, ca. 1950), Adolf Nichtenhauser History of Motion Pictures in Medicine Collection, MS C 380, Archives and Modern Manuscripts Program, History of Medicine Division, National Library of Medicine, Bethesda, MD.

14. Snow to Storey, June 30, 1920.

15. This happened in the case of *Fit to Win*, which was an adaptation for civilian use of *Fight to fight* (1918), the first film produced for the military.

16. Harry E. Kleinschmidt, "Educational Prophylaxis of Venereal Diseases," *Journal of Social Hygiene* 5, no. 1 (1919): 27–40, 28.

17. Ibid., 29.

18. Ibid., 29–30.

19. Ibid., 31.

20. Hugo Münsterberg, *Das Lichtspiel: Eine psychologische Studie [1916] und andere Schriften zum Kino*, ed. Jörg Schweinitz (Wien: Synema, 1996), 65–67. The term "emotion machine" established by Ed S. Tan originates in the ideas presented by Münsterberg at the beginning of the twentieth century. Ed S. Tan, *Emotion and the Structure of Narrative Film: Film as an Emotion Machine* (Mahwah, NJ: Erlbaum, 1996). Recent studies of feature film theory deal with the emotional experience of film audiences. Some have tried to research how specific takes, sequences or entire films generate empathetic or sympathetic response or how specific emotions like fear are reproduced and evoked in films. See Carl Plantinga and Greg M. Smith, eds., *Passionate Views: Film, Cognition, and Emotion* (Baltimore: John Hopkins University Press, 1999); Christine Brinkmann, "Die Rolle der Empathie im Dokumentarfilm," in *Kinogefühle: Emotionalität und Film*, ed. Matthias Brütsch et al. (Marburg: Schüren 2005), 333–60; and other authors. Others like Thomas Elsaesser have explored emotions in the wider context of the cinematic experience ("Kinoerfahrung"). Thomas Elsaesser, "'Zu spät, zu früh': Körper, Zeit und Aktionsraum in der Kinoerfahrung," in *Kinogefühle: Emotionalität und Film*, 415–39.

21. For Münsterberg films could stimulate different or the same emotions in the audience as displayed in the films. Münsterberg concentrated on the later ones and their mimetic potential. Especially in the context of delinquency the mimetic effects of film watching were widely discussed in the beginning of the twentieth century. For the history of the mimetic concept and its widely influence within the human sciences and film history see Lee Grieveson, "Cinema Studies and the Conduct of Conduct," in *Inventing Film Studies*, ed. Lee Grieveson and Haidee Wasson (Durham NC: Duke University Press 2008), 3–37.

22. See Hugo Münsterberg, *Grundzüge der Psychotechnik* (Leipzig, 1914). For him results of psychological research should be applied to different social spheres. Thus Münsterberg regarded psychology as in service of the modern world and its demands. For a wider discussion of Hugo Münsterberg and his perspectives on emotions, see Anja Laukötter, "How Films Entered the Classroom: The Sciences and the Emotional Education of Youth through Health Education Films in the US and Germany, 1910–1930," *Osiris* 31 (2016): 181–200.

23. Before he had seen a film at all in 1914 also Hugo Münsterberg had promoted the idea that films have an "unhealthy influence" on people and led to criminality and immoral pleasures. See Hugo Münsterberg, *Psychology: General and Applied* (New York: Appleton, 1914), 454.

24. Eberwein, *Sex Ed*, 16.

25. See for example Andreas Killen, "Weimar Psychotechnics between Americanism and Fascism," *Osiris* 22, no. 2 (2007): 48–71.

26. See Curtis, "Dissecting the medical Training Film," 162f. And Scott Curtis, "Images of Efficiency: The films of Frank B. Gilbreth," in *Films That Work: Industrial Film and the Productivity of Media*, ed. Vinzenz Hediger and Patrick Vonderau (Amsterdam: Amsterdam University Press, 2009), 85–101. See also A. Baumgart and D. Neuhauser, "Frank and Lillian Gilbreth: Scientific Management in the Operating Room," *Quality and Safety in Health Care* 18 (2009): 413–15. In this sense the Gilbreths had turned the questions of efficiency also to the medical realm, specifically to the work of surgeons in the operating room. Here they used film as a device to improve the work environment. Nevertheless it was Watson and Lashley to answer the question of whether and how educational films worked effectively to persuade the wider public in a comprehensive way.

27. John B. Watson, "Psychology as the behaviorist views it," *Psychological Review* 20 (1913): 158–77.

28. George Mandler, *A History of Modern Experimental Psychology: From James and Wundt to cognitive science* (Cambridge, MA: MIT Press, 2007), 99.

29. John B. Watson and J. J. B. Morgan, "Emotional Reactions and Psychological Experimentation," *American Journal of Psychology* 28, no. 2 (1917): 163–74, 163. Emphasis according to the quotation within the article by Watson.

30. John B. Watson, "A Schematic Outline of the Emotions," *Psychological Review* 26, no. 3 (1919): 165–96.

31. In a wider sense there had already been pioneering works on cinema audiences, such as Emelie Altenloh's 1911 sociological study on the social structure of cinema audiences in Mannheim (Germany), relying on a questionnaire survey. Emilie Altenloh, "Zur Soziologie des Kinos: Die Kino-Unternehmung und die sozialen Schichten ihrer Besucher" (PhD diss., Ruprecht-Karls-Universitaet zu Heidelberg,

Jena: E. Diederichs, 1914). An American example is Ray Leroy Short's 1916 study on one thousand Iowa City schoolchildren, who were submitted a questionnaire about their preferences in moving pictures ("love stories," "tragedies," "scenic," and "clearly educational" films). Garth S. Jowett, "Giving Them What They Want: Movie Audience Research before 1950," in *Current Research in Film: Audiences, Economics, and Law*, ed. Bruce A. Austin (Norwood, NJ: Ablex Publishing Corporation, 1985), 23.

32. John B. Watson, General Director, American Social Hygiene Association to Thomas A. Storey, US Interdepartmental Social Hygiene Board, May 20, 1919, RG 90 130/65/2/5-6 Interdepartmental Social Hygiene Board, General Records, box 3, National Archives, Washington, DC.

33. Thomas A. Storey, US Interdepartmental Social Hygiene Board to C. C. Pierce, April 13, 1920, RG 90 130/65/2/5-6 Interdepartmental Social Hygiene Board, General Records, box 3, National Archives, Washington, DC.

34. The study quantifies the probands of the socially stratified groups, ranging from 40 to 400 people; the "small-town-studies" count about 2,308 people.

35. Karl S. Lashley and John B. Watson, *A Psychological Study of Motion Pictures in Relation to Venereal Disease Campaigns* (Washington, DC: US Interdepartmental Social Hygiene Board, 1922).

36. Lashley and Watson, *A Psychological Study*, 4.

37. Ibid., 4.

38. Storey to Pierce, April 13, 1920.

39. Though not representative, the objection formulated by physician Bertha C. Downing, who strongly criticized the fact that two German- and Freudian-oriented researchers, namely Adolph Meyer and S. F. Franz, were involved in this project, is worth mentioning for its political impact. Bertha C. Downing to Carter Glass, Secretary of the Treasury, Washington, August 8, 1919, RG 90 130/65/2/5-6 Interdepartmental Social Hygiene Board, General Records, box 3, National Archives, Washington, DC: "Two German minds to one Anglo-Saxon to pass judgment on vital problems of Hygiene for our future U.S. Will not the reaction to this work be German? . . . Someone is asleep in Wash. and will waken some day to find our race a race of neurasthenics because the Germans made it so . . . War is not ended."

40. John B. Watson and Karl S. Lashley, "A Consensus of Medical Opinion upon Questions Relating to Sex Education and Venereal Disease Campaigns," *Mental Hygiene* 4, no. 4 (October 1920): 769–84, 769.

41. Including the American Psychopathological Association, the American Association of Genito-Urinary Surgeons, and the American Gynecological Society. See Watson and Lashley, "A Consensus," 770.

42. Watson and Lashley, "A Consensus," 772, 780.

43. Ibid., 830, 839.

44. Ibid., 843.

45. Ibid., 844–47.

46. Ibid., 844–46.

47. Ibid., 845. Each aspect is evaluated in seconds as for example 453 seconds are devoted to the subject of continence.

48. Lashley and Watson, *A Psychological Study*, 33.

49. Davis, "Social Hygiene and the War," 557. Contrary to Davis's argument, Martin S. Pernick describes both women as "innocent": Martin S. Pernick, *The Black*

Stork: Eugenics and the Death of "Defective" Babies in American Medicine and Motions Pictures since 1915 (New York: Oxford University Press, 1996), 148; and Pernick, "More than Illustrations," 19–35.

50. Davis, "Social Hygiene and the War," 533.

51. Eberwein, *Sex Ed*, 32.

52. Ibid., 22–23.

53. In this part of their study only the film *Fit to Win* was discussed, although in the following parts process the film *The End of the Road* was also included.

54. Lashley and Watson, *A Psychological Study*, 7.

55. Ibid., 14–15.

56. Ibid., 16.

57. Ibid., 11.

58. Ibid., 12–13, 37–38.

59. Also Hugo Münsterberg used these techniques in experiments on himself. For example he measured his pulsebeat in different situations. This form of self-experimentation belonged to comprehensive psycho-physiological experiments starting from the late nineteenth century on. See Otniel Dror, "The Scientific Image of Emotions: Experience and Technologies of Inscription," *Configurations* 7, no. 3 (1999): 355–401.

60. Wolfgang Schönpflug, "Aus den Anfängen der experimentellen Emotionspsychologie" in *Experimentelle Emotionspsychologie: Methodische Ansätze, Probleme, Ergebnisse*, ed. Wilhelm Janke et al. (Lengerich, Westfalen: Pabst Science Publishers, 2008), 47–62. See extensive works by Otniel Dror as, for example, Dror, "The Scientific Image."

61. Lashley and Watson, *A Psychological Study*, 41–42.

62. Brenton J. Malin, "Mediating Emotion Technology, Social Science, and Emotion in the Payne Fund Motion-Picture Studies," *Technology and Culture* 50, no. 2 (2009): 366–90, 387.

63. Lashley and Watson, *A Psychological Study*, 36–37.

64. Ibid., 26. This "average person" as an imagined parameter was also a focal point of censorship debates in Germany in 1920. Hermann Liepe, *Das Reichslichtspielgesetz vom 12. Mai 1920* (Berlin and Leipzig: de Gruyter, 1920).

65. Lashley and Watson, *A Psychological Study*, 39.

66. Ibid., 40.

67. Ibid.

68. Ibid., 80.

69. Ibid., 67.

70. Ibid., 50.

71. Ibid., 52. Capital letters in the source.

72. Ibid., 53.

73. Ibid., 58.

74. Ibid., 58.

75. Ibid., 59.

76. Ibid., 87.

77. Ibid.

78. Ibid., 88.

79. Major Dudnam, Medical Corps, US to H. M. Neeb, Major-General, New York, January 25, 1924, RG 112 290/44/24/00 General Correspondence Files, 1917–27, box 421, National Archives, Washington, DC. From August 1918 onward screening of the War Department film *Fit to Fight* for soldiers accompanied by a lecture of a medical corps member was compulsory throughout the country. See Adjutant General of the Army to all Department, Camp and Cantonment Commanders, July 8, 1919, RG 112 290/44/24/00 General Correspondence Files, 1917–27, box 421, National Archives, Washington, DC; and RG 407 370/79/20/3 Central Decimal Files, 1917–25 (726.1-1), box 1099, National Archives, Washington, DC. The Secretary of War, Adjutant General of the Army to all Department, Camp and Cantonment Commanders, July 8, 1918. This "*picture which deals frankly with prostitution and social disease and the importance of wiping them out of civilian life if we are to have an army fit to fight*" was shown to "big crowds" up to "fully 3000 men" a night or up to 67, 000 men a week. See "Battle Opens Here," August 31, 1918; and Walter Clarke, Captain, Sanitary Corps, US to Surgeon General of the Army, Report for week ending September 12, 1918, September 19, 1918, RG 112 290/44/24/00 General Correspondence Files, 1917–27, box 421, National Archives, Washington, DC. The screening to "*2000 men clerks of the leading retail store*" in Boston in September 1918 hints to the repeatedly used argument that the disease hit the industry. See "Strong Social Health Force," Newspaper Clip, August 30, 1918, RG 112 290/44/24/00 General Correspondence Files, 1917–27, box 421, National Archives, Washington, DC.

80. Surgeon General, US Public Health Service, attention of Doctor William A. Wilson, New York, April 8, 1919, and Royce R. Long, Captain, Sanitary Corps, US, Report for week ending 27th, 1919, RG 112 290/44/24/00 General Correspondence Files, 1917–27, box 421, National Archives, Washington, DC.

81. Edwards does not indicate a source for these numbers. Edwards, Health Pictures, 133–38, 137. He also mentions numbers for other films, claiming that *Working for Dear Life* was screened by 4 million viewers and *One Scar or Many* by 1.5 million viewers.

82. Jean B. Pinney, "The Motion Picture and Social-Hygiene Education," *Journal of Educational Sociology* 10, no. 3 (November 1936): 161.

83. Pinney, "The Motion Picture," 158.

84. Colwell, "The End of the Road," 110.

85. Ibid., 110.

86. J. E. Rush, "Critical Comment on Current Methods of Public Education in Venereal Disease," *American Journal of Sociology* 27, no. 3 (1921): 325–33, 329.

87. Colwell, "The End of the Road," 112.

88. Stanley P. Pavies, Captain, Sanitary Corps, US to the Surgeon General of the Army, February 8, 1919, RG 112 290/44/24/00 General Correspondence Files, 1917–27, box 421, National Archives, Washington, DC.

89. Pavis to Surgeon General of the Army, February 8, 1919. A letter of inquiry regarding the authorization for revisions was turned down by the director Edward Griffith. See Royce R. Long, Captain, Sanitary Corps, US to Major Swayer, February 19, 1919, and W. A. Swayer, Major, Medical Corps, Social Hygiene Division to Captain Long, February 22, 1919, NARA/RG 112 290/44/24/00 General Correspondence Files, 1917–27, box 421, National Archives, Washington, DC.

90. Opening the Road, review of *The End of the Road*, directed by Lieutenant Griffith, Plymouth Theater, New York, *New York Times*, March 2, 1919.

91. Thomas C. Edwards, "Health Pictures and Their Value," *The Annals of the American Academy of Political and Social Science* 128, *The Motion Picture in its Economic and Social Aspects* (November 1926): 133–38, 133–36. Also Charlotte Perkins Gilman, "Public Library Motion Pictures," *The Annals of the American Academy of Political and Social Science* 128, *The Motion Picture in its Economic and Social Aspects* (November 1926): 143–45, 145; Floyde E. Brooker, "Motion Pictures as an Aid to Education," *The Annals of the American Academy of Political and Social Science* 254, *The Motion Picture Industry* (November 1947): 103–9; Jean B. Pinney, "The Motion Picture and Social-Hygiene Education," *Journal of Educational Sociology* 10, no. 3 (*The Motion Picture in its Educational and Social Aspects*) (November 1936): 158–67.

92. See for example the German reception by the influential health educator Bruno Gebhard: Bruno Gebhard, "Karl S. Lashley, and John B. Watson, Psychologische Studien über die Wirkung von Filmen in der Bekämpfung der Geschlechtskrankheiten," *Hygienischer Wegweiser* 4 (1927): 123–25.

93. For an overview of other studies focussed on the mimetic influence of film on the audience see Grieveson, "Cinema Studies," 15–24. One example for a set of experiments on movies in the classroom is the study by Frank N. Freeman in 1924 where he comparatively researched the effects of books, images and films on students. Frank N. Freeman, *Visual Education: A Comparative Study of Motion Pictures and Other Methods of Instruction* (Chicago, 1924). See also Laukötter, "How Films Entered the Classroom."

94. Patrick Vonderau, "Bruenett bevorzugt: 'Erfahrung' in der Zuschauerforschung Hollywoods," *Montage AV* 19, no. 1 (2010): 135–60.

95. Vonderau, "Bruenett bevorzugt," 139. See also Stephan Durrer, "Emotional 'possession' im Kino: Sozialwissenschaftler auf den Spuren der Gefühle des Filmpublikums," *Traverse: Zeitschrift für Geschichte = Revue d'Historie* 14, no. 2 (2007): 85–99. For the invention of the lie detector, see for example, Geoffrey C. Bunn, "The Lie Detector, Wonder Woman and Liberty: The Life and Work of William Moulton Marston," *History of the Human Sciences* 10, no. 1 (1997): 91–119.

96. Arthur R. Jarvis, "The Payne Fund Reports. A Discussion on their Content, Public Reaction and Affect on the Motion Picture Industry, 1930–1940," *Journal of Popular Culture* 25, no. 2 (Fall 1991): 127–40; Malin, The Payne Motion-Picture Studies.

97. Marjorie Fiske and Leo Handel, "Motion Picture Research: Response Analysis," *Journal of Marketing* 11, no. 3 (January 1947): 273–80, 273–76.

98. Samuel Renshaw, Vernon L. Miller, and Dorothy P. Marquis, *Children's Sleep* (New York: The Macmillan Company, 1933).

99. Wendell S. Dysinger and Christian A. Ruckmick, *The Emotional Responses of Children to the Motion Picture Situation* (New York: Macmillan, 1933).

100. Vonderau, "Bruenett bevorzugt," 143, 149.

Chapter Ten

Truffle Hunters and Parachutists

In Search of the Audience for British Health Education Films, 1919–45

Tim Boon

How do films and their consumers interact? And what, if anything, can we know about this interaction if it has taken place in the past?

—Annette Kuhn

Introduction

"There [was] a vague feeling" in the 1920s "that places of public entertainment [were] responsible in some way for the spread of infection," as Allen Daley, MOH for Blackburn put it.[1] Droplet infections, strained eyes, and unsuitable and dangerous amorous liaisons were all on the bill. At the same time, voluntary health associations were falling over themselves to make health education films, to the extent that more than 350 were made and shown in Britain in the interwar period, and at least 50 during the Second World War.[2] So, while the public health professions might often have distrusted and feared the disease-spreading behavior of cinema audiences, others perceived them as peculiarly receptive to cinematic health teaching. Perhaps the audience was simply seen as susceptible to germs or to education. Certainly, health education films attracted substantial audience numbers: over three thousand were said to have attended a single showing of VD and TB films in the 1920s.[3] Dangerous or docile? It should provoke little surprise amongst historians of the interwar period to witness such divergent views of the "masses," here gathered together as audiences.

Most historical work on health education films has focused on their production at the expense of their consumption.[4] Serious study of this subgenre of films, anticipated by Rachael Low,[5] really began with Annette Kuhn's 1988 study, *Cinema, Censorship and Sexuality*.[6] This, like other studies of specific medical conditions including tuberculosis,[7] focuses on individual films within a broader account, although it gives more attention to who might have been watching than other studies do.[8] The current volume is eloquent testimony to the ways in which the field has opened up in the last quarter century, with more scholars making this subgenre a field of focused endeavor. Martin Pernick's 1996 book *The Black Stork* made a single film the core concern of a broad study of eugenics and euthanasia in America.[9] Subgenre studies have also appeared, including Kirsten Ostherr's work on notions of global contagion[10] and Elizabeth Lebas's study of British Municipal Cinema.[11] Some of this work has appeared as part of studies of medical films more broadly, including *Signs of Life* from 2005 and the 2007 collection *Medicine's Moving Pictures*. In both of these significant contributions to the literature, audiences are consistently alluded to but, with the exception of a useful two pages in the introduction to the latter, they are rarely the central concern.[12] These works touching on the history of health education films have been supplemented by the beginnings of work in cognate fields such as instructional and educational filmmaking.[13] Many of these authors acknowledge that serious issues surround questions of audiences and some suggest how differing kinds of access to their experience might be achieved. But focused concern with the study of audiences has been elsewhere, the principal concern of quite different groups of scholars, especially those in media, communications, and cultural studies concerned with the influence of the mass media in the later twentieth century.[14] To adopt the language of these writers, publications on the history of health education filmmaking have been dominated by the "text" at the expense of the audience.

The belief that the audience experience is beyond capture, in terms of both hard data and available analytical tools, has been widespread; Sylvia Harvey has commented that "there has been a tendency [for studies of film language and production] to be accompanied by an ill-considered and unhelpful assumption that all attempts at sociological research into the conditions of reception or consumption of filmic texts can only be manifestations of the rashest empiricism."[15] But unlike many movies, health education films were envisaged as instrumental; they were not made primarily for the sake of box office takings, or even of artistic expression, but to influence the health behaviors of viewers. Accordingly, there is a special case for audience studies here. But we need to beware anachronism. As we shall see, the people committed to the production of health education films, whether voluntary health associations or filmmakers, most often simply assumed that film was a powerful medium. The editors of the *Health Education Yearbook* stated in 1939, "The value of the Film as an impressive visual medium of education needs no emphasis."[16] For sure, the effects of the cinema on public behavior were part of the way that films were considered in our period, but this expressed itself more as a concern with general moral effects on impressionable groups than with detailed concern over the effects of individual films. This is visible in both the 1917 report, *The Cinema: Its Present Position and Future Possibilities,* which concluded that worries about the moral influence of films were overstated[17] and in Cyril Burt's 1925 publication *The Young Delinquent.*[18] Participants in health education judged the success of films in terms of audience numbers, not by any surveillance via opinion surveys, or of consequent attendance at clinics, or any of the techniques that are now the common sense of public health practice.[19] Accordingly, to ask about effectiveness in this sense risks wanting to know what contemporaries did not ask and therefore could not have known. For health educators, this would be the key question, but historians should be concerned with the operation of culture in the past, not with its evaluation.

Yet the sheer numbers of health education films produced in the period discussed here demands attention to reception, even if it is difficult; there are positive reasons to overcome doubts and to study the health education audience, and these have provoked the current essay.[20] In other words, there is a need to move the health education "text" from the center of analysis and to pay attention also to what the films actually meant to people. To do so respects all the participants on the historical ground, rather than privileging the producers. It offers the prospect of a "thicker" understanding of a culture becoming more infused with science and transformed by new communications media, including the cinema. It promises to illuminate the action of biomedical knowledge by asking questions about acceptance, assimilation, and resistance. In total, studying audiences may provide an opportunity to assess biomedicine's place in broader culture.[21]

This essay is a methodological contribution to the current collection; it proposes a series of approaches that scholars might take to the study of audiences for films of the kind discussed throughout the volume. Problems of lack of evidence are at their most acute for the early period covered here; this very starkness may be seen as helpful in revealing questions of audience more broadly. Unlike most of this book's other contributions, this essay uses its chosen corpus of films in illustration of my broader themes rather than as the main focus of the essay. Of the hundreds of health education films in distribution in the period explicitly considered, I have opted here to use as my principal examples the more than two hundred that fall into the style I have referred to as the "moral tale" genre, simply because it was so widely adopted by health educators. These fictional stories presented as entertainment films using moral narratives (featuring sequences of innocence, temptation, transgression, punishment, and atonement) were used by the majority of organizations that made or distributed health education in the period; the stories were intended to convey a health implication and an incitement to modify behavior. There were, for certain, other genres of health film in circulation at the time, including factual films in an instructional mode, such as the Eugenics Society's 1938 *Heredity in Man,* and health documentary films that were descriptions of areas of concern, such as *Enough to Eat?* (1936),[22] but the majority of films intended to change health behavior did take the moral tale approach. Within this broad category, in this essay I refer to the subset produced and promoted by the British Social Hygiene Council (BSHC), which were almost exclusively intended to counter the spread of venereal diseases, the core concern of the council. They used the genre from the time of *Whatsoever a Man Soweth* (1917), the first film they distributed, and throughout the 1930s.[23] The BSHC subcorpus provides a good case for analysis, partially because of the films' strong exemplification of the genre and partially because the good survival of BSHC archives and publications provides the best opportunity available to study this phenomenon. In addition, because of the perceived urgency of the VD problem, these films were close to British state policy, which meant that the council was able to finance production from government sources across most of the period under consideration in ways that no other organization could, resulting in a larger corpus than for other similar voluntary health associations. Survival of prints (in the BFI National Archive) is also appreciably better than for other organizations, with a selection available on DVD.[24]

The venereal diseases had been a significant concern of the medical profession since before the Contagious Diseases Acts of the 1860s. There had been an International Conference on Prostitution and Venereal Disease at Brussels in 1899, and in the same year the BMA had urged the prime minister to mount an enquiry into the prevention of VD in the civilian population. A Royal Commission into venereal disease had been launched by Herbert Asquith in November 1913, which reported three years later; the problem was considered to be so significant that, unusually, measures for health education were included in its recommendations. In parallel, the National Council for Combating Venereal Disease (NCCVD) had been formed as a side concern of the Eugenics Society. (It adopted the new name British Social Hygiene Council in 1925.) By the end of 1916, overwhelmed by the duties of establishing the VD clinics recommended by the commission, the Local Government Board (predecessor of the Ministry of Health) delegated responsibility for VD health education to the NCCVD, de facto providing them with 75 percent Treasury and 25 percent Local Authority funding for the purpose.[25] Until the Local Government Act of 1929, the BSHC continued to receive Treasury funds via the Ministry of Health for the production of propaganda, a substantial proportion of which was spent on the production and distribution of films. Thereafter, and more problematically, it drew 100 percent of its funding from the local authorities. Like other voluntary health associations, including the National Association for the Prevention of Tuberculosis or the Health and Cleanliness Council, the BSHC also used a wide range of health education media, including lectures, leaflets, posters, and stands at Local Authority health weeks, though all organizations tended to consider film to be the most powerful medium.[26]

The current essay shares with Annette Kuhn in *An Everyday Magic: Cinema and Cultural Memory*, her 2002 work on 1930s cinema audiences, the wish to go beyond abstractions to gain insights into "the historical social audience."[27] I review a wide range of first empirical and then theoretical approaches, looking for ways to access the audience experience, or of moving from "text" to audience, so as to piece together a better sense of how people in the past responded to the authority encoded in my chosen corpus of health education films. I employ for my analysis Le Roy Ladurie's familiar metaphor of the truffle hunter and the parachutist—exemplars of two approaches within historical method and the humanities in general. Truffle hunters dig out tasty morsels of evidence, whilst parachutists look down on the scenery from above, seeing the patterns that are not perceptible on the ground.[28] This is a congenial metaphor for organizing the material in the essay and has the advantage of not elevating one approach over the other.

Truffle Hunters

This first section, taking evidential approaches first, looks at context, numbers, and the first anthropological/sociological approaches to cinema in Britain, ending with a brief consideration of the potential of oral history.

Context

Health, and especially VD, propaganda films were distinguished from ordinary cinema entertainments in several ways.[29] First, they were often explicitly sponsored by the BSHC, with high-profile launches involving civic and public health dignitaries. The opportunity of public showings was also used for the distribution of health education leaflets. The second distinguishing factor is censorship: the fact that the British Board of Film Censors (BBFC) from 1919 issued a blanket statement that no propaganda films would be granted certificates on the grounds that the cinema was a place of entertainment, not education, and as the Home Office agreed, that its audience was "less intelligent and educated" than that for the theater and "includes more children and young people."[30] But the BBFC was a trade body, and it was up to the local authorities whether to allow particular films to be shown. In those areas such as Blackburn, where Medical Officers of Health were active in health education, the decision was more likely to be in favor of showing than in abiding by BBFC strictures. Where they were shown in cinemas in lieu of conventional films, attendance was often boosted not just by sensationalist publicity, but also by practices intended to ensure decorum, such as separate showings to men and to women and insisting that they were for adult audiences only. As an observer commented in 1934, "One has only to listen to the conversations of many of these people [queuing for the films] who believe they are going to see something frankly pornographic."[31] The difficulty in controlling the context of showings contributed to the view of many VD health educators that the right place for their films was not in the cinema at all but as part of explicit health education events. A BSHC lecturer, for example, argued that "unless the film was accompanied by an address 95 per cent of the potential good was lost."[32] Cinema managers, via their trade organization, the Cinema Exhibitors Association, often rejected the imposition of cinematic propaganda within their programs.[33] Although less than half of managers belonged to the association,[34] if we take their reluctance with the BSHC's preference for showing films accompanied by lecturers, we can understand how it came about that most of these films were not shown in cinemas. Rather, they were projected in town or church halls, mechanics institutes, and other civic spaces, particularly as features of local authority health weeks. And they were often shown free of charge, which may have been highly significant, especially during the Depression, and especially in working-class districts.

From this section on the context of showings of health education films we may assume that their audience was composed of the same individuals who at other times made up the normal cinema audience. They were the same audience but in a different mode. We may suspect that some may have had a particular reason to want to see a VD film—hypochondria or concern about symptoms, perhaps—but apart from a proportion of the dignitaries who attended the gala openings and who may have been quoted in reportage, from the evidence of the context of showings we cannot know.

Numbers

In relation to the empirical ground of audience numbers, one contemporary statistical publication, from 1934, by Simon Rowson is frequently cited. The headline figure he quotes is of 18 million per week visiting the ordinary cinemas.[35] This is the source of the 1930s data quoted by Philip Corrigan in the 1983 essay which opened up the historical study of cinema's audiences, a subject which he stated at that stage was "almost completely undeveloped, even unconsidered."[36] He sketched out the conventional demographic categories: regional, age, gender, and class differences. But the fault here is the assumption that such studies could be extended across the whole history of cinema whereas, in fact, before 1937 the British cinema audience was not the site of sociological investigation, and the data for such an analysis do not exist in any consistent form.[37] All we know is that these very significant numbers attended cinemas and that attendance was perceived at the time to be predominantly working class.

If this is true of the cinema audience in general, what hope for the much smaller health education film audience? There are, in fact, detailed reports of showings in the papers of the British Social Hygiene Council. For example, the Council's Cinemotor lorry—a traveling projection outfit—traveled to Southport in September 1922, where a total of 1,700 people saw films at three venues. "At each meeting the halls were full, many having to be turned away. In many cases it was necessary to admit the public an hour before the beginning of the showing."[38] And because of the BSHC's policy of sometimes targeting propaganda films separately at men and women, there are disaggregated data about the gender split of audiences, which *could* be mapped onto the geographical reports; for example, at Stoke on Trent in February 1923, 3,834 men and 4,274 women watched VD films in a period of a fortnight.[39]

Perhaps the most impressive figures relate to the Canadian film *Damaged Lives,* in whose British distribution the BSHC shared. It was made by the German director Edgar Ulmer, then new in Hollywood. The film was described in the journal *Public Health* as "an excellent demonstration of the influence to be wielded on public opinion by visual education."[40] The documentary filmmaker Paul Rotha was less glowing; he commented that "technically, the film is only interesting in that it marks the level below which poor photography and ineffectual direction cannot sink."[41] But between August 1933 and May 1934, the BSHC claimed a total audience of "approximately four million persons" spread over 357 towns for this film and the distribution of over 126,000 pamphlets giving details of treatment centers.[42] These very large figures were achieved by working with a commercial film distributor and persuading cinema managers to show the film. This figure may well have been dwarfed by the eighteen million per week going to ordinary cinema shows, but even allowing for exaggeration, it is highly significant within the history of health education.

The conclusion we can draw from the numerical approach is that there are data in the archives and, in the case of VD films, there are sufficient data to make comparisons.[43] But at the best, we can only say how many men and women saw particular films in particular places at particular times. We are not getting close to any detailed sense of impact. This leads us to the conclusion that the main thing we know about these audiences is what we don't know; these people are anonymous.

Sociological Investigations

The first organization in Britain to apply sociological technique to the cinema audience was Mass Observation, the home-brew social anthropology organization founded by a journalist, a documentary filmmaker, and an anthropologist in 1937 with the avowed aim of undertaking an "anthropology of our own people."[44] Their method was to recruit observers to make notes of public behavior, and for diarists to record details of their own lives, often responding to thematic "directives" from the organizers. A research program outlined in 1937 directed observers to record details of the size, composition, appearance and behavior of cinema audiences, reaction to films, and overheard conversations. A questionnaire was also circulated to cinema audiences in the spring of 1938.[45] None of this study was directed to health education films; rather, it traced responses to the ordinary diet of cinemagoers, which from at least 1925 was 95 percent Hollywood product.[46] One can be too pedantic, of course, and the generality of the responses does give a sense of the context within which audience members might have placed the health education films they saw. For example, the questionnaire responses show that the most popular category of film, namely, musical romance, was liked best by 44 percent of women and 24 percent of men. Drama and tragedy, into which category we might place the majority of the VD dramas, was the next most popular category, with 21 percent of women and 17 percent of men placing it as their favorite. So we may conclude that the VD film producers had selected a popular genre, but we can't say that the audiences believed VD films to be particularly fine examples.

During the war, Mass Observation did contract work for the Ministry of Information, especially centered around questions of civilian morale. A special study was made of Ministry of Information short propaganda films. The report explains that "the object of this investigation was to find out what effects, if any, these films had."[47] This is the sort of question that had scarcely been asked earlier, one that we might like to ask of health education films. However, to be pedantic, no health films were included in these studies.[48] Once again, the evidence is oblique and suggestive rather than specific. One gets a glancing sense of the atmosphere of cinemas during the showing of propaganda films, for example, in the suggestion that "if we classify these films into 'short stories' and 'strict documentaries,' and compare the audience response . . . we find a consistently higher degree of response to the documentary."[49] One might conclude that the "moral tale" approach to health education filmmaking was inappropriate—even though this was the style favored by the Central Council for Health Education, which was then briefly in charge of film production.[50] But this was October 1940, after the Blitz had stirred up the doldrums of the "phoney war"; a very different England from that of the 1920s and 1930s. More generalizable, perhaps, is a comment on an antirumor film that "a large part of the response was laughter, and it is not certain how much of such laughter means the registration of a message about *rumour*."[51] This may back up the assumption that films were often scarcely received in an air of sobriety and reflection. The judgment of MO's historians on this work is salutary; they conclude that MO "were never able ultimately to determine how, if at all, films influenced people's behaviour and attitudes, arguably the *raison d'être* of their MOI work."[52] The American context provided more explicit evidence of this kind in the 1919–22 study of VD films conducted by the founders of behaviorism, Karl Lashley and John B. Watson, in one of the first studies of media effects. Different audiences were shown the film *Fit to Win*; the mixed audience showed responses including ribald laughter and embarrassment, while an audience of doctors "was frankly bored throughout the picture," finding it exaggerated and falsely dramatic."[53] There was nothing like this in Britain, and I have found no evidence that British health educators were aware of the study.

The Wartime Social Survey (WSS) was another organization that used social survey techniques to assay the mental state of the population in wartime, including the cinema audience. Their concerns were similar to those of MO, as was the relative absence of enquiries relevant to health questions. And when the WSS did ask whether those responding to the diphtheria immunization campaign had seen the associated films, the answer was expressed quantitatively, and the quantity was small. Only one percent of families with diphtheria-immunized children cited the film when answering the question "how did you learn about the immunisation scheme."[54]

One empirical way around the absence of contemporary witness and data might be—for just a few more years, while participants survive—to employ oral history. Memory is not the same as contemporary evidence—it may be highly constructed and conventionalized—and so should be considered as complementary to sources contemporary with the films themselves. Annette Kuhn uses a sophisticated approach of this kind in her *An Everyday Magic*, which situates the cinemagoing recollections of seventy-eight respondents within the broader context of memory studies and supplements its ethnohistorical core with studies of contemporary publications and close study of particular film "texts."[55] All the same, as a means of accessing the historical experience and impact of the minority genre of health education films, this approach could only be expected to deliver at the level of broad context; such minority genres as this disappear in the mass of more popular fare, especially Hollywood films, which dominated cinema in Britain in this period.

In sum, the absence up to the end of the war of sociological concern with the questions we might wish them to have asked about the audience for health education is a significant absence.[56] No one was terribly concerned to ask about the subjectivity of audiences exposed to health education films. As long as an audience for health education existed, then to count them was sufficient. Even the poor response to the diphtheria film did not dent participants' belief in the power of films within health education. And oral history is unlikely to furnish a substantial retrospective proxy for what the absent contemporary studies cannot supply.

Parachutists

The truffle hunting approaches give a foundation, but they are able to shed little light on the experiences of the millions of people who saw films of this kind over this period. But there is a range of theoretical approaches that can be used to survey this subject, like parachutists seeing possible patterns; these may allow us—at least in principle—to think about what the audience experience might have been like. I have selected some of these approaches that come from critical study of films and other media over the last forty years, from art history, narratology, medical sociology, and studies of cultural consumption. I have adopted a fairly agnostic approach to these different approaches so as to reveal how they may illuminate the central concerns of this essay; other writers have more to say in distinguishing their strengths and shortcomings.

"Film studies" is the name given to a new disciplinary grouping that arose, mainly in literature faculties, in the 1970s, responding to and rejecting the concerns of connoisseurial traditions of film criticism, exemplified by established reviewers, critics, and advocates of particular film genres. From the early decades of the film studies community, it is immediately possible to see how new agendas could generate new kinds of insights into audiences. In its first decades, this was generally achieved by looking at films as texts and at audiences as ideal spectators posited by, or "inscribed in," these film texts. At the beginning, it adopted an essentially ahistorical, psychoanalytic, and semiotic approach to film, with a sprinkling of Althusserian Marxism.[57] This work is useful in its emphasis on the relationship between the viewer and the film narrative. The film studies community often turned to psychoanalysis in seeking to come closer to the spectator. For example, for Christian Metz, watching films was a type of voyeurism. He suggested that in the theater, the voyeur is not secretive and "the performance of the play deliberately sets out to be a collective experience." By comparison, in the cinema, "all the viewer requires . . . is that the actor should behave as though he is not being seen, and so cannot see him, the voyeur." He proceeds along conventional Freudian lines of ego, id, primal scene, and the rest.[58] The route to establishing a firm historical sense of the usefulness of such an approach would, however, be to look at how psychoanalytic and psychological understandings were deployed in relation to the cinema *at the time.* All the same, whether or not the detail of this is useful, the notion of the spectator as voyeur does illuminate what we know of VD films' partial reputation as pornography. And it is unproblematic to accept that there could be something voyeuristic—in the general sense—in choosing to see films that promise sight of others' lives, of disease conditions, or of medical practice which would normally be outside viewers' experience.[59] *Any Evening After Work* (1930), for example, was built around the viewing experience of the central figure—scarcely a "hero"—who has contracted a sexually transmitted disease through a casual liaison. Dithering before deciding not to visit a doctor, he visits a BSHC lecture and film show, where he witnesses the stories of a sailor, a farm worker, a lorry driver, a clerk, and a steelworker whose lives and those of their families have been blighted by untreated gonorrhoea or syphilis. The impact of these stories on him is also the path to his salvation; the lecturer arranges an appointment for him at the clinic. The viewer, in the Metz interpretation, would be a voyeur of the misfortunes of the main character and of the five men in the stories within a story. Certainly the reaction shots of the protagonist suggest a voyeuristic discomfort.

Reference to Metz's views alerts us to a major difference in how film studies sees the audience compared with the truffle hunters already discussed. For Metz and his fellow travelers, the audience is no longer a series of demographic abstractions. Instead we have a different level of abstraction; the audience here is made up of individuals having individual experiences. As Sheila Johnston stated in 1985, "on the one hand there is the empirical spectator whose interpretation of film will be determined by all manner of extraneous factors like personal biography, class origins, previous viewing experience, the variables of conditions of reception etc." But in the end, she says, "empirical audience research is unable to account fully for the viewing experience, and for the relations between film narrative and spectator."[60] So "on the other hand" there is "the abstract notion of a 'subject position,' which could be defined as the way in which a film solicits, demands even, a certain closely circumscribed reading from a reader by means of its own formal operations."[61]

This "subject position" is an ideal-typical audience member, which is said to be manipulated by cinematic technique. The individual cinemagoer's isolation from the remainder of the audience is reinforced by the narrative conventions of cinema, particularly those which became established during the 1920s, known as "the classic narrative system."[62] This operates by establishing for the viewer a believable world in both spatial and temporal terms. The suspension of the viewers' disbelief, their capacity to forget they are in the cinema and to "get lost" in the narration depends on particular narrative codes of editing to achieve an illusion of continuity and camera angles that, for example, use close-ups to specify significant details or have characters in conversation looking toward opposite sides of the screen (in film language, not "crossing the line"). In this world, the fictional characters, who are given character traits, motivations, and so on, propel forward the action of the film until narrative closure is reached at its conclusion. It is by means of techniques such as this that viewers come to identify with the protagonists of onscreen dramas. This is clearest in those cases where the camera takes the position of one character, as for example when conversations are edited so that the on-screen speaker addresses an unseen listener, but at some level is perceived by viewers as speaking to them.[63] We see a variant of this deployed at the end of *A Test for Love* (1937), where a long close-up of Betty, the film's central character, is held while the VD clinic nurse delivers a long speech about the effectiveness of the treatment and the dangers of "running after adventure"; the address, like a moralizing lecture, might as well be direct to the woman in the audience.

A specific way this is said to have functioned was via what Bill Nichols termed "mode of address."[64] For our purposes, this may be taken to describe the tone of voice in which a film speaks to its audience. Different genres of film, by using different modes of address, *assert* particular relationships to exist between the audiences and the individuals seen and heard in the film. Mode of address may be "direct" as is found in most instructional and documentary films, where an individual—only sometimes seen on the screen—speaks directly to people viewing. In the "moral tale" VD films, the mode of address is "indirect," where the viewer follows the action of the film through identification with the characters on the screen.[65] Each of these modes implies a position for the viewer in relation to the film and its authors: active in the case of the direct address of the documentary, and passive in the case of the indirect address of the fiction film. A rare BSHC example of the former is *The Mystery of Marriage* (1932), not a moral tale in the sense of following the normal narrative arc already discussed but in the sense of lessons conveyed by a series of comparisons between vegetable and animal forms of "marriage" (shot by the doyen of natural history filmmakers, Percy Smith) and human relationships. In this case, the comparisons are drawn out by a humorous and facetious commentary; in describing homemaking, for example, there is a sequence of a stickleback building a nest. The commentator advises "and here is the completed bijou residence with old Ma stickleback in residence, and Pa at the door"; shortly we see the human protagonists negotiating for a new house signposted Bijou Baronial Halls. Indirect address is seen in all the majority "moral tales" discussed elsewhere in this essay, where a moral predicament caused by the contraction of a sexually transmitted disease is acted out by a protagonist. For example, the naval wireless officer in *Deferred Payment* (1929) who, having been "transferred to home service [having picked up VD abroad], and anxious to marry his old sweetheart with a clean bill of health, visits a quack doctor to whom he makes heavy payments for so-called 'treatment.'" Despite later medical intervention, failure to comply with treatment leads to inherited syphilis for his son; "through treatment the little boy's sight is saved, but so weakened that it will affect his choice of profession. The father realises that the child will continue to pay indefinitely for his fault."[66]

Concentrating on mode of address directs our attention to the choices of cinematic technique made by the makers of health films and to the way that has led to the construction of a cinematic "voice of public health." Mode of address, in the case of health education films, embodies the voice of medicine to potential patients; it is a vehicle of the power relations of medicine. By their choice of film genre, voluntary associations such as the BSHC and filmmakers may be seen to be making assumptions about their audience's degree of active engagement in health issues. While the address of documentary was said and believed to imply the active engaged citizen making rational health choices, the "moral tale" health education film implied an acquiescent audience in a passive state which could be exploited to convey health "messages."[67] Via this kind of scholarship, our view of the audience has been broadened: should we think of it as a mass, or should we think of it as a congruence of individuals? The film studies answer is an ideal-typical spectator.

Much activity in the consideration of audiences undertaken within cultural studies has been in relation to television, notably in the study of viewers of current affairs and soap operas, in a spate of work described by Virginia Nightingale as the "cultural studies audience experiment."[68] Abercrombie and Longhurst explain the genealogy of this research, identifying three overlapping paradigms. The 'effects' model, exemplified by the Lashley and Watson study and Mass Observation wartime investigations already mentioned, continued to be developed for many decades. The "uses and gratifications" model, which was first proposed in the 1940s, placed much more emphasis on the uses made by audiences of media, producing a much less top-down model than the first. The third, "encoding/decoding" model, was developed by Stuart Hall and others at the Birmingham Centre for Contemporary Cultural Studies in the 1980s in reaction to these earlier approaches, both of which Hall described as "behaviourist."[69] In David Morley's influential work within this new approach on the audience for the current affairs program *Nationwide,* deeper understanding of "text-viewer relations" and "knowing through television" was generated through group discussions following video screening of programs. Morley used Hall's encoding/decoding approach, which established a dominant meaning of the program "text" and then ethnographically assayed the "readings" of carefully selected viewing groups.[70] Such an approach would evidently be impossible for the remote past of the 1920s and 1930s. But the Morley School approach could be used to provoke questions of the historical findings we do have. For example, it might well be valuable to consider the value of his scale of different kinds of "reading" of the program—the "dominant," the "negotiated," and the "oppositional." In these, viewers respectively fully accept the program's "preferred reading"; accept but modify it, reflecting their position and interests; or reject it and substitute an alternative frame of interpretation.[71] It is interesting to note, as Nightingale identifies, that this approach relied on a model of "communication as a compartmentalised and linear process" of sender—message—receiver, which—though deployed in a more sophisticated manner than the earlier behaviorist approaches—would have been familiar to the producers of the much older health education films, where the model of communication, as we saw with *Any Evening after Work*, is of the lecture.[72]

Historians looking for a way to historicize the film theorist's abstract spectator could turn to the work of the art historian Michael Baxandall, whose notion of "the period eye" is advanced in his influential *Painting and Experience in Fifteenth Century Italy* (1985). Here he suggests that audiences in the past for whom cultural products were intended may be considered to have possessed a "period eye." In his study, for example, experience of buying or riding horses made contemporaries' appreciation of how these animals were depicted in paintings much richer than would be possible for the majority of modern viewers. Or it may be that knowledge of the high price of blue pigment affected how they saw representations of the Virgin Mary, traditionally represented in this color. This kind of study could be applied via close studies of health education films as texts revealing the shared cultural assumptions of makers and audiences in the past. By this route, we might gain a sense of what contemporary audiences would have known that we don't which would have affected how they received the film.[73] One example in *A Test for Love* is of George, the unsuitable man—and gonorrhoea carrier—who drives an expensive American car, which would not be evident to most modern viewers but which would have been to contemporaries.[74] Similarly, we may assume that the clothing worn by particular characters would signify more about them than would be visible to any current viewers unless they were fashion historians.

A further approach that can illuminate the experience of generic spectators employs the insights of narratology. I have proposed in an essay on tuberculosis health education that "by using an approach to tuberculosis that focuses on the storied nature of lay understandings of disease it may be possible to gain a broad grasp of its place in the culture of the past."[75] The argument is intended to address the reception of all "moral tale" films, not simply those concerned with TB. In brief, the essay argues that we can understand the likely impact of health education narratives if we concede that audiences already carry a narrative sense of life events (including disease) when they encounter films of the kind we have been discussing, and that the conflicting film narrative, though intended to "sugar the pill" of instruction, might in fact make it less digestible. This possibility may well be reinforced from the internal evidence of many of the BSHC's films of noncompliance with treatment and a preference for quack "cures," as in *Any Evening after Work* or *Deferred Payment.*

The Sick Role

We have, so far, considered approaches to audiences as if they were watching *any* film. But it is important to consider the quasi-medical nature of health education. Just as voluntary associations were content with sheer numbers as an index of success, so were they not often explicit about whom they expected to attend. Napier Burnett of the Red Cross argued that the population as a whole was possessed of "abysmal ignorance in regard to health questions," voicing an anticipation of what would later be called the deficit theory of public communication.[76] But the established sociological literature can provide us with useful categories in helping us to distinguish these films from others, especially Parson's notion of the "sick role." Levine and Kozloff in their literature review on this subject distinguish three stages leading from a well state via impairment and coping to the sick role proper.[77] The Parsonian model of the sick role relies on what Uta Gerhardt describes as a "two-rights-two-obligations" structure: rights to be exempted from normal social responsibilities and to be spared from blame for the condition; and obligations to get better (for the sake of the social system) and to accept the physician's authority.[78] It looks as though, in Parsonian terms, the individual member of the health education audience has the responsibilities of the sick role—to accept the authority of biomedicine so as to get better—but without the right of being excluded from blame, which sickness would enable. This is indeed one of the characteristics of the health education films under discussion here; their scenarios encode obedience to social authority represented by medical figures, often literally, with long authoritarian speeches and with camera angles encoding deference to authority. This is visible, for example, in *A Test for Love,* in which we see Betty the patient sitting, looking up at the doctor as he berates her for her irresponsibility.[79] Further, if we accept that fiction films work by identification of the audience member with the protagonist of the film, then it would be difficult for them not to feel some of the shame, and accept some of the blame, for the irresponsible actions that are the mainstay of VD dramas.

Let us also look at this in the context of Jewson's notion that the modern medicine of the Paris school, based on pathological anatomy, had by about 1870 replaced a previous "person-orientated cosmology" with one that was object-orientated (that is, one focusing on organs, tissues, and cells), leading to the "disappearance" of the "sick man" with his idiosyncratic personal experiences from medical cosmologies. Within public health discourse, the ostensibly well target of the discourse also had little personhood; he or she was principally the potential carrier of pathology.[80] But to the extent that audience members might have been able to identify with the more extensively characterized figures in the moral tale films, it is arguable that health education technique had at least the potential to override some of the reductionism of modern medicine.

Authority and Cultural Consumption

If the truffle hunters and the parachutists provide a thesis and an antithesis in our argument, then a really satisfactory account will need to synthesize the virtues of both approaches, just as there has been a rapprochement between film history and film studies. Such a synthesis would have to respect both the specificity of the truffle hunters' data and the patterns visible to the parachutists. Michel de Certeau's *The Practice of Everyday Life* (1984) can take us some way to such a resolution. His chapter "Walking in the City," explicitly addresses the differences between the behaviors of consumers and the patterns that a parachutist might perceive. Here he compares the individual routes of urban pedestrians—the consumers of urban spaces—with how those patterns might seem to someone looking down from a tall building. This is one of several ways that he addresses the nature of cultural consumption: of cities, books, magazines, and many more categories. He characterizes the consumer as being a poacher on someone else's land, intent on stealing a "rabbit" for himself. Closer to our territory, he states "once the images broadcast by television [for example] and the time spent in front of the TV set have been analyzed, it remains to be asked what the consumer *makes* of these images and during these hours." This is a type of question that we have not yet encountered. He continues, "The thousands of people who buy a health magazine, the customers in a supermarket, the practitioners of urban space, the consumers of newspaper stories and legends—what do they make of what they "absorb," receive, and pay for? What do they do with it?" But this is not, as he shows, quite the right question: "In reality . . . production is confronted by an entirely different kind of production, called 'consumption' and characterised by its ruses, its fragmentation . . . its poaching, its clandestine nature, its tireless but quiet activity, in short by its quasi-invisibility, since it shows itself not in its own products . . . but in an art of using those imposed on it."[81] This is where Napier Burnett's assertion that health education should "bridge the hygienic knowledge of the medical profession and the abysmal ignorance of the population as a whole" is set in stark relief.[82] The assumption among the historical actors I have described is that the individual audience member's mind was a tabula rasa ready to absorb health propaganda, whereas, from the viewpoint of de Certeau, consumption is a creative act, and consumers would "poach" only what they required from the territory of health educators. To put de Certeau's insight into the language of media studies, cultural consumers render a consumed text "polysemic," that is, capable of several interpretations. As John Fiske notes of television, "although it works within cultural determinations, it also offers freedoms and the power to evade, modify, or challenge these limitations and controls."[83] To take examples from our corpus, we can imagine that the viewer of *Any Evening after Work* might take strength in his avoidance of the doctor from the protagonist's dithering. Or we could imagine the keen gardener taking away valuable insights on the growth of sweet peas from a viewing of *The Mystery of Marriage* while disregarding the "message" about human relations.

We can apply de Certeau's model of consumption in the context of the Parsonian health education film audience who, as we suggested, were expected to display obedience to medical authority. Our synthetic account might effectively be marshaled around questions of authority, both historical and theoretical. Social hierarchy was at the heart of the interwar health education project. From its foundation in 1919, senior Ministry of Health officials defined a position aloof from the public and delegated health education to "the medical, scientific, and better educated classes of the community," which included the voluntary health associations such as the BSHC.[84] In a Foucauldian sense, this makes the professional classes instruments of governmentality. Stuart Hall, equally, in formulating his encoding/decoding approach, criticized the earlier "effects" and "uses and gratifications" approaches to audiences in part because of their failure to treat "issues of social and political power and economic relations." His resource in responding to this was a model of the hegemony by which a dominant class secured and expanded its mastery over society.[85]

Returning to approaches from historical context, we may note that the mode of address of the health education films produced by voluntary associations drew on long traditions of the class authority associated with aristocratic power and nineteenth-century charitable activity. This carried implications of an older deferential politics. The BSHC, typical of the voluntary health associations, was a coalition of groups responding in different ways to the changing political landscape of the period: aristocrats seeking to retain a political role in a period of decline;[86] aspirant middle class professionals—including doctors and lawyers—finding a quasi-political role asserting a class ideal,[87] perhaps a particular view of medicine; and women finding a political role across the period in which they acquired the vote on the same terms as men in 1928. A grouping such as this would, in Hall's account of hegemony, constitute a dominant class seeking to extend its influence over society.

De Certeau explicitly addresses the potential of resistance by people such as the audiences of health education films in the play of power between elites and the public:

> Inclined to believe that its own cultural models are necessary for the people in order to educate their minds and to elevate their hearts, the élite . . . always assumes that the public is moulded by the products imposed on it. To assume that is to misunderstand the act of "consumption." This misunderstanding assumes that "assimilating" necessarily means "becoming similar to" what one absorbs, and not "making something similar" to what one is, making it one's own, appropriating or reappropriating it.[88]

Similarly, in its developing sense of the relative power of "text" and audience, the encoding/decoding approach came to exhibit a continuum of approaches from those that stress the dominance of the text to those that emphasize the dominance of the audience. John Fiske, for example, argues that "people can and do make their own culture, albeit within conditions that are not of their own choosing. How much power is available within this terrain [is a matter] of considerable debate, in which I align myself with those who propose that ideological and hegemonic theories of popular culture have overestimated the power of determinations and underestimated that of the viewer."[89] Now, the film theorist Christian Metz found it significant that the cinema "was born much later than the theatre, in a period when social life was strongly marked by the notion of the *individual*."[90] We may note that this resonates with the major shifts in public health in the same period, as George Newman, the Chief Medical Officer, said, making his argument for public education in health: "In every direction the prevention of disease is becoming a personal concern. . . . Public provision . . . cannot make particular men, women or children feel well day by day. It is neglect of this personal aspect which is now restricting the operations and results of Preventive Medicine in many fields; and it is this personal aspect which accentuates the need for a greater degree of public education."[91] In this sense, both personal public health and cinema were creatures of their age. We are speaking of a period of expansion of the reach of medicine into the larger population via medical services, from the 1870s mainly via the local authorities and from 1911 by the establishment of National Health Insurance and the Ministry of Health in 1919. Insofar as health education is concerned with prevention of sickness among the ostensibly well, then it is also typical of the extension of medicine into previously unmedicalized spheres of life. And here is the paradox at the heart of health education: as the public health establishment became more powerful and expansive, it carried with it class attitudes to its subject population, its potential clients, that viewed them as an undifferentiated mass highly susceptible to health education, while at the same time opting for modes of intervention which spoke of the individual subject and of her or his everyday behavior. In that sense, perhaps the choice of "moral tales" as the genre for health education was more apposite than the voluntary health associations could have known, with its capacity to engage hundreds or thousands of people in a single audience through identification with the characters, as though they were receiving an attuned, personalized, address. What we don't know is how resistant the "readings" of the "film texts" were. Here the parachutist needs to ally with the truffle hunter and, de Certeau-like, go onto the territory of the past to "poach" a few choice morsels of evidence.

Notes

Epigraph: Annette Kuhn, *An Everyday Magic: Cinema and Cultural Memory* (London: I. B. Tauris, 2002), 3.

1. W. A. Daley, "The Sanitation of Places of Public Entertainment," *Journal of the Royal Sanitary Institute* 43 (1922): 34–42, 34. Similar sentiments are explored in A. M. Chalmers, MOH Glasgow, "The Kinema as a Means of Health Propaganda (read at kinematograph trade conference, June 24th 1919)," *Medical Officer* 22 (1919): 23–24.

2. Interwar examples are tabulated in Timothy Boon, "Films and the Contestation of Public Health in Interwar Britain" (PhD diss., University of London, 1999).

3. George Newman, *Public Education in Health* (London: HMSO, 1925 (rev. ed.; original 1924), 16.

4. This generalization includes my own thesis on the production of British interwar health education films. Boon, *Films and the Contestation.*

5. Rachael Low, *Films of Comment and Persuasion of the 1930s* (London: George Allen and Unwin, 1979), 152–59.

6. Annette Kuhn, *Cinema, Censorship and Sexuality, 1909–1925* (London: Routledge, 1988).

7. Lynda Bryder, *Below the Magic Mountain: A Social History of Tuberculosis in Twentieth-Century Britain* (Oxford: Clarendon Press, 1988), e.g., 145.

8. Esp. 114–25 (though the audience here is considered as a problem perceived by elites). See also below.

9. Martin S. Pernick, *The Black Stork: Eugenics and the Death of 'Defective' Babies in American Medicine and Motion Pictures since 1915* (New York: Oxford University Press, 1996).

10. Kirsten Ostherr, *Cinematic Prophylaxis: Globalization and Contagion in the Discourse of World Health* (Durham, NC: Duke University Press, 2005).

11. Elizabeth Lebas, *Forgotten Futures: British Municipal Cinema 1920–1980* (London: Black Dog, 2011).

12. Leslie J. Reagan, Nancy Tomes, and Paula A. Treichler, eds., *Medicine's Moving Pictures: Medicine, Health, and Bodies in American Film and Television* (Rochester, NY: University of Rochester Press, 2007), esp. 8–10; Graeme Harper and Andrew Moor, eds., *Signs of Life: Cinema and Medicine* (London: Wallflower Press, 2005). Gudrun Loehrer has also written a thesis on an aspect of the American scene. Gudrun Loehrer, "Cinematic Governmentality: A Cultural History of Tuberculosis and Malaria Health Films in the United States of the 1940s" (PhD diss., University of East London, 2009).

13. Vinzenz Hediger and Patrick Vonderau, eds., *Films that Work: Industrial Film and the Productivity of Media* (Amsterdam: Amsterdam University Press, 2009); Devin Orgeron, Marsha Orgeron, and Dan Streible, eds., *Learning with the Lights Off: Educational Film in the United States* (New York: Oxford University Press, 2012); Charles Acland and Haidee Wasson, eds., *Useful Cinema* (Durham, NC: Duke University Press, 2012).

14. Helpful summaries include Nicholas Abercrombie and Brian Longhurst, *Audiences: A Sociological Theory of Performance and Imagination* (London: Sage, 1998), and Virginia Nightingale, *Studying Audiences: The Shock of the Real* (London: Routledge, 1996). Several of these are discussed in the second part of this essay.

15. Quoted in David Morley, *The Nationwide Audience: Structure and Decoding* (London: British Film Institute, 1980), 22.

16. Central Council for Health Education, ed., *Health Education Yearbook* (London: CCHE, 1939), 111.

17. Kuhn, *Cinema, Censorship and Sexuality*, 43; Luke McKernan, "The Cinema: Its Present Position and Future Possibilities," *The Bioscope*, May 31, 2007, http://thebioscope.net/2007/05/31/the-cinema-its-present-position-and-future-possibilities/.

18. Luke McKernan, "(I'm Not a) Juvenile Delinquent," *The Bioscope*, July 16, 2008, http://thebioscope.net/2008/07/16/im-not-a-juvenile-delinquent/.

19. An interesting exception to this general principle, in the American context, was Karl S. Lashley and John B. Watson, *A Psychological Study of Motion Pictures in Relation to Venereal Disease Campaigns* (Washington, DC: United States Interdepartmental Social Hygiene Board, 1922).

20. This work was initiated for the conference organized by Roger Cooter, "Health Promotion in Historical and Contemporary Context," University of East Anglia, Norwich, UK, April 27, 2001, and has been completely overhauled for this publication. This work shares some territory with other strands of my research that originated at this time, including my "Lay Disease Narratives, Tuberculosis and Health Education Films," in *From Urban Penalty to Global Emergency: New Approaches to the History of Tuberculosis*, ed. Flurin Condrau and Michael Worboys (Montreal: McGill-Queens University Press, 2008), 24–48; and "A Walk in the Museum with Michel de Certeau: A Conceptual Helping Hand for Museum Practitioners," *Curator* 54 (October 2011): 419–29. It can be seen as an expansion of the audience coverage in my "Health Education Films in Britain, 1919–1939: Production, Genres and Audiences," in *Signs of Life: Cinema and Medicine*, ed. Graeme Harper and Andrew Moor (London: Wallflower Press, 2005), 45–57, 52–5. It has benefited significantly from the insights of the editors and my colleague Jean-Baptiste Gouyon.

21. As I argue of medical films in general in Timothy Boon, "Medical Film and Television: An Alternative Path to the Cultures of BioMedicine," in *Oxford Handbook of the History of Medicine*, ed. Mark Jackson (Oxford: Oxford University Press, 2011), 617–34.

22. For these, see Boon, *Films of Fact*, chap. 3.

23. They stopped producing films by the start of the war, when the Central Council for Health Education, then the Ministry of Information, took charge of health education filmmaking.

24. See, for example, *The Birds and the Bees: 60 Years of British Sex Education Films* (London: British Film Institute, 2011). This and other films are available from the BFI store at http://shop.bfi.org.uk/.

25. Bridget A. Towers, "Health Education Policy, 1916–1926: Venereal Disease and the prophylaxis dilemma," *Medical History* 24 (1980): 70–87, 78–79.

26. Boon, *Contestation*, chap. 3.

27. Kuhn, *An Everyday* Magic, 4–5.

28. For citation, see John H. Elliott, *Spain, Europe and the Wider World, 1500–1800* (New Haven, CT: Yale University Press, 2009), 20n11.

29. Kuhn, *Cinema, Censorship and Sexuality*, 64–72, is good on this territory.

30. Home Office official quoted by Kuhn, *Cinema, Censorship and Sexuality*, 67.

31. Dorothy Knowles, quoted in Kuhn, *Cinema, Censorship and Sexuality*, 68.

32. I. Feldman, "Address on the use of films (BSHC Branch Conference, March 15th 1928)," *Health and Empire* 3 (March 1928): 168.

33. This dates back at least as far as 1920: "[In Worcester] Mr Gray, finding that the Cinema Exhibitors Association had banned the film [*The End of the Road*], had exhibited it in halls or buildings other than recognised cinema theaters." NCCVD propaganda committee minutes, October 18, 1920, Wellcome Library SA/BSH/C. The issue is explored in relation to documentary films by Paul Swann, *The British Documentary Film Movement, 1926–1946* (Cambridge: Cambridge University Press, 1989), 120–22.

34. Kuhn, *Cinema, Censorship and Sexuality*, 68.

35. S. Rowson, "A Statistical Survey of the Cinema Industry in Great Britain in 1934," *Journal of the Royal Statistical Society* 99 (1936): 67–129.

36. Though he does pay due attention to those who, from the very late thirties, began the sociological study of audiences (see n. 57 below). Philip Corrigan, "Film Entertainment as Ideology and Pleasure: A Preliminary Approach to a History of Audiences," in *British Cinema History*, ed. John Curran and Vincent Porter (London: Wiedenfeld and Nicolson, 1983), 24.

37. See next section.

38. BSHC Propaganda Committee meeting, October 16, 1922, Wellcome Library SA/BSH/C, 29.

39. Ibid., March 19, 1923, Wellcome Library SA/BSH/C, 111.

40. Anon, "Damaged Lives," *Public Health* 1933, 46, 384–85.

41. Rewinder (nom de plume of Paul Rotha), "Damaged Lives," *Sight and Sound*, Autumn 1933, 100.

42. BSHC Annual Report for 1933–34, 24–25.

43. Similar studies are possible in the archives of, for example, the National Association for the Prevention of Tuberculosis, also held in the Wellcome Library.

44. These were, respectively, Charles Madge, Humphrey Jennings, and Tom Harrison.

45. Jeffrey Richards and Dorothy Sheridan, eds., *Mass-Observation at the Movies* (London: Routledge, 1987), 4.

46. Corrigan, "Film Entertainment as Ideology and Pleasure," 26.

47. Richards and Sheridan, eds., *Mass-Observation*, 445.

48. With the possible exception of *Food for Thought*, a nutrition film, and *Westward Ho!*, an evacuation film (this was a MH responsibility).

49. Richards and Sheridan, eds., *Mass-Observation*, 426.

50. This can be followed in the relevant files for the Central Council at the National Archives, Kew, London; relevant classes include MH82/6 and MH82/18.

51. Richards and Sheridan, eds., *Mass-Observation*, 434.

52. Ibid., 11.

53. Luke McKernan, "*Fit to Win*," *The Bioscope*, September 20, 2009, http://thebioscope.net/2009/09/20/fit-to-win/; Lashley and Watson, *A Psychological Study*.

54. WSS, *Diphtheria Immunisation Enquiry*, National Archives, Kew, RG23/23, 16.

55. Kuhn, *An Everyday Magic*, 7–12.

56. In Britain, the first significant synthetic work on the sociology of cinema audiences was Jacob Peter Mayer, *Sociology of Film: Studies and Documents* (London: Faber, 1946). Tellingly, David Schrire's article from 1933 under the title "The Psychology of Film Audiences" turns out to be an argument for the value of documentary as opposed to story films; *Sight and Sound* 2, no. 8 (Winter 1933): 122–23.

57. Most of this section derives from Pam Cook, ed., *The Cinema Book* (London: BFI, 1985 and subsequent editions, 1999 and 2007). The relationship of the film studies community to others who work on films was vexed; Katherine and Phillip Dodd, for example, argued that the film studies approach "deliberately cut itself off from the knowledges provided by the more traditional disciplines of History and Literature, in an attempt . . . to establish its own disciplinary credentials and autonomy." Katherine Dodd and Phillip Dodd, "Engendering the nation: British

documentary film, 1930–1939," in *Dissolving views: Key Writings on the British Cinema*, ed. Andrew Higson (London: Cassell, 1996), 38. Since the 1990s, there has been a rapprochement between film studies and historical perspectives—or between "textual" and "contextual" approaches—see, for example, Andrew Spicer, "Film Studies and the Turn to History (Review Article)," *Journal of Contemporary History* 39, no. 1 (2004): 147–55.

58. Christian Metz, *Psychoanalysis and Cinema: The Imaginary Signifier* (London: Macmillan, 1982), 95, 97.

59. And deliberately so; doctors were keen to preserve the sanctity of the doctor-patient relationship. Although this did not arise explicitly in this period, partially because of censor control, it did arise in the late 1950s in the context of the BBC series *Your Life in Their Hands*; see Boon, "On the Varieties of Medical Filmmaking," 625–27.

60. Sheila Johnston, "Film Narrative and the Structuralist Controversy," in *The Cinema Book* (London: BFI, 1985), 246.

61. Ibid., 245.

62. Annette Kuhn, "The History of Narrative Codes" in *The Cinema Book* (London, 1985), 41–48.

63. Kuhn, "History of Narrative Codes," 212–15.

64. Bill Nichols, "Documentary Theory and Practice," *Screen* 17 (1976–77): 34–48.

65. Speech by an actor not visible in the scene has very particular meanings within fiction films, usually denoting narration or thought processes.

66. Tom Crew, *Health Propaganda, Ways and Means* (Leicester, UK: Bell, 1935), 42.

67. The crucial distinction used by Nichols, which is essential to the argument of this study, was evidently well established by 1935. See my argument in "Health Education Films in Britain, 1919–1939," 54. Still more simply put was Sidney Low's statement that "the drama appeals to the emotions and the instincts, not to the reasoning faculty," Sidney Low, "Propaganda Films and Mixed Morals," *Fortnightly Review* 113 (May 1920): 727.

68. Nightingale, *Studying Audiences*, 21–22.

69. Abercrombie and Longhurst, *Audiences*, 3–15.

70. Morley, *The Nationwide Audience*. See John Corner's discussion in "Meaning, Genre and Context: The Problematics of 'Public Knowledge' in the New Audience Studies," in *Studying Media: Problems of Theory and Method* (Edinburgh: Edinburgh University Press, 1998), 112–13.

71. Morley, *Nationwide Audience*, 26–28, 134–38, and Corner, "Meaning, Genre and Context," 114.

72. Nightingale, *Studying Audiences*, 3, 27.

73. Michael Baxandall, *Painting and Experience in Fifteenth Century Italy: A Primer in the Social History of Pictorial Style* (Oxford: Oxford University Press, 1988).

74. This was pointed out to me by Alex Hayward, then a transport curator at the Science Museum.

75. Boon, "Lay Disease Narratives."

76. Sir Napier Burnett of the Joint Committee of the Red Cross and St John's Ambulance wanted to undertake an initiative in health education. "He described the fundamental health problems before the country as something that should bridge the hygienic knowledge of the medical profession and the abysmal ignorance of the

population as a whole in regard to health questions." George Newman to Minister, November 3, 1920, National Archives, Kew, MH55/27 For a discussion of the deficit theory, see Patrick Sturgis and Nick Allum, "Science in Society: Re-evaluating the Deficit Model of Public Attitudes," *Public Understanding of Science* 13 (January 1, 2004): 55–74.

77. S. Levine and M. A. Kozloff, "The Sick Role: Assessment and Overview," *Annual Review of Sociology* 4 (1978): 317–43, 319–20.

78. Uta Gerhardt, "Parsons, Role Theory and Health Interaction," in *Sociological Theory and Medical Sociology*, ed. Graham Scambler (London: Tavistock, 1987), 110–33; Levine and Kozloff, "The Sick Role," 317–18. Armstrong states that Brackenbury's 1935 book on the doctor-patient relationship identified obedience to the doctor and the will to get better within the patient role; David Armstrong, *Political Anatomy of the Body* (Cambridge: Cambridge University Press, 1983), 115.

79. Boon, *Films and the Contestation*, 156–59.

80. Nick Jewson, "Disappearance of the sick-man from medical cosmologies, 1770–1870," *Sociology* 10 (1976): 225–44; Armstrong, *Political Anatomy*, 116.

81. Michel de Certeau, *The Practice of Everyday Life* (Berkeley: University of California Press, 1984), 31. This is similar in effect to the approach associated with the television scholar James Halloran that "we should ask not what the media does to people, but what people do to the media" in his *The Effects of Television* (London: Panther, 1970).

82. In a modern setting, Rosemary McKechnie was able to address such issues of supposed ignorance ethnographically. As she comments, "The common starting-point is not individuals' lack of knowledge of scientific 'facts' or processes, but how people reflect on the status of their own knowledge and situate themselves *vis à vis* science *vis à vis* others in relation to science." Rosemary McKechnie, "Insiders and Outsiders: Identifying Experts on Home Ground," in *Misunderstanding Science? The Public Reconstruction of Science and Technology*, ed. Alan Irwin and Brian Wynne (Cambridge: Cambridge University Press, 1996).

83. Quoted in Abercrombie and Longhurst, *Audiences*, 23.

84. This phrase seems first to have been used by Aubrey Symonds (assistant secretary in the Ministry of Health) in a minute to Chief Medical Officer George Newman on August 30, 1920, MH55/27, but the principle it enshrines became a touchstone of official policy. It was used in Newman, *Public Education in Health*.

85. Stuart Hall, "The Rediscovery of 'Ideology': Return of the Repressed in Media Studies," in *Culture, Society and the Media*, ed. Michael Gurevitch, Tony Bennett, James Curran, and Janet Woollacott (London: Methuen, 1982), 81. Quoted in Abercrombie and Longhurst, *Audiences*, 13.

86. David Cannadine, *The Decline and Fall of the British Aristocracy* (London: Papermac, 1992).

87. Harold Perkin, *The Rise of Professional Society* (London: Routledge, 1989).

88. De Certeau, *Practice of Everyday Life*, 166.

89. John Fiske, "Moments of Television: Neither the Text nor the Audience," in *Remote Control: Television Audiences and Cultural Power*, ed. Ellen Seiter, Hans Borchers, Gabriele Kreutzner, and Eva-Maria Warth (London: Routledge, 1989), 57, quoted in Abercrombie and Longhurst, *Audiences*, 23.

90. C. Metz, *Psychoanalysis and Cinema*, 95.

91. Newman, *Public Education in Health,* 4. David Armstrong's Foucauldian view takes up the same refrain, comparing the regime of personal hygiene with the preceding regime of sanitary science; David Armstrong, "Public Health Spaces and the Fabrication of Identity," *Sociology* 27 (1993): 401.

Contributors

Christian Bonah, MD, PhD, is professor of the history of medical and health sciences and a member of the Institute of Advanced Studies at the University Strasbourg. He has worked on comparative history of medical education and social and cultural studies of science and technology, including notably the history of medicaments and the history of human experimentation. Recent works include research on risk perception and management in drug scandals and courtroom trials as well as studies on medical and health film. He is the author and editor of the audio-visual database dedicated to health film: medfilm.fr. Selected publications include "Packaging BCG: Standardizing an Anti-tuberculosis Vaccine in Interwar Europe," *Science in Context* 21, no. 2 (2008): 279–310; with David Cantor and Mathias Dörries, *Meat, Medicine and Human Health in the Twentieth Century* (London: Pickering & Chato, 2010); *L'expérimentation humaine: Discours et pratiques en France, 1900–1940* (Paris: Les Belles Lettres 2007); and "'Health Crusades': Environmental Approaches as Public Health Strategies against Infections in Sanitary Propaganda Films, 1930–1960," in *Environment, Health and History*, edited by Virginia Berridge and Martin Gorsky (London: Palgrave Macmillan, 2011), 152–75. Christian Bonah is also the principle investigator of the ERC Advanced Grant "BodyCapital, The Healthy Self as Body Capital: Individuals, Market-based Societies and Body Politics in Visual Twentieth Century Europe (2016–2021)," proposing a social history of media and health from a utility visual perspective.

Tim Boon is head of research and public history for the Science Museum and a historian of the public culture of science. He is responsible for developing the Museum's research program and for its public history program, which is concerned with investigating the lay historical imagination as it relates to science and technology. His published research (more than twenty-five articles) is concerned with the history of science in documentary films and television, museum history, and sound studies. His doctoral thesis is "Films and the Contestation of Public Health in Interwar Britain" (1999). His first book, *Films of Fact*, was published in 2008, and he recently published an account of the origins and early years of the BBC program, *Horizon*. He is coeditor (with Frode Weium) of *Artefacts: Material Culture and Electronic Sound* (Washington, Smithsonian Institution Scholarly Press: 2013). His exhibitions include *Health Matters* (1994),

Making the Modern World (2000), *Treat Yourself* (2003, with Ken Arnold), *Films of Fact* (2008), and *Oramics to Electronica* (2011).

David Cantor is a historian in the Office of History at the National Institutes of Health, Bethesda, Maryland, and teaches in the School of Public Health, University of Maryland, College Park. He is the editor of *Reinventing Hippocrates* (Aldershot, Hampshire, UK: Ashgate, 2002) and *Cancer in the Twentieth Century* (Baltimore: Johns Hopkins University Press, 2008), coeditor (with Christian Bonah and Matthias Dörries) of *Meat, Medicine, and Human Health in the Twentieth Century* (London: Pickering and Chatto, 2010) and coeditor (with Edmund Ramsden) of *Stress, Shock, and Adaptation in the Twentieth Century* (Rochester, NY: University of Rochester Press, 2014). He is series editor (edited collections) of Social Histories of Medicine, published by Manchester University Press.

Ursula von Keitz, PhD, is professor of film research and media education at the Filmuniversität Babelsberg "Konrad Wolf" and director of the Filmmuseum Potsdam. She is also coleader of the long-term research project "The History of Documentary Film in Germany 1945–2005," supported by the German Research Foundation (DFG). Her main fields of work are film history, film and literature, modes of screenplay writing, theory and aesthetics of documentary film, cinema as a space of experience, and problems of critical film edition. Publications (partial listing) include *Im Schatten des Gesetzes: Schwangerschaftskonflikt und Reproduktion im deutschsprachigen Film* (Marburg, Germany: Schüren 2005); "Between Dramatization and Epicization: The Portrayal of Nazi Crimes in Exemplary German Films from the Late 1940s to the 1970s," *New German Critique* 102 (Fall 2007): 45–60; and "*The Shining*—Frozen Material: Stanley Kubrick's Adaptation of Stephen King's Novel" in *Stanley Kubrick*, ed. Hans Peter Reichmann and Ingeborg Flagge, 2nd ed. (Frankfurt am Main: Deutsches Filmmuseum, 2015), 184–97. She also coedited several books and theme issues such as *Kinogefühle: Emotionalität und Film*, 2nd ed. (Marburg, Germany: Schüren, 2010); *Mediale Transformationen des Holocausts*, 2nd ed. (Berlin: Avinus, 2014); and *Alles dreht sich . . . und bewegt sich: Der Tanz und das Kino* (Marburg, Germany: Schüren 2017).

Anja Laukötter, PhD, is a researcher in the department of the History of Emotions at the Max Planck Institute for Human Development in Berlin, where she is working on a book concerning the transnational history of knowledge and emotions in health educational films in the twentieth century. She studied history, political science, and anthropology in Cologne, Berlin, and New York. Her first book, *Von der "Kultur zur 'Rasse'—vom Objekt zum Körper? Völkerkundemuseen und ihre Wissenschaften zu Beginn des 20. Jahrhunderts*" (2007) is on the history of anthropology and anthropological museums at the turn of the twentieth century. She is the author of various publications in the field of the history of science and knowledge, postcolonial studies, visual media (including the history of educational films), and history of emotions throughout the nineteenth and twentieth centuries including several recently coedited volumes and theme issues such as

"History of Science and the Emotions" (*Osiris*, 2016, together with Otniel Dror, Bettina Hitzer, and Pilar Leon-Sanz); "Screening Sex Hygiene Films in the first Half of the 20th Century" (*Gesnerus*, 2015, together with Christian Bonah) and "*Learning How to Feel: Children's Literature and the History of Emotional Socialization,* 1870–1970" (Oxford: Oxford University Press, 2014, together with U. Frevert, P. Eitler, S. Olsen, U. Jensen, M. Pernau et al.) and she is coeditor of the bilingual platform *History of Emotions—Insights into Research,* https://www.history-of-emotions.mpg.de/en (since 2013, together with Margrit Pernau). Anja Laukötter is codirecting with Christian Bonah the ERC Advanced Grant "BodyCapital: The Healthy Self as Body Capital; Individuals, Market-Based Societies and Body Politics in Visual Twentieth-Century Europe."

Elizabeth Lebas was senior lecturer (and later reader) in the history of art and architecture at Middlesex University as well as senior tutor at the Architectural Association. Her work focused on health, housing reform, and urban policy in the 1920s–70s, a period that fascinated her because of its commitment to a collective future. She was the coauthor, editor or translator of many books on cities, architecture, and art, including editing and translating several of the works of French sociologist Henri Lefebvre, including his *Writings on Cities* (Oxford: Blackwell, 1996). She carried out original research on municipal filmmaking and discovered, catalogued, and rescued the extraordinary public information films that progressive local governments made between 1920 and 1978. Her 1995 paper "When Every Street Became a Cinema" in *History Workshop Journal* was highly influential in opening up the historical study of public health films at the same time as it conveyed her infectious excitement at discovering the Bermondsey Borough Council films. In 2012 she was involved in putting together an exhibition at the Wellcome Collection in London, *Here Comes Good Health,* which focused on her beloved Bermondsey films; her work in this area culminated in her book *Forgotten Futures: British Municipal Cinema, 1920–1980,* published by Black Dog Publishing in 2011. Dr. Lebas died in 2014.

Vincent Lowy is the director of the Ecole Nationale Superieur Louis-Lumière, Paris, France. As a professor in film and media studies, he specializes in film history, visual propaganda, and nonfiction cinema. After a pioneering study on Nazi camps and Holocaust movies, *L'histoire Infilmable: Les Camps d'extermination Nazis à l'écran* (Paris: L'Harmattan, 2001), he published several articles on Media/Social and Political Violence/Film, a landmark study on pacifism on screen, *Guère à la guerre: Le Pacifisme dans le Cinéma Français, 1936–1940* (Paris: L'Harmattan, 2006), a reference biography of documentary filmmaker *Marcel Ophuls* (Lormont, France: Le Bord de l'Eau, 2008) and an extended essay on globalization and cinema *Cinéma et Mondialisation: Une Esthétique des Inégalité* (Lormont, France: Le Bord de l'Eau, 2011). Since 2009, he has been in charge of several book collections for film and media studies at Le Bord de l'Eau Editions and has published more than twenty authors, including filmmakers Jean-Luc Godard, Marcel Ophuls, and the Dardenne brothers.

Kirsten Ostherr, PhD, MPH, is a media scholar and health researcher at Rice University in Houston, Texas. Dr. Ostherr is the author of two books, *Medical Visions: Producing the Patient through Film, Television and Imaging Technologies* (New York: Oxford University Press, 2013) and *Cinematic Prophylaxis: Globalization and Contagion in the Discourse of World Health* (Durham, NC: Duke University Press, 2005), coeditor of *Science/Animation*, a special issue of the journal *Discourse* 38, no. 3 (Detroit, MI: Wayne State University Press, 2016), editor of the collection *Applied Media Studies* (New York, NY: Routledge, forthcoming 2018) and numerous articles. She was awarded a New Directions Fellowship from the Andrew W. Mellon Foundation in 2012 to pursue an MPH in health media and communication. Her current research is on information and communication technologies in aging and end-of-life care, patient narratives in EHRs, and the role of simulation as a mediator between human and technological forms of medical expertise. Her current book project is called "Quantified Health: Making Stories from Data in the Algorithmic Age." She is director of the Medical Futures Lab and has spoken to audiences at TEDx, the mHealth Summit, Medicine X, the Louisville Innovation Summit, the World Health Organization, the National Library of Medicine, and other universities and conferences worldwide.

Miriam Posner is assistant professor in the Information Studies department at the University of California, Los Angeles. She frequently writes and speaks on digital humanities, as well as on the history of technology, particularly the history of medical imaging. Her PhD, from Yale University, is in film studies and American studies.

Alexandre Sumpf is assistant professor at the Faculty of History, University of Strasbourg, France. His research interests are in Russian and Soviet history of the first half of the twentieth century, techniques of mass mobilization and propaganda, history of the world wars, and nonfiction cinema. After his first monograph *Bolcheviks en campagne: Paysans et éducation politique dans la Russie des années 1920* (CNRS, 2010), he published several articles on Russian and Soviet cinema, a study on the social history of Soviet Union (Gallimard, 2013), a monograph on the First World War in Russia (Perrin, 2014), and *Révolutions russes au cinema: Naissance d'une nation, URSS 1917–1985* (Armand Colin, 2015). In 2015 he also commissioned with Valerie Pozner and Vanessa Voisin the exhibition *Filmer la guerre: Les Soviétiques face à la Shoah* (Mémorial de la Shoah, Paris).

Index

An italicized page number indicates a table or graphic. Years in parentheses indicate a film's first showing.

www.ingramcontent.com/pod-product-compliance
Ingram Content Group UK Ltd.
Pitfield, Milton Keynes, MK11 3LW, UK
UKHW040857081026
15587UKWH00016B/690

9 781580 469166